# Planar Chromatography-Mass Spectrometry

# CHROMATOGRAPHIC SCIENCE SERIES

## *A Series of Textbooks and Reference Books*

Editor:
Nelu Grinberg

Founding Editor:
Jack Cazes

# Planar Chromatography-Mass Spectrometry

Edited by
Teresa Kowalska
Mieczysław Sajewicz
Joseph Sherma

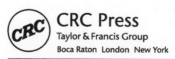

CRC Press
Taylor & Francis Group
Boca Raton London New York

CRC Press is an imprint of the
Taylor & Francis Group, an **informa** business

CRC Press
Taylor & Francis Group
6000 Broken Sound Parkway NW, Suite 300
Boca Raton, FL 33487-2742

First issued in paperback 2020

© 2016 by Taylor & Francis Group, LLC
CRC Press is an imprint of Taylor & Francis Group, an Informa business

No claim to original U.S. Government works

ISBN 13: 978-0-367-57527-4 (pbk)
ISBN 13: 978-1-4987-0588-2 (hbk)

**Visit the Taylor & Francis Web site at**
**http://www.taylorandfrancis.com**

**and the CRC Press Web site at**
**http://www.crcpress.com**

# Dedication

*This book is dedicated to the memory of Friedrich ("Fritz")
Geiss, who passed away on February 14, 2015, nine days before
his 83rd birthday. Excellent reviews of Dr. Geiss' education
and work history, as well as contributions to the field of thin-
layer chromatography (TLC), were given in editorials on the
occasion of his 80th birthday published in the* Journal of Planar
Chromatography—Modern TLC *(25(3), 193, 2012) and* Acta
Chromatographica *(24(2), 143–144, 2012). We would like to
focus here on the two indispensible TLC books that he wrote.*

*In 1972, Dr. Geiss' book* Die Parameter der
Duennschictchromatographie *was published by Vieweg in German,
and the second edition in English titled* Fundamentals of Thin-
Layer Chromatography (Planar Chromatography) *was published
in 1987 by Huethig. In the preface to the German edition, Dr.
Geiss wrote that during his work in TLC that began in 1960
with attempts to separate a mixture of hydrocarbons, he and his
colleague Helmut Schlitt were concerned for many years with
the problem of factors that influence TLC. His aim for the book
was to build a bridge between the laboratory handbooks of
TLC and the fundamental books of chromatography available
at that time in order to translate the fundamentals into daily
practice and realize TLC's real potential to become a reliable
and nonempirical method. He addressed for the first time the
theory and fundamentals necessary to understand the layer–
analyte–mobile phase interactions and predict the most favorable
conditions for successful and reproducible TLC separations.*

*In the preface to the English edition, Dr. Geiss stated that he found the information on fundamentals and reproducibility obsolete, incorrect, or misleading in TLC books available in 1987, and that he was writing a book that "is not theoretical but describes what happens in TLC, or what the practitioner should know that happens, and how he can control what happens." He provided information he believed was needed to understand and predict optimal conditions for TLC in order to provide adequate and reproducible separations and reliable quantification. He was the only author up to that time to attempt to explain the complex situation occurring inside the TLC development tank with multicomponent mobile phases.*

*In his foreword to Dr. Geiss' English edition, Lloyd R. Snyder, author of the renowned fundamentals book* Principles of Adsorption Chromatography, *wrote that among Dr. Geiss' accomplishments in his two books was to develop and make available a better understanding of the complex phenomena occurring in the "simple" technique of TLC, organize the first practical theory of TLC, improve conventional TLC, provide information leading to important new TLC techniques based on his studies of pre-equilibration of the TLC plate and mobile-phase demixing, and present the first valid equation and practical instructions for the safe transfer of separation from layer to column. Dr. Snyder noted that in the updated edition were comprehensive accounts of method development and selectivity optimization in TLC and high-performance TLC (HPTLC), interrelationship of separation by TLC and column HPLC, importance of band broadening in TLC, and instrumentation needed for quantitative work.*

*Over the last few years, Dr. Geiss was considering an updated and expanded third edition of his book to include the latest technical innovations, such as modern instrumentation and chemometrics and embrace all possibilities and enhanced potentials of modern TLC. He kept up to date on these advances by regularly attending numerous chromatography meetings even after stopping experimental work upon retirement. One of the technical advances Dr. Geiss would have undoubtedly included enthusiastically in his new edition is TLC–mass spectrometry, the topic of this book. Sadly, the new edition was not realized as a further invaluable and lasting contribution of Dr. Geiss to the field.*

*Dr. Geiss' books have had enormous impact on the TLC work of the editors during our careers, and we are pleased to dedicate this book as a heartfelt, although inadequate, token of thanks for the critical contributions on behalf of all chromatographers of this brilliant colleague.*

**Teresa Kowalska**
**Mieczysław Sajewicz**
**Joseph Sherma**

# Contents

## SECTION I  Materials, Instrumentation, and Techniques of Planar Chromatography-Mass Spectrometry

## SECTION II    Practical Applications of Planar Chromatography-Mass Spectrometry Methodology

# Preface

This book is devoted to a relatively new approach to chemical analysis in general, and to separation science in particular, the combination of thin-layer chromatography (TLC) and high-performance TLC (HPTLC), among the simplest, most cost-effective, and yet very well-performing techniques for determining complex mixtures of compounds, with mass spectrometry (MS), a sophisticated and relatively expensive spectrometric technique that enables rapid identification of separated chemical species. TLC–MS coupling can significantly facilitate identification of mixture components, which is particularly important, for example, in forensic studies; identification of drug metabolites, breakdown products, and impurities; and identification of biologically active components in phytochemical samples, especially in cases when analytical standards are for certain reasons unavailable (e.g., they are not traded commercially or are too expensive). Quantification of identified compounds can also be obtained by using the TLC–MS combination.

As one- and two-dimensional gel electrophoresis are often classified as planar chromatographic techniques and are increasingly more exploited in proteomic and molecular biology studies, and for medical diagnostic purposes as well, the book also covers electrophoretic–MS methods and applications.

The book consists of 19 chapters that provide general information about the existing possibilities of coupling TLC with MS, as well as a selection of important and diverse practical applications of the TLC–MS technique to a variety of analytical separation/identification/quantification problems written by worldwide experts in the field from the United States, Europe, Asia, and South America. It is the first published book on the topic of TLC–MS, and it comprehensively covers all aspects of the hyphenated method for separation/identification/quantification of a wide variety of analytes in a wide range of sample matrices. It contains information on principles, methods, and instrumentation of all offline and online modes of TLC–MS as well as practical examples of applications originating from laboratories in which it has been in use for some time. It provides necessary information for the use of TLC–MS in laboratories that have appropriate MS equipment but have not yet employed it to enhance the analytical power of TLC. The use of a relatively inexpensive commercial TLC–MS interface/mass spectrometer system is also described for those laboratories without the benefit of MS instrumentation at this time. The contents of the book are especially useful for those laboratories that employ TLC for rapid screening of herbal nutritional supplement and medicinal samples in order to confirm the identity, origin, or possible adulteration by use of "fingerprinting" with TLC–MS. It encourages adoption or greater use of the hyphenated method with enhanced analytical capabilities by graduate students, industry professionals, researchers, academics, and regulatory analysts, and it introduces the field to junior and senior undergraduate students.

The editors would like to thank Barbara Glunn, senior editor, chemistry, and Jill Jurgensen, senior project coordinator, editorial project development, for their support during all aspects of the proposal and editorial processes. We also thank the chapter authors for their invaluable contributions.

**Teresa Kowalska**
**Mieczysław Sajewicz**
**Joseph Sherma**

# Editors

**Teresa Kowalska** earned an MSc in chemistry from the former Pedagogical High School in Katowice, Poland, in 1968, a PhD in physical chemistry from the University of Silesia, Katowice, Poland, in 1972, and a DSc in physical chemistry from the Maria Curie-Skłodowska University in Lublin, Poland, in 1988. In the 1974–1975 school year, Professor Kowalska stayed for 12 months as a British Council postdoctoral fellow at the Chemistry Faculty of Salford University, Salford, Lancashire, United Kingdom, under the supervision of the late Professor Hans Suschitzky, head of the Organic Chemistry Department there.

Professor Kowalska has authored and coauthored approximately 300 original research and review papers in approximately 30 different peer-reviewed chemistry journals, 16 invited book chapters, and approximately 500 conference papers (both lectures and posters) included in the programs of scientific conferences at home and abroad (also on numerous personal invitations). Moreover, Professor Kowalska coedited with Professor Joseph Sherma *Preparative Layer Chromatography* and *Thin Layer Chromatography in Chiral Separations and Analysis*, and with Professor Monika Waksmundska-Hajnos and Professor Sherma *Thin Layer Chromatography in Phytochemistry*, all published in the Chromatographic Science Series by CRC Press/Taylor & Francis Group. Last, Professor Kowalska (together with Professor Mieczysław Sajewicz) acts as coeditor-in-chief of the international chromatography journal *Acta Chromatographica*, published by Akademiai Kiado, Budapest, Hungary. She also acts as an editorial board member for several chromatography journals, including the *Journal of Chromatographic Science* (published by Oxford University Press), the *Journal of Planar Chromatography—Modern TLC* (published by Akademiai Kiado), and the online journal *Chromatography Research International* (published by Hindawi Press). On an invitation of approximately 20 internationally recognized analytical chemistry and separation science journals, Professor Kowalska has prepared several hundred peer reviews of manuscript submissions.

Professor Kowalska's main research interests focus on the applications of the thin-layer, high-performance liquid and gas chromatography to physicochemical problems (such as extraction of thermodynamic information from gas chromatographic data, enantioseparations mechanisms, and tracing the nonlinear chemical reactions with the aid of liquid chromatographic techniques). She is also interested in analytical applications of liquid chromatographic techniques to food chemistry (mainly to the chemistry of medicinal plants and meat products). In the field of nonlinear reaction mechanisms, Professor Kowalska has established fruitful collaboration with the world's leading research group in this area, headed by Professor Irving R. Epstein from the Chemistry Department of Brandeis University, Waltham, Massachusetts.

In parallel with her research, Professor Kowalska has been an academic teacher for over four decades and in this capacity she has taught undergraduate courses in general chemistry and undergraduate and postgraduate courses in fundamentals and applications of the chromatographic techniques. Professor Kowalska has supervised approximately 80 MSc and 13 PhD theses (in the field of analytical chemistry and chromatographic science), and also served as a jury member for approximately 40 doctorates at home and abroad. She is actively involved in the EU undergraduate students international exchange program Socrates, encouraging her own students to pursue a one-semester training experience in a foreign institution, and also hosting foreign undergraduate students and postdoctoral fellows in her laboratory. For her continuous and dedicated engagement in teaching chemistry, Professor Kowalska has been awarded many times at the local and national levels.

**Mieczysław Sajewicz** earned an MSc and a PhD in chemistry from the University of Silesia, Katowice, Poland, in 1978 and 1989, respectively. The main area of his MSc and PhD studies was analytical chemistry and, more precisely, application of gas chromatography to studying factors governing separation quality (e.g., isomerism of analytes, polarity of stationary phases, and working parameters of gas chromatographic system as a whole). In 2013, Professor Sajewicz earned a DSc in pharmacy from Collegium Medicum, Jagiellonian University, Kraków, Poland. His DSc dissertation focused on spontaneous nonlinear processes (oscillatory chiral conversion and oscillatory condensation) running in aqueous and nonaqueous solutions of profen drugs and the other low-molecular-weight chiral carboxylic acids (derived from acetic, propionic, and butyric acid).

Professor Sajewicz has authored and coauthored over 150 original research papers and over 350 conference papers, presented at conferences and congresses at home and abroad. Moreover, he has coauthored one encyclopedia entry in *Encyclopedia of Chromatography* (2nd edition revised and expanded; 2005) and two book chapters (Chapter 2 in *Preparative Layer Chromatography*, edited by Teresa Kowalska and Joseph Sherma with CRC Press/Taylor & Francis Group in 2006, and Chapter 9 in *Thin Layer Chromatography in Chiral Separations and Analysis*, also edited by Teresa Kowalska and Joseph Sherma with CRC Press/Taylor & Francis Group in 2007). Since 1992, Professor Sajewicz has been an editorial board member for *Acta Chromatographica*, and in 2002, he became coeditor-in-chief of the same journal. He also acts as an editorial board member for the analytical chemistry section of *The Scientific World Journal*.

Since 1980, Professor Sajewicz has been a member of the Organizing Committee of the annual all-Polish Symposium on Chromatographic Methods of Investigating the Organic Compounds, organized by the Institute of Chemistry, University of Silesia, Katowice, Poland, and has been cochairman of the Scientific and Organizing Committee of the same scientific event since 2002.

Professor Sajewicz has wide teaching experience at the undergraduate and graduate university levels. He has run courses in chemical calculus, several laboratory courses in planar, high-performance liquid and gas chromatography, and MSc lecture courses on selected chromatographic techniques and on applications thereof to environmental analysis. He has supervised and cosupervised approximately 70 MSc theses, and he has cosupervised 4 PhD theses. For his continuous and dedicated engagement in teaching chemistry, Professor Sajewicz has been awarded at the local and national levels.

**Joseph Sherma** earned a BS in chemistry from Upsala College, East Orange, New Jersey, in 1955 and a PhD in analytical chemistry from Rutgers, The State University, New Brunswick, New Jersey, in 1958 under the supervision of the renowned ion exchange chromatography expert Wm. Rieman III. Professor Sherma is currently John D. and Francis H. Larkin professor emeritus of chemistry at Lafayette College, Easton, Pennsylvania; he taught courses in analytical chemistry for more than 40 years, was head of the Chemistry Department for 12 years, and continues to supervise research students at Lafayette. During sabbatical leaves and summers, Professor Sherma did research in the laboratories of the eminent chromatographers Dr. Harold Strain, Dr. Gunter Zweig, Professor James Fritz, and Professor Joseph Touchstone.

Professor Sherma has authored, coauthored, edited, or coedited more than 750 publications, including research papers and review articles in approximately 55 different peer-reviewed analytical chemistry, chromatography, and biological journals; approximately 30 invited book chapters; and more than 65 books and U.S. government agency manuals in the areas of analytical chemistry and chromatography.

In addition to his research in the techniques and applications of thin layer chromatography (TLC), Professor Sherma has a very productive interdisciplinary research program in the use of analytical chemistry to study biological systems with Bernard Fried, Kreider Professor Emeritus of Biology at Lafayette College, with whom he wrote *Thin Layer Chromatography* (1st–4th editions) and edited the *Handbook of Thin Layer Chromatography* (1st–3rd editions), both published by Marcel Dekker, Inc., as well as editing *Practical Thin Layer Chromatography* for CRC Press. Professor Sherma wrote with Dr. Zweig a book titled *Paper Chromatography* for Academic Press and the first two volumes of the *Handbook of Chromatography* series for CRC Press, and coedited with him 22 more volumes of the chromatography series and 10 volumes of the series Analytical Methods for Pesticides and Plant Growth Regulators for Academic Press. After Dr. Zweig's death, Professor Sherma edited five additional volumes of the chromatography handbook series and two volumes in the pesticide series. The pesticide series was completed under the title Modern Methods of Pesticide Analysis for CRC Press with two volumes coedited with Dr. Thomas Cairns. Three books on quantitative TLC and advances in TLC were edited jointly with Professor Touchstone for Wiley-Interscience. For the CRC/ Taylor & Francis Group Chromatographic Science Series, Professor Sherma coedited with Professor Teresa Kowalska *Preparative Layer Chromatography* and *Thin Layer Chromatography in Chiral Separations and Analysis*; with Professor Kowalska and Professor Monika Waksmundska-Hajnos, *Thin Layer Chromatography in Phytochemistry*; with Professor Waksmundska-Hajnos, *High Performance Liquid Chromatography in Phytochemical Analysis*; and with Professor Lukasz Komsta and Professor Waksmundska-Hajnos, *Thin Layer Chromatography in Drug Analysis*. A volume titled *High Performance Liquid Chromatography in Pesticide Residue Analysis,* coedited with Professor Tomasz Tuzimiski in the Chromatographic Science Series, was published in 2015.

Professor Sherma served for 23 years as editor for residues and trace elements of the *Journal of AOAC International* and is currently that journal's acquisitions editor. He has guest edited with Professor Fried 16 annual special issues on TLC of the *Journal of Liquid Chromatography & Related Technologies* and regularly guest edits special sections of issues of the *Journal of AOAC International* on specific subjects in all areas of analytical chemistry. For 12 years he also wrote an article on modern analytical instrumentation for each issue of the *Journal of AOAC International*. Professor Sherma has written biennial reviews of planar chromatography published in the American Chemical Society journal *Analytical Chemistry, Journal of AOAC International,* and *Central European Journal of Chemistry* since 1970 and biennial reviews of pesticide analysis by TLC since 1982 in the *Journal of Liquid Chromatography & Related Technologies* and the *Journal of Environmental Science and Health, Part B*. He is now on the editorial boards of the *Journal of Planar Chromatography—Modern TLC*; *Acta Chromatographica*; *Journal of Environmental Science and Health, Part B*; and *Journal of Liquid Chromatography & Related Technologies.*

Professor Sherma was the recipient of the 1995 ACS Award for Research at an Undergraduate Institution sponsored by Research Corporation. The first 2009 issue, Volume 12, of the journal *Acta Universitatis Cibiensis, Seria F, Chemia* was dedicated in honor of Professor Sherma's teaching, research, and publication accomplishments in analytical chemistry and chromatography.

# Contributors

**Alen Albreht**
Laboratory for Food Chemistry
National Institute of Chemistry
Ljubljana, Slovenia

**Anna Bodzoń-Kułakowska**
Department of Biochemistry and
  Neurobiology
AGH University of Science and
  Technology
Kraków, Poland

**Amadeu Cardoso Jr.**
Contraprova Análises
Ensino e Pesquisas Ltda.
Rio de Janeiro, Brazil

**Michał Cegłowski**
Department of Supramolecular
  Chemistry
Adam Mickiewicz University in
  Poznań
Poznań, Poland

**Sychyi Cheng**
Department of Chemistry
National Sun Yat-Sen University
Kaohsiung, Taiwan

**Anna Drabik**
Department of Biochemistry and
  Neurobiology
AGH University of Science and
  Technology
Kraków, Poland

**Beate Fuchs**
Institute of Medical Physics and
  Biophysics
University of Leipzig
Leipzig, Saxony, Germany

**Agnieszka Godziek**
Institute of Chemistry
University of Silesia
Katowice, Silesia, Poland

**Hans Griesinger**
Merck KGaA
Darmstadt, Hesse, Germany

**Tim T. Häbe**
Institute of Nutritional Sciences
  and Interdisciplinary Research
  Center (IFZ)
Justus Liebig University Giessen
Giessen, Hesse, Germany

**Urszula Hubicka**
Collegium Medicum
Jagiellonian University
Kraków, Poland

**Suresh Kumar Kailasa**
Department of Applied Chemistry
S. V. National Institute of Technology
Surat, Gujarat, India

**Teresa Kowalska**
Institute of Chemistry
University of Silesia
Katowice, Silesia, Poland

**Jan Krzek (Deceased)**
Collegium Medicum
Jagiellonian University
Kraków, Poland

**Katharina Lemmnitzer**
Institute of Medical Physics and
  Biophysics
University of Leipzig
Leipzig, Saxony, Germany

**Anna Maciejowska**
Institute of Chemistry
University of Silesia
Katowice, Silesia, Poland

**Anna Maślanka**
Collegium Medicum
Jagiellonian University
Kraków, Poland

**Katerina Matheis**
Merck KGaA
Darmstadt, Hesse, Germany

**Przemysław Mielczarek**
Academic Centre for Materials and
   Nanotechnology
AGH University of Science and
   Technology
Kraków, Poland

**Gertrud E. Morlock**
Institute of Nutritional Sciences
   and Interdisciplinary Research
   Center (IFZ)
Justus Liebig University Giessen
Giessen, Hesse, Germany

**Joanna Ner**
Department of Biochemistry and
   Neurobiology
AGH University of Science and
   Technology
Kraków, Poland

**Michaela Oberle**
Merck KGaA
Darmstadt, Hasse, Germany

**Claudia Oellig**
Institute of Food Chemistry
University of Hohenheim
Baden-Württemberg, Stuttgart, Germany

**Yulia Popkova**
Institute of Medical Physics and
   Biophysics
University of Leipzig
Leipzig, Saxony, Germany

**Fred Rabel**
ChromHELP, LLC
Woodbury, New Jersey

**Jigneshkumar V. Rohit**
Department of Applied Chemistry
S. V. National Institute of Technology
Surat, Gujarat, India

**Wanderson Romão**
Department of Chemistry
Federal University of Espírito Santo
Vitória, Espírito Santo, Brazil

**Bruno D. Sabino**
Institute of Criminalistic Carlos Éboli
and
Contraprova Análises
Ensino e Pesquisas Ltda.
Rio de Janeiro, Brazil

**Mieczysław Sajewicz**
Institute of Chemistry
University of Silesia
Katowice, Silesia, Poland

**Jürgen Schiller**
Institute of Medical Physics and
   Biophysics
University of Leipzig
Leipzig, Saxony, Germany

**Grzegorz Schroeder**
Department of Chemistry
Adam Mickiewicz University in
   Poznań
Poznań, Poland

**Michael Schulz**
Merck KGaA
Darmstadt, Hasse, Germany

**Wolfgang Schwack**
Institute of Food Chemistry
University of Hohenheim
Baden-Württemberg, Stuttgart,
  Germany

**Joseph Sherma**
Department of Chemistry
Lafayette College
Easton, Pennsylvania

**Jentaie Shiea**
Department of Chemistry
National Sun Yat-Sen University
Kaohsiung, Taiwan

**Jerzy Silberring**
Department of Biochemistry and
  Neurobiology
AGH University of Science and
  Technology
Kraków, Poland

and

Centre of Polymer and Carbon
  Materials
Polish Academy of Sciences
Zabrze, Poland

**Marek Smoluch**
Department of Biochemistry and
  Neurobiology
AGH University of Science and
  Technology
Kraków, Poland

**Jacob Strock**
Department of Chemistry
Lafayette College
Easton, Pennsylvania

**Rosmarie Süß**
Institute of Medical Physics and
  Biophysics
University of Leipzig
Leipzig, Saxony, Germany

**Piotr Suder**
Academic Centre for Materials and
  Nanotechnology
AGH University of Science and
  Technology
Kraków, Poland

**Irena Vovk**
Laboratory for Food Chemistry
National Institute of Chemistry
Ljubljana, Slovenia

**Hui-Fen Wu**
Department of Chemistry
National Sun Yat-Sen University
Kaohsiung, Taiwan

**Barbara Żuromska-Witek**
Collegium Medicum
Jagiellonian University
Kraków, Poland

# Section I

Materials, Instrumentation, and Techniques of Planar Chromatography-Mass Spectrometry

# 1 Overview of the Field of TLC–MS and Contents of the Book

*Teresa Kowalska, Mieczysław Sajewicz, and Joseph Sherma*

## CONTENTS

## 1.1 OVERVIEW OF THIN-LAYER CHROMATOGRAPHY–MASS SPECTROMETRY

Although the history of thin-layer chromatography (TLC) dates back to the analysis of plant tinctures on aluminum oxide layers with methanol mobile phase by Ismailov and Shraiber in 1938 as chronicled by Sherma and Morlock in a published chronology [1], the first report on TLC coupled with mass spectrometry (MS) was not until 1977 by Issaq [2]. He eluted separated zones on a layer using the CAMAG Eluchrom instrument, designed and described in the literature in 1975 [1], and eluates were introduced into a mass spectrometer through a Pyrex inlet probe.

It is useful to comment on correct use of nomenclature in the field of liquid chromatography (LC). The acronym HPLC is almost universally used to denote column high-performance liquid chromatography, but high-performance TLC (HPTLC) involves the use of a liquid mobile phase and technically belongs to the category of HPLC. Similarly, the acronym LC–MS is almost always used for hyphenation of column LC (HPLC, ultra-performance liquid chromatography [UPLC, used for Waters Corp. Acquity systems with columns containing <2 μm sorbent particles], or ultra-high-performance liquid chromatography [UHPLC, used for systems from other manufacturers with columns containing <2 μm sorbent packings]) with MS, but it should be realized that TLC–MS is also correctly included in the category of LC–MS because of its use of a liquid mobile phase. TLC and HPTLC are included within the category of planar chromatography, in which the stationary phase (sorbent) is in the form of a (flat) plane such as a layer on a glass plate, aluminum or plastic sheet, or a piece of paper (paper chromatography).

The combination of TLC with MS both online and offline allows obtaining the maximum amount of information from the chromatograms on a plate about

3

identification of separated zones, which is very important for studies in many areas including, but not limited to, identification and confirmation of drugs and their break-down products and metabolites, analytes in forensic samples, biologically active components in phytochemical samples (TLC fingerprinting combined with MS), fast screening of foodstuffs, and analysis of environmental samples. The availability of MS is especially critical when analytical standards are not available for the usual methods of zone identification and confirmation, that is, comparison of $R_f$ values, similar detection characteristics with dip and spray reagents, cochromatography, and comparison of *in situ* UV–visible spectra with the spectral mode of a densitometer. Quantification of identified compounds can also be obtained by TLC–MS to replace or complement densitometric quantification. It is among the simplest, cost-friendly, and well-performing techniques for analysis of complex mixtures, especially when part of "super-hyphenations" such as HPTLC-UV/visible/fluorescence detection and densitometry-bioactivity-MS [3].

The earliest comprehensive descriptions of TLC–MS coupling were in three book chapters by Busch [4–6], and research papers reporting instrumentation, methodology, and applications are included in biennial reviews of planar chromatography by Sherma, the latest of which was published in 2014 [7].

A scheme for classification of the approaches for hyphenation of TLC/HPTLC with MS was given by Morlock and Schwack in a review paper [8]. Elution-based approaches were subdivided into microcapillary arrow, surface sampling probe, overrun chromatography on a TLC strip, forced flow techniques (overpressured layer chromatography [OPLC] and rotation planar chromatography [RPC]), and elution-head-based interfaces. The second major classification was desorption-based techniques, which was subdivided into desorption by fast atom bombardment (FAB); desorption by ion bombardment (secondary ion mass spectrometry [SIMS]); desorption by laser light (matrix-assisted laser desorption/ionization [MALDI] with the option of imaging MS, surface-assisted laser desorption/ionization [SALDI], electrospray-assisted laser desorption/ionization [ELDI], laser ablation inductively coupled plasma mass spectrometry [LA-ICPMS], and laser-induced acoustic desorption electrospray ionization mass spectrometry [LIAD–ESI–MS]); desorption by a spray beam (desorption electrospray ionization [DESI], and easy ambient sonic spray ionization mass spectrometry [EASI]); and desorption by an excited gas beam (direct analysis in real time [DART] and flowing afterglow-atmospheric pressure glow discharge [FA-APGD]). The ionization process of each of these MS methods was described in the review paper by Morlock and Schwack [8] and three extensive reviews [9–11], and four book chapters [12,13] covering many of the MS techniques coupled with TLC have been published.

Coupling of gel electrophoresis to MS is also discussed in this book even though it is not a chromatography method according to the purest definition of the term; the separation occurs on a plane like in TLC, but the flow of a mobile phase is not involved in the separation mechanism. This combined method is being increasingly used in proteomic and molecular biology studies and for medical diagnostic purposes.

Despite all of the TLC–MS combinations given above, only three commercially available TLC–MS hyphenations were documented by Morlock [13], that is, an elution-head interface used exclusively thus far for ESI–MS and two others for HPTLC–MALDI–MS and HPTLC–DART–MS. Use of the CAMAG elution-head interface has been most widely reported in the literature by far, and a dedicated chapter is, therefore, devoted to it in this book (Chapter 3). The MALDI–MS system is available from Bruker-Daltonics for application using laser light as a largely automated, software-supported package (TLC/HPTLC–MALDI–MS software in Compass 1.3 with FlexControl and FlexAnalysis components for direct readout of zones). A DART–MS interface based on a gas beam for desorption is available from IonSense, Inc.

An example application of the commercial MALDI–MS system is in the paper by Torretta et al. on the qualitative and quantitative profiling of glycosphingolipids [14]. Aluminum-backed HPTLC silica gel plates were developed with chloroform/methanol/water (110:40:6) mobile phase, dried, placed into a Bruker Daltonics ImagePrep device for matrix (DHB: 2.5-dihydroxybenzoic acid) deposition, and then mounted on a Bruker Daltonics MTP TLC adapter (Figure 1.1) for transfer of analyte zones into the mass spectrometer. In addition, Brucker Daltonics has published two application notes on lipid determination [15,16], and Fuchs reviewed determination of phospholipids and glycolipids [17] using the commercially available TLC–MALDI–MS system.

The first commercial coupling of HPTLC with DART was reported by Morlock and Ueda in 2007 using a silica gel $60F_{254}$ HPTLC plate and an IonSense excited gas stream DART installed on a JMS-T100LC (AccuTOF-LC, JEOL) for qualitative analysis of isopropylthioxanthone and caffeine [18]. Later, Dytkiewitz and Morlock [19] used the IonSense TLC–DART MS interface for the identification of lubricant additives in mineral oil. Developed RP chemically bonded diol (C2) $F_{254}$ and silica

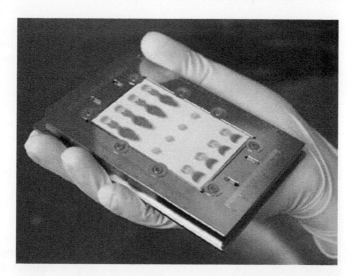

**FIGURE 1.1** MTP TLC–MALDI adapter target for $50 \times 75$ mm TLC silica gel aluminum plates. After TLC separation and matrix coating, the plate is ready for MALDI analysis. (Adapted from Bruker Daltonics, Billerica, MA.)

gel $60F_{254}$ plates were cut at marked positions with a CAMAG smartCUT based on zone detection under 254 nm ultraviolet (UV) light, and the zone of interest was positioned in the excited gas stream of an IonSense DART interface with a 1-cm sampling distance from an Agilent single quadrupole mass spectrometer. The technology of the coupling of TLC with DART through the IonSense interface was explained by Morlock and Chernetsova [20] and is available on the IonSense website, http://www.ionsense.com/dart_technology. Wood et al. used the IonSense DART ion source coupled to a JEOL AccuTOF mass spectrometer operated in the positive-ion mode and controlled by Mass Center software version 1.3.4 m (JEOL) for forensic analysis of pharmaceutical preparations on silica gel GHLF 250 μm Analtech plates [21]. A laser ablation TLC plasma (DART) ionization system described by Zheng et al. included an IonSense DART ion source; it was successfully applied in the analysis of a dye mixture, drug standards, and tea extract on silica gel plates with a limit of detection of 5 ng mm$^{-2}$ [22]. Crawford and Musselman reviewed the four commercial IonSense interfaces (DART 100, 2006–2009; DART 100 and SVP, 2006–present; DART SVP at Angle, 2009–present; and Laser Ablation DART, 2012–present) and the vertical on-edge, horizontal, 45° angle, and laser ablation procedures for TLC–MS [23]. Figure 1.2 shows the current DART 100.

A fourth commercial hyphenation system was used for liquid extraction surface analysis (LESA) of hydrophobic TLC plates coupled to chip based nanospray high-resolution MS as described by Himmelsbach et al. [24]. A mixture of lipid standards (triacylglycerols and phospholipids) was separated on an HPTLC C18 glass plate using chloroform/methanol/acetonitrile (2:1:1) mobile phase and detected with primuline dye reagent. Sample zones were analyzed using a TriVersa NanoMate system (Advion Inc., Figure 1.3) that was equipped with the LESA feature using the following briefly described procedure. The TLC plate is mounted onto a universal

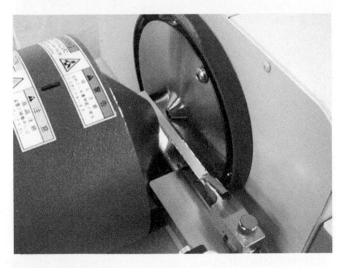

**FIGURE 1.2**   IonSense DART 100 TLC–MS interface. (Courtesy of JEOL Ltd., Aksihima, Japan.)

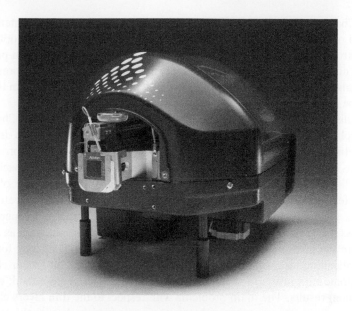

**FIGURE 1.3** TriVersa NanoMate chip-based ESI system coupled to TLC; see http://www.advion.com/products/triversa-nanomate/ for details on the technology, chip, and software. (Adapted from Advion Inc., Ithaca, NY.)

adaptor plate, and a robotic arm picks up a conductive pipet tip, moves to a solvent reservoir, and aspirates a defined volume. The tip moves to the analyte zone center position on the layer and dispenses an adjustable volume of the extraction solvent. The microjunction created allows extraction of the analyte into a small volume of solvent before it is aspirated back into the pipet tip, which is then moved to the ESI chip to generate a nanoelectrospray directed toward the inlet of the mass spectrometer (APEX III FTICRMS from Bruker Daltonics). Depending on zone size to be sampled, 5–9 μL was dispensed and consequently 1–4 μL aspirated. The optimized extraction solvent composition was methanol/chloroform/water/formic acid (52:24:24:0.2), and nanospray voltage was 1.6 kV and gas pressure 0.2 psi in all experiments. Use of the Advion TriVersa Nanomate system was also reported for identification of proteins and/or modifications [25] and in the areas of food and beverage, cosmetic active ingredients, and pharmaceutical ingredients [26].

## 1.2 ORGANIZATION OF THE BOOK

The book comprises 19 chapters that are divided into Sections I and II. Section I contains Chapters 1 through 9, which provide an overview of chromatographic thin layers, special instrumentation for the TLC–MS coupling, and various different mass spectrometric techniques that can be directly or indirectly combined into the planar chromatography–MS methodologies. Gel electrophoretic layers are additionally included in this book because they formally fall within the scope of the definition of a thin layer and can be coupled offline with mass spectrometric detectors. Section II

contains Chapters 10 through 19 and presents practical applications of methodologies based on planar chromatography-mass spectrometry and gel electrophoresis–
mass spectrometry to a wide variety of practical separation/identification problems
from such diverse research fields as medicine, pharmacy, biochemistry, forensic science, chemistry of enantiomers, etc. The characteristics of each chapter in the book
will now be given briefly.

After this introductory chapter beginning Section I of the book, Chapter 2,
titled "Applicability of Commercial and Noncommercial Thin Layers for Mass
Spectrometric Detection," provides critical information for current and prospective
users of this hyphenated approach. Coupling of these two analytical approaches considerably differing in several crucial points (e.g., relatively low degree of instrumentation for planar chromatography versus fully instrumental mass spectrometric
techniques, generally lower sensitivity of planar chromatography compared with
that of mass spectrometry, and operation under different conditions such as ambient
temperature and pressure for planar chromatography versus high vacuum for MS) is
quite a challenging task. In this chapter, a strong accent is laid on proper choice of
the appropriate thin layers to secure the best possible identification (and, possibly,
quantification) results. The main problems with respect to the thin layers chosen to
couple with mass spectrometers are the noise signals (which obscure the signals of
interest and originate from various different sources of layer contamination) and
the layer thickness (as mass distribution in the separated chromatographic bands
reaches to the depth of the layers, whereas transfer of substances from the bands to
the mass spectrometric sources goes predominantly from a shallow layer surface,
which negatively affects the quantification results). The author provides expert and
largely complete information on commercial and noncommercial thin layers, with
particular attention paid to the advantages and disadvantages of each one of them
when employed in the analytical thin-layer–mass spectrometry combination.

Chapter 3 is titled "The CAMAG TLC–MS Interface" and provides detailed
description of this unique device known as the TLC–MS interface, developed in order
to elute separated chromatographic bands from the chromatogram and to introduce
the eluates to the mass spectrometric source. The authors remind readers of the preliminary attempts in this direction and describe the prototype of the device further
improved to reach to its present form. The multipurpose versatility of this device is
emphasized by pointing out possibilities of its coupling with IR and NMR spectrometers as well, thus enabling hyphenation of TLC with IR and NMR spectrometry.
Finally yet importantly, the authors give a selection of the most interesting practical
applications of the TLC–MS interface to solving diverse analytical problems.

In Chapter 4, titled "Principles of Mass Spectrometry Imaging Applicable to Thin-
Layer Chromatography," the authors first introduce a budding analytical approach
known as imaging mass spectrometry (IMS) strategy and then present some successful examples of its practical applications. Then, they introduce in detail three
mass spectrometric techniques as those routinely used within the framework of IMS.
These are secondary mass spectrometry (SIMS), matrix-assisted laser desorption/
ionization (MALDI–IMS), and desorption electrospray ionization (DESI). Finally,
the authors discuss the advances and bottlenecks of these techniques when applied
to TLC.

In Chapter 5, titled "Mass Spectrometry Applicable to Electrophoretic Techniques," the authors discuss hyphenation of protein separations on electrophoretic gel layers under the influence of an electric field with offline mass spectrometric detection. Different types of electrophoretic gels and different techniques of running the electrophoretic separation process in the one-dimensional (1D) and the two-dimensional (2D) separation mode are presented. The authors introduce different visualization techniques applicable to the separated peptides in the electropherograms (that predominantly are different staining techniques, but also isotope labeling). All of these techniques allow localization of individual peptides or peptide fractions on the gel layers. Thus far, no interface is available for online coupling of electropherograms with mass spectrometers, so that the separated protein bands have to be excised from the gel layer prior to the mass spectrometric analysis. This crucial step of the discussed tandem approach can also be accomplished with the aid of dedicated robots. As a wide variety of different mass spectrometric techniques are applicable to the analysis of proteins, less attention is paid to these techniques (which, on the other hand, are extensively discussed in Chapters 6 and 7). Summing up, Chapter 5 furnishes an interesting overview of the approaches utilized for the analysis of proteins in biotechnological and biochemical laboratories, which provide an invaluable source of information for proteomics.

Chapter 6, titled "Selection of Ionization Methods of Analytes in the TLC–MS Techniques" provides an overview of mass spectrometric techniques that can be coupled with TLC and act as specific detectors in this hyphenated approach. The mass spectrometric techniques discussed in this chapter are secondary mass spectrometry (SIMS), liquid secondary ion mass spectrometry (LSIMS), fast atom bombardment (FAB), matrix-assisted laser desorption/ionization (MALDI), atmospheric pressure matrix-assisted laser desorption/ionization (AP–MALDI), electrospray ionization (ESI), desorption electrospray ionization (DESI), electrospry-assisted laser desorption/ionization (ELDI), easy ambient sonic spray ionization (EASI), direct analysis in real time (DART), laser-induced acoustic desorption/electrospray ionization (LIAD/ESI), plasma-assisted multiwavelength laser desorption/ionization (PAMLDI), atmospheric-pressure chemical ionization (APCI), and dielectric barrier discharge ionization (DBDI). For the sake of illustration, the authors introduce practical examples of implementing TLC separations with detection carried out by means of individual mass spectrometric techniques for the systematically arranged compounds belonging to different chemical classes.

Chapter 7, titled "Interfacing TLC with Laser-Based Ambient Mass Spectrometry," provides an overview of mass spectrometric techniques that can be coupled with TLC under the most convenient working conditions, that is, at room temperature and atmospheric pressure. The authors introduce readers to electrospray laser desorption ionization (ELDI), plasma-assisted multiwavelength laser desorption/ionization (PAMLDI), laser desorption atmospheric pressure chemical ionization (LD–APCI), laser desorption-dual electrospray and atmospheric pressure chemical ionization I (LD – ESI + APCI), laser-induced acoustic desorption electrospray ionization (LIAD–ESI), and laser-induced acoustic desorption–dielectric barrier discharge ionization (LIAD–DBDI). Chapters 6 and 7 are largely complementary because in the former one, main attention is paid to practical applications of a wide number of ambient mass spectrometric techniques, and the latter focuses more on the operating and theoretical principles thereof. Moreover, Chapter 7 presents an abundant overview of the contributions made by the Chinese teams of authors to laser-based ambient mass spectrometric detection in TLC.

Chapter 8, titled "TLC-MS Analysis Using Solvent Elution of Compounds from Chromatographic Media," is written as a comprehensive guide leading the reader from the early 1960s of the twentieth century, when MS was first introduced in an offline mode to enhance the analytical potential of TLC to modern applications with the use of an online solvent elution, facilitated by the CAMAG TLC–MS interface. At the beginning, MS was applied for the purely qualitative purpose of identification of the separated analytes, while nowadays an encouraging and relatively rapid progress of the TLC–MS technique employing solvent elution makes this approach an increasingly more quantitative analytical tool. The authors present the development stages of the method in a systematic manner, and, even today, practical application of the earlier elaborated approaches (e.g., manual scraping of individual chromatographic bands from the plate, washing the compounds out from the adsorbent, and an offline introduction of the resulting solution to mass spectrometer) on many occasions can be successfully applied.

Chapter 9, titled "Recording of Mass Spectra from Miniaturized Layers (UTLC–MS)," closes Section I of the book. The chapter focuses on various technical aspects of the thin layers and instrumentation applicable to the development of the hyphenated planar chromatography-mass spectrometry modes. In fact, Chapters 2 and 9 are complementary in the sense that they jointly provide an exhaustive overview of the thin layers that are best suited for coupling with mass spectrometric detection. While Chapter 2 focuses on commercial and noncommercial thin layers applicable to TLC/HPTLC (with a relatively brief entry concerning the UTLC layers), Chapter 9 provides virtually complete information on a novel and promising trend within planar chromatography, which is the miniaturized thin-layer chromatography (UTLC) with different types of ultrathin layers. Although this novel trend remains mostly at the infancy stage, the authors provide a nicely structured overview of the subject matter, in separate chapters, handling different concepts of manufacturing ultrathin layers, different technical possibilities of coupling these layers with mass spectrometers, and the best examples of successful practical applications of the UTLC–MS technique.

Chapter 10, titled "Strategies of Coupling Planar Chromatography to HPLC–MS," presents a 2D operating mode, with the possibility of enhancing the separation potential of TLC/HPTLC by introducing the HPLC intermediary system as a second and orthogonal separation dimension. This rather easily available setup (in either the online or the offline version) proves particularly inevitable in such cases when thin-layer modifiers (e.g., impregnation agents) obscure the 1D TLC/HPTLC–MS results, or when planar chromatography plays a preliminary cleanup role as a specific solid-phase extractor (SPE) with the complex analyte mixtures. The authors illustrate their text with attractive practical examples taken mostly from the fields of food and drug analysis and provide very well chosen and comprehensive figures and tables.

Chapter 11, titled "Drug Analysis by TLC–DESI MS," introduces basic information on technical solutions needed for an efficient coupling of TLC with the DESI MS detection. The authors attribute primary importance to the quality of the TLC plates recommended for an efficient TLC–DESI MS coupling, and at the same time, they offer valuable advice regarding the geometry of the ion source and the solvents best suited for the DESI technique. The strength of the chapter lies in presentation of the most favorable working parameters needed for an efficient application of the TLC–DESI MS technique to the analysis of drugs (and the other low-molecular-weight analytes as well).

Chapter 12, titled "Application of TLC and Plasma-Based Ambient MS in Bioanalytical Sciences," provides detailed discussion of TLC separations assisted by plasma-based ambient ionization MS modes as specific detection techniques, and emphasizes practical advantages of such couplings. Among the examples of relevant mass spectrometric techniques, DART is mentioned in the first instance, but also its modification known as DART SVP-A (DART ion source with desorption at an angle), then PAMLDI, DBDI, and FAPA (flowing atmospheric pressure afterglow). Coupled TLC–MS approaches of this type can be applied to a wide range of practical tasks, like detection of warfare agents, control of chemical reactions, mass spectrometry imaging, identification of polymers, food safety monitoring, drug and pharmaceutical analysis, medical diagnostics, forensic research, biochemical analyses, etc. The authors present an interesting selection of well-chosen practical examples of the aforementioned hyphenated techniques.

Chapter 13, titled "TLC–MALDI MS for the Analysis of Lipids," is devoted to a challenging issue of lipid separation and identification with use of a hyphenated analytical technique that combines TLC with MALDI MS detection. In fact, the main interest of the researchers is focused on the applications of the aforementioned technique to the analysis of glycerophospholipids (GPLs) and sphingolipids (SLs), due to their respective biological importance. GPLs play an important role as constituents of cellular and subcellular membranes, and are generated by esterification of glycerol with two (normally different) fatty acids. SLs (and particularly glycosylated sphingolipids, GSLs) are nowadays regarded as highly important molecules that are involved in the pathogenesis of different serious diseases, such as cancer. The authors introduce the physiological importance of analytical research carried out within the framework of the aforementioned subject matter, followed by an up-to-date overview of practical applications of TLC–MALDI MS to these studies.

Chapter 14, titled "Application of TLC–MS to Drug Photodegradation Studies," is in the first instance a mini review of the authors' interesting contribution to this very important area of drug analysis, focusing on photosensitivity of selected drugs and tracing the directions of their photolytic decay. Photostability testing of drugs under the defined working conditions is recommended by the International Conference on Harmonization (ICH) guidelines, and the authors present the TLC–MS methods developed in their own laboratory as a kind of model approach applicable to the analogous stability indicating studies with other drugs. With photolabile compounds, the photodegradation products often prove harmful (e.g., toxic, allergogenic, or carcinogenic), so that thorough photodegradation studies can ensure timely warning to the pharmaceutical industry and drug regulatory agencies. MS (in combination with the thin-layer separations) proves a particularly helpful analytical tool in photostability tests, which yield photodegradation products mostly at low concentrations, and in that way MS largely facilitates their identification.

Chapter 15, titled "Combination of Thin-Layer Chromatography with Laser Desorption Ionization and Electrospray Ionization–Mass Spectrometric Techniques for Screening of Organic Compounds," addresses a selection of practical applications of the TLC separation technique implemented with the ESI and LDI mass spectrometric detection systems. The authors present well-chosen examples dealing with lipids, gangliosides, drugs, and various other organic compounds of general interest, and the chapter is additionally enriched with a tabulated overview of the working TLC and MS parameters, and with references valid for the selected TLC–MS applications.

Chapter 16, titled "Application of TLC–MS to Analysis of Drugs of Abuse," presents an interesting insight into this sector of forensic sciences, which is oriented on investigation of such drugs. For obvious reasons, forensic procedures based on chemical analysis require reliable, high throughput, and at the same time low-cost analytical methods of identification and quantification of suspicious materials. TLC separations combined with mass spectrometric detection perfectly satisfy all these forensic demands. In this tandem approach, a particular role is played by TLC, which ensures minimum or no sample preparation, satisfactory sensitivity, high throughput, and relatively low equipment cost, and, hence, it can be considered a very cost-friendly analytical option. The authors, who are the renowned experts in the TLC–MS analysis of drugs of abuse, present in their chapter an overview of such methods applied to identification and quantification of cannabinoids, opiates, LSD, cocaine, and some other accompanying compounds of significant biological importance.

Chapter 17, titled "TLC–MS Analysis of Carotenoids, Triterpenoids, and Flavanols in Plant Extracts and Dietary Supplements," provides a thorough and up-to-date overview of the TLC–MS techniques applied to the analysis of selected secondary metabolites, abundantly present in botanical materials of considerable nutritional, but also curative, importance. Chemically, some carotenoids are recognized as vitamin A precursors, certain naturally occurring triterpenoids exert a well-proven anticancer activity, whereas flavanols are the well-established antioxidant agents, preventive against various different neurodegenerative conditions (e.g., Alzheimer and Parkinson diseases). Owing to particular versatility and robustness of the TLC systems, TLC has gained a firm position in phytochemical analysis long before the emergence of the online planar chromatography-mass spectrometry couplings. Consequently, in Chapter 18, a detailed coverage is provided of the offline and online TLC–MS systems applied to the analysis of carotenoids, triterpenoids, and flavanols, contained in botanical materials.

Chapter 18, titled "TLC–MALDI MS of Carbohydrates," provides up-to-date information regarding the TLC analysis of carbohydrates supported with MALDI MS. The contents of this chapter are particularly relevant because carbohydrates—owing to their chemical structure and the resulting physicochemical properties—represent a class of organic compounds that are quite difficult to analyze. Consequently, the literature including applications of TLC–MS to the investigations of carbohydrates is not very abundant. However, the authors did their very best to cover the existing literature on the subject and to critically evaluate the advantages and limitations of the TLC–MALDI MS technique applied to the analysis of carbohydrates.

The last chapter in the book, Chapter 19, is titled "Spontaneous Chiral Conversion and Peptidization of Amino Acids Traced by Means of TLC–MS" and presents an interesting application of MS to the TLC investigation of spontaneous chiral inversion of amino acids dissolved in the abiotic aqueous and organic solvents. Chiral inversion of amino acids (and other low-molecular-weight chiral carboxylic acids) is an example of a nonlinear process that still needs thorough investigation. In the course of this process, an optically pure amino acid of a given configuration (L or D) undergoes spontaneous inversion to its own mirror image (D or L, respectively). In the first instance, this inversion can be confirmed with the use of optically pure L and D standards and the respective retention parameters thereof (i.e., the $R_F$ values) However, reproducibility of the TLC retention parameters is known as a somewhat sensitive issue. Therefore, an additional confirmation of chiral conversion with use of the CAMAG TLC–MS interface enabling registration of mass spectra of the chromatographically separated enantiomer pairs can be considered a particularly useful complementary approach.

In conclusion, it can be stated that this book devoted to planar chromatography-mass spectrometry provides a comprehensive insight into a wide variety of technical possibilities and practical applications of planar chromatographic and gel electrophoretic separations supported with mass spectrometric detection, offered by leading experts in the individual research areas covered in this volume. To our best knowledge, this is the first monograph in the field that is meant to introduce researchers from many different fields of investigation to this versatile tandem methodology known as TLC–MS (in fact, implemented with a wide variety of different MS modes) and, at the same time, to encourage them to benefit from its multiple advantages in their future studies.

## REFERENCES

1. Sherma, J. and Morlock, G. 2008. Chronology of thin layer chromatography focusing on instrumental progress, *J. Planar Chromatogr.-Mod. TLC*, 21: 471–477.
2. Issaq, H., Schroer, J.A., and Barr, E.W. 1977. A direct online thin layer chromatography–mass spectrometry coupling system, *Chem. Instrum.*, 8: 51–53.
3. Morlock, G. and Schwack, W. 2010. Hyphenations in planar chromatography, *J. Chromatogr. A*, 1217: 6600–6609.
4. Bush, K.L. 1991. Thin layer chromatography coupled with mass spectrometry, in *Handbook of Thin Layer Chromatography*, Sherma, J. and Fried, B., Eds., CRC Press/Taylor & Francis Group, Boca Raton, FL, Chapter 8.
5. Bush, K.L. 1996. Thin layer chromatography coupled with mass spectrometry, in *Handbook of Thin Layer Chromatography*, 2nd ed., Sherma, J. and Fried, B., Eds., CRC Press/Taylor & Francis Group, Boca Raton, FL, Chapter 9.
6. Bush, K.L. 2003. Thin layer chromatography coupled with mass spectrometry, in *Handbook of Thin Layer Chromatography*, 3rd ed., Sherma, J. and Fried, B., Eds., CRC Press/Taylor & Francis Group, Boca Raton, FL, Chapter 9.
7. Sherma, J. 2014. Biennial review of planar chromatography, *Cent. Eur. J. Chem.*, 12: 427–452.
8. Morlock, G. and Schwack, W. 2010. Coupling of planar chromatography to mass spectrometry, *Trends Anal. Chem.*, 29: 1157–1171.

9. Berry, K.A.Z., Hankin, J.A., Barkley, R.M., Spraggins, J.M., Caprioli, R.M., and Murphy, R.C. 2011. MALDI imaging of lipid biochemistry in tissues by mass spectrometry, *Chem. Rev.*, 111: 6491–6512.

10. Meisen, I., Mormann, M., and Muething, J. 2011. Thin layer chromatography, overlay technique and mass spectrometry: A versatile triad advancing glycosphingolipidomics, *Biochim. Biophys. Acta,* 1811: 875–896.

11. Monge, M.E., Harris, G.A., Dwivedi, P., and Fernandez, F.M. 2013. Mass spectrometry: Recent advances in direct open air surface sampling/ionization, *Chem. Rev.*, 113: 2269–2308.

12. Srivastava, M., Ed., *High Performance Thin Layer Chromatography (HPTLC)*, Springer, Heidelberg, Chapters 15–17.

13. Morlock, G. 2012. High performance thin layer chromatography–mass spectrometry for analysis of small molecules, in *Applied Mass Spectrometry Handbook*, Lee, M., Ed., John Wiley & Sons, New York, Chapter 49.

14. Torretta, E., Vasso, M., Fania, C., Capitanio, D., Bergante, S., Piccoli, M., Tettamanti, G., Anastasia, L., and Geifi, C. 2014. Application of direct HPTLC-MALDI for the qualitative and quantitative profiling of neutral and acid glycosphingolipids: The case of NEU3 overexpressing C2C12 murine myboblasts, *Electrophoresis,* 25: 1319–1328.

15. Bruker Daltonics Application Note # MT-101, High resolution lipid profiling and identification by hyphenated HPTLC–MALDI-TOF/TOF, Billerica, MA.

16. Bruker Daltonics Application Note # MT-94, Direct read-out of thin layer chromatography (TLC) using MALDI-TOF, Billerica, MA.

17. Fuchs, B. 2012. Analysis of phospholipids and glycolipids by thin layer chromatography-matrix assisted laser desorption and ionization mass spectrometry, *J. Chromatogr. A*, 1259: 62–73.

18. Morlock, G. and Ueda, Y. 2007. New coupling of planar chromatography with direct analysis in real time mass spectrometry, *J. Chromatogr. A,* 1143: 243–251.

19. Dytkiewitz, E. and Morlock, G.E. 2008. Analytical strategy for rapid identification and quantification of lubricant additives in mineral oil by high performance thin layer chromatography with UV absorption and fluorescence detection combined with mass spectrometry and infrared spectroscopy, *J. AOAC Int.,* 91: 1237–1243.

20. Morlock, G.E. and Chernetsova, E.S. 2012. Coupling of planar chromatography with direct analysis in real time mass spectrometry, *Cent. Eur. J. Chem.*, 10: 703–710.

21. Wood, J.L. and Steiner, R.R. 2011. Purification of pharmaceutical preparations using thin layer chromatography to obtain mass spectra with direct analysis in real time and accurate mass spectrometry, *Drug Test. Anal.*, 3: 345–351.

22. Zhang, J., Zhigui, Z., Yang, J., Zhang, W., Bai, Y., and Liu, H. 2012. Thin layer chromatography/plasma assisted multiwavelength laser desorption ionization mass spectrometry for facile separation and selective identification of low molecular weight compounds, *Anal. Chem.*, 84: 1496–1503.

23. Crawford, E. and Musselman, B. 2014. Planar chromatography meets direct ambient mass spectrometry: Current trends, *HPTLC 2014*, Lyon, France, July 2–4, Abstract O-9.

24. Himmelsbach, M., Varesio, E., and Hopfgartner, G. 2014. Liquid extraction surface analysis (LESA) of hydrophobic TLC plates coupled to chip based nanoelectrospray high resolution mass spectrometry, *Chimia*, 68: 150–154.

25. Morschheuser, L., Biller, J., Reim, V., Trusch, M., and Rohn, S. 2014. A further look at protein analysis—Useful applications of nano-ESI–MS for the identification of proteins and possible modifications, *HPTLC 2014*, Lyon, France, July 2–4, Abstract P-35.

26. Oberle, M., Griesinger, H., Minarik, S., Matheis, K., and Schulz, M. 2014. HPTLC-nanospray-MS using the Advion NanoMate system, *HPTLC 2014*, Lyon, France, July 2–4, Abstract P-31.

# 2 Applicability of Commercial and Noncommercial Thin Layers for Mass Spectrometric Detection

*Fred Rabel*

## CONTENTS

## 2.1  INTRODUCTION

Over the years, the manufacturers of thin-layer plates have followed advances in this field of thin-layer chromatography and developed improved products to meet newer demands, such as purity, substrates, and chemistries. Sometimes these advances came from researchers developing new applications or uses of these products. Other times, it was independent or in conjunction with the manufacturers of thin-layer equipment such as spotting devices, developing method, or detection devices. This chapter will detail the thin layers available commercially and those other researchers have made or designed for use in mass spectrometric detection.

After separation, the components have to be characterized, which was easily automated with gas chromatography (GC) and high-performance liquid chromatography/ultra-high-performance liquid chromatography (HPLC/UHPLC) over the years. Although it has its advantages, thin-layer chromatography/high-performance thin-layer chromatography (TLC/HPTLC) has always been hands-on and more difficult to automate. Still, this disadvantage has not deterred researchers and companies from continuing to bring knowledge and products to help TLC to be competitive with other analytical tools that have led to this text.

Obviously, the most important criteria for the chromatographer are the reproducibility of the silica gels, chemicals, and solvents used in any protocol. It is also important that these materials be available over a long period of time so a revalidation is not required. Because many of the companies making TLC products had been supplying large particle size silica gels for column chromatography, the TLC line became a natural extension. However, a considerable product development time was needed to produce the thin layers taken for granted today. The silica gel had to be paired up with the support, suitable binder, and additive to be coated, dried, and packaged before it got to the customers.

## 2.2  THE SUPPORTS

Classically, glass has been the support of choice for thin-layer plates. Most chromatographers are not aware of the special requirements of the glass holding the layer. It has to be absolutely flat to give a reproducible layer, so "float" glass has to be used, where the molten glass is cast onto molten metal for its manufacture. It is also thinner (~1.2 mm) than the usual windowpane glass to save on weight when shipped. The glass plates have to be rigorously cleaned of any oily residues and thoroughly dried before they can be coated. The most used sizes of standard glass-backed TLC plates are the $20 \times 20$ cm and $5 \times 20$ cm sizes, but each manufacturer has many other sizes available.

Because of the weight and space requirements for glass-backed prepared plates, the manufacturers found flexible supports for their thin layers. Thus, thin layers coated on plastic (polyterephthalate for its chemical resistance, 200 μm thick) and aluminum (100 μm thick) were offered. These had the added advantage that they were much easier to cut to any size needed with any sharp blade/straight edge or with scissors. In 1998 when Chen et al. [1] began to do surface-assisted laser desorption/ionization (SALDI) work, the use of silica gel layers on the plastic support allowed them to cut samples from $2 \times 2$ mm to $1 \times 1$ cm to place in their mass spectrometry (MS). Early work with matrix-assisted laser desorption ionization time-of-flight (MALDI TOF) also required silica gel layers on aluminum, which allowed the sample to be cut from the developed plate but also provided electric conductivity necessary for ionizing the sample [2].

HPTLC prepared plates are mostly available on glass in $10 \times 20$ cm, $10 \times 10$ cm, and $5 \times 5$ cm sizes because of the shorter developing distances required. A couple, however, are available with the aluminum support (often called an aluminum foil). These are $5 \times 7.5$ cm in size and are used in MS techniques as described previously. One such paper by Himmelsback et al. [3] used the HPTLC silica gel on aluminum to separate various mixtures, cut the plate with a $60°$ angle point in front of the band, placing it in front of the MS orifice, and a spectra was obtained after a spray solvent was applied to the thin layer.

Since more HPTLC layers are available on glass than on plastic, CAMAG offers a smartCut glass plate cutter, unless one practices with other glass-cutting devices.

## 2.3  BINDING AGENTS

On its own, a slurry of a sorbent coated and dried on a thin layer support would fall off when the plate is moved. Thus, it is necessary to include a binder to adhere the sorbent to the support. Presumably, because of its well-known nature, calcium sulfate hemi-hydrate, or plaster of Paris (or the G designation for gypsum) was initially used by anyone making thin-layer silica gel plates. On drying, it forms the dihydrate and keeps the soft layer intact as long as the plate is carefully handled. This binder is in the range of 10%–15% by weight. The gypsum-bound silica gel TLC plate over time became the de facto standard in most TLC protocols because it was the only available prepared plate. Because of its fragile nature, special packaging had to be developed to keep one soft layer from touching any plate below or above. Hence, the usual box of twenty-five $20 \times 20$ cm plate ended up in a cube of slightly larger dimensions. Still, depending on the handling of these packages, some damage to a percentage of the soft layer plates often occurred.

Because of this problem, research was done by the TLC manufacturers to find a suitable organic binder that could be used to form a more durable thin layer. Most thin layer sorbents are slurried in water (or water/alcohol mixtures) for coating onto the supports. Thus, the search concentrated on water-soluble organic monomers that would crosslink with air or oven drying to form a polymer to bind the sorbent to the support. Of primary concern was that it does (1) not interfere with the chromatography, (2) not allow irreversible binding of any sample component placed on the thin layer, and finally (3) not interfere with the detection or visualization steps that might be required. These binders are proprietary for each manufacturer but are similar to polyvinyl alcohol, polyvinyl pyrollidone, or acrylates. Their concentration need only be 1%–2% by weight.

These organic binders used on silica gel prepared layers have been well received because of the resulting hard layer and ease of use. The binders do impart a barrier to moisture and these plates absorb less moisture with time after heat activation (which keeps absorbed moisture content less with time). In addition, if an aqueous-based visualization reagent is sprayed on this hard layer plate after development and drying, the visualization solution is not immediately absorbed and runs down over the surface. The solution is to incorporate 5%–10% methanol or ethanol to the aqueous reagent formulation to decrease their surface tension allowing penetration into the layer.

Since some silica gel or bonded reversed phase (RP) thin-layer plates might be developed with water-rich mobile phases, different binders or concentrations had to be found to allow the layer to remain intact and not swell or lift during the development process. A designation for water-tolerant binder is noted in the naming of these thin layers with the letter, W, in their description. If lifting or swelling of the layer is observed on a standard binder plate (non-W-type plate), the aqueous portion of the mobile phase can be replaced with 1 M sodium chloride, which prevents swelling of the binder [4]. A pretreatment below details prepared layer heat activation, a step that can also help cross-linked any monomeric binder that was not well cross-linked during manufacturer thus might be considered an additional preparation step whether using a silica gel or bonded silica gel layer.

Depending on the support and the intended layer thickness, the binder or its concentration might vary. A flexible support must be able to bend to a certain degree as it is used, and the layer must not lift and fall from the support. With a glass support, the need for flexibility is unnecessary.

If the sorbent and separated component needs to be scrapped from a hard layer/polymer bound plate, it is best done after a light spraying with methanol or ethanol to soften the layer to prevent "flaking" and loss of sample.

## 2.4  FLUORESCENT INDICATORS

Unless the chromatographer is working with plant extracts, as was Tswett, then compounds being separated on thin layer plates will not be visible. There are visualization reagents based on organic spot tests, which allow them to be derivatized *in situ*. Before this is done, however, it is possible to first look under a UV light at short (254 nm) or long (366 nm) wavelengths to see whether there is any native fluorescence from one or more sample components.

To aid in initial detection, the TLC plate manufacturers have included different inorganic fluorescent indicators in the sorbent slurries that can be made to fluoresce with UV light. Inorganic indicators need to be used so that they will not be moved with any solvent used for development. They allow detection of compounds that do not fluoresce but absorb the UV light. If they absorb the UV light, the fluorescent indicator is not activated, and the separated compound appears as a dark band or spot against the green, light blue, or white fluorescence. These fluorescent indicators also allow quantitation with densitometry as described in the TLC text [5].

One fluorescent indicator used is an alkali earth wolframate, which is acid stable and fluoresces pale blue or white. It is indicated by the letters and numbers UV254s/F254s, meaning it is activated by 254 nm UV light and is acid stable. The other widely used fluorescent indicator is manganese-activated zinc silicate, which fluoresces green and is not acid stable. It is indicated by the letters and numbers UV254/

F254; again, activation is with 254 nm UV light. There are other indicators such as Ultraphor PAN and a few others that are activated at 366 nm, and fluoresce blue, green, or red that might also be found in prepared plates.

Regarding the acid stability mentioned above, it means that the indicator will or will not continue to fluoresce after spraying with a visualization reagent that contains acid. If the plate used does have the fluorescent indicator that degrades, it is likely not a problem because this UV visualization is first after separation and any results recorded before any spraying with a visualization reagent.

Every manufacturer uses one or the other of these fluorescent indicators in their F-type plates. They will be in different concentrations resulting in different fluorescent intensities. Some newer TLC products are available with a higher concentration of the fluorescent indicator yielding a brighter fluorescence. Depending on the chromatographer's preference and needs, one might give better results compared to the other. Also to be considered is that the intensity does not overwhelm the detection of low concentration components. The only way to determine suitability is to compare the results with the samples being analyzed on the different products during method development.

To get the best results of fluorescence quenching, after developing the plate it should be thoroughly dried to remove all solvents, acids, or bases, which might have been in the mobile phase. Some of these may have quenching or UV absorbing properties, so the full effect of the fluorescent indicators could be masked. Many of these chemicals will not have the volatility of organic solvent and are retained longer or they may actually form chemical bonds with the silanols present. More complete drying can be done in a hood with a hair dryer, a forced air oven at temperature between 60°C and 80°C, or a special thin layer plate heater available from CAMAG with a programmable surface. Such forced heating assumes that any compounds on the thin layer will not volatilize or degrade under these conditions.

Most chromatographers prefer to purchase the TLC or HPTLC plates with a fluorescent indicator because it is there if needed but does not interfere with other steps in the protocol.

## 2.5 THIN-LAYER CHROMATOGRAPHY VERSUS HIGH-PERFORMANCE THIN-LAYER CHROMATOGRAPHY VERSUS ULTRATHIN-LAYER CHROMATOGRAPHY

One of the basic principles of chromatography is that smaller particles give increased efficiency and separation in a shorter amount of time. This has been the focus for many advances over the years for many chromatography products including TLC. Since the late 1950s, the standard TLC sorbent was irregular silica gel with an average particle size of 15 μm, with a particle size range of 5–20 μm. Standard TLC-prepared plates typically have a thickness of 250 μm on glass, 200 μm on a flexible layer, and thicker layers from 500 to 1000 μm on glass for preparative work.

In the mid-1970s, the smaller particle HPTLC prepared plates came onto the market. These are coated with irregular silica gel with an average particle size of 5 μm, with a particle size range of 4–8 μm. The HPTLC plates offered have a thickness of between 50 and 200 μm depending on the support and their intended use, to be discussed later. Also, rather than the larger size prepared plates up to $20 \times 20$ cm, only a $20 \times 10$ cm HPTLC prepared plate is available but to be developed in the 10-cm direction to take advantage of the fast development and accomodating many more samples and standards. Most HPTLC users order the $5 \times 5$ cm or $10 \times 10$ cm size plates. The general properties of these different silica gels are shown in Table 2.1

Note that for the best resolution, smaller sample amounts are placed on these layers, best with a streaking device, and lower limits of detection are found compared to TLC layers.

Many manufacturers of TLC plates also had been manufacturing supports for HPLC column. From the early 1970s, they began to switch from packing columns with irrregular silica gels to solid spherical silica gels, which had performance advantages of greater speed, efficiency, and less backpressure. With the knowledge of producing spherical particles, they could use these to also produce HPTLC plates with the same spherical sorbent such as LiChrospher® 60 (Merck [EMD] Millipore, Darmstadt, Germany) with 5–7 μm particle sizes, on different supports with 100–200 μm layer thicknesses. A comparison of HPTLC silica gel 60 and LiChrospher separation parameters are shown in Table 2.2.

At times, as mentioned previously, a researcher or company not in the TLC plate manufacturing business develops a device or procedure that requires a TLC product with different specifications. One such instance is the development of the automatic multiple development (AMD, CAMAG) device, which required thinner layer HPTLC plates for best results. AMD layers are available in 50 and 100 μm thicknesses from Merck (EMD) Millipore and Macherey-Nagel. Also offered by Merck (EMD) Millipore are HPTLC with irregular or spherical thinner layer plates (100 μm or 200 μm) for applications to determine polyaromatic hydrocarbons (PAH), peptides, and for Raman spectroscopy. Sources to a more detailed information on the world's leading manufactures of the pre-coated TLC/HPTLC plates are provided in Table 2.3.

---

**TABLE 2.1**

**Specifications of Classical TLC Compared to HPTLC Plates**

|                                          | TLC                   | HPTLC                 |
| ---------------------------------------- | --------------------- | --------------------- |
| Average particle size                    | 10–12 μm              | 5–7 μm                |
| Particle size distribution               | 5–20 μm               | 4–8 μm                |
| Layer thickness                          | 250 μm (200 μm)       | 200 μm (100 μm)       |
| Typical plate height                     | 30 μm                 | 12 μm                 |
| Typical developing distance              | 10–15 cm              | 3–6 cm                |
| Typical separation time                  | 20–200 min            | 3–20 min              |
| Number of sample most often applied to plate | <10               | <36                   |
| Range of sample volume                   | 1–5 μL                | 0.1–0.5 μL            |
| Adsorption limits of detection           | 1–5 ng                | 100–500 pg            |
| Fluorescence limits of detections        | 50–100 pg             | 5–10 pg               |

*Source:*   Adapted from Merck Millipore/EMD Millipore websites (Table 2.3).
*Note:*   Thinner layers are often coated on flexible and special use plates.

---

**TABLE 2.2**

**Comparison of Analysis Times—Irregular HPTLC Silica to HPTLC LiChrospher Plates**

| Eluent | Developing Distance | HPTLC Silica Gel 60 $F_{254s}$ | LiChrospher Silica Gel 60 $F_{254s}$ (min) |
|---|---|---|---|
| Toluene | 4 cm | 5 min, 45 s | 4 |
| Ethyl acetate/toluene (95:5) | 5 cm | 7 min, 50 s | 6 |
| Methyl ethyl ketone/1-propanol/water/ acetic acid (40:40:20:5) | 5 cm | 26 min, 30 s | 20 |
| n-Hexane/toluene/acetone (70:20:10) | 7 cm | 19 min | 13 |

*Source:*   Adapted from Merck Millipore/EMD Millipore websites (Table 2.3).

**TABLE 2.3**

**Major TLC/HPTLC Prepared Plate Manufacturers**

| Company | Web URL |
|---|---|
| Analtech | www.ichromatography.com |
| Dynamic Adsorbents | www.dynamicadsorbents.com |
| Macherey Nagel | www.mn-net.com |
| Merck Millipore | www.merckmillipore.com |
| EMD Millipore | www.emdmillipore.com |

*Note:*   J.T. Baker and Whatman no longer make TLC plates. Dynamic Adsorbents and Analtech can supply some of the Whatman TLC products.

Recently, Griesinger et al. [6] examined TLC–MS of lipids with positive ion MALDI-TOF on various thickness silica gel layers: 200, 100, and 60 μm. As the layer thickness decreases, there was less matrix background and increased sensitivities for the compound studied, with the best results on the 60-μm layer. This was true whether the sorbent bed was made up of TLC or HPTLC size particles.

For even faster and lower limits of detection, there has been an increasing interest in ultrathin-layer chromatography (UTLC). Only one of these layers made with monolithic silica was marketed but has since been discontinued. There is continued interest in UTLC since newer methods of preparation of these layers have been investigated and are discussed in Section 2.9.5.

## 2.6   PLATES WITH PREADSORBENT ZONES, CHANNELS, PRESCORING, OR GOOD LABORATORY PRACTICE NUMBERING

Through the years, the TLC plate manufacturers have added some features to their prepared layers that can help the chromatographer in some manner. Although they may not offer any specific advantage when doing any TLC–MS work in general, they will briefly be described.

*Preadsorbent zones*: This is a thin-layer plate designed with an area below the silica or bonded silica sorbent that is made up of diatomaceous earth or a wide pore silica gel. The purpose of this preadsorbent area is to allow fast sample application even with a crude spotting device with no absorption or separation of the sample components. After drying, when the development begins, the sample dissolves and concentrates onto itself to form a narrow band before it moves onto the active sorbent for separation. These sample bands improve the resulting separation compared to spots placed on the active layer, as streaking the sample does on any TLC plate. These plates are particularly well suited for dirty or biological samples where this area acts to preclean the sample, rather like an initial filtration.

*Channeled plates*: To keep samples and standards in their own space on the thin-layer plate, some manufacturers have scored away some of the layer so 1-cm-wide channels from bottom to top of the plate are available. Often two channels are spotted with the same mixture. After development, one channel is used for visualization and the other for use with MS work, whether *in situ* or extraction. This concept would be particularly valuable if on a flexible support but the channeled plates now sold are only on glass.

*Prescored plates*: To aid in breaking a larger TLC glass plate into smaller sizes, some manufacturers have scored the back of these plates so they can more easily be broken to a smaller size if encountering a smaller number of samples and standards.

*GLP (good laboratory practice) plates*: Each TLC or HPTLC prepared layer is laser etched with item/batch/individual plate number. This aids in the documentation of the separation.

Each of these plate variations is illustrated in Figure 2.1.

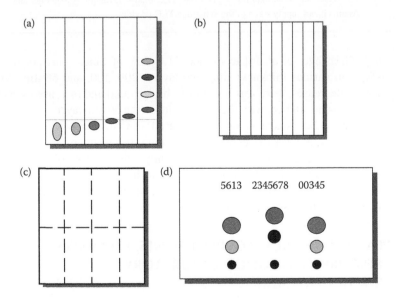

**FIGURE 2.1** Illustration of the plates/layers described in Section 2.6. (a) Preadsorbent plate, (b) channeled plate, (c) prescored plate, and (d) GLP plate.

## 2.7 PRETREATMENT OF THE THIN-LAYER CHROMATOGRAPHY/HIGH-PERFORMANCE THIN-LAYER CHROMATOGRAPHY PLATE

If doing simple TLC work where only cursory observation of purity or completeness of a reaction is required, taking a prepared TLC plate from the box, spotting, drying, developing, and visualizing can be done without any pretreatment. If quantitative analytical work is to be done, then greater detail is required to ensure reproducible results.

First, visually check the TLC or HPTLC prepared plate to see that there are no imperfections. These might arise during manufacture or while being stored if the package had been opened previously. The plate is held up to a sunlit window or some source of bright light to see that it is evenly coated, with no light or dark areas or streaks of heavier or lighter coating. If fluorescent quenching is to be done, then examining it under the appropriate wavelength UV light should be done to ensure an even background is seen. Any dark or light areas mean that the denser fluorescent indicator has settled out during manufacture.

The layer thickness near the edges of the plate is important to ensure even solvent travel up the TLC plates. Some chromatographers remove a 1-mm strip from both right and left edges of the thin-layer plate, the so-called "edging," with a straight edge and flat spatula. Likewise, remove any sorbent on the 1.2-mm glass plate edges with a paper towel, which will also improve the solvent travel on the plate. For safety reasons, all of these operations should be done in a hood and with proper protective gear.

Once a thin-layer plate has passed these initial inspections, then it should be prewashed because it may have absorbed impurities from the manufacture, storage, or packaging. This is especially true if the package or box has been opened and stored in an open environment for any amount of time and if a silica gel layer is being used because of their very absorptive nature. Bonded phases, as mentioned previously, are less prone to absorbing impurities and moisture. They do present another source of impurities, however, because remains of bonding reagent often migrate out of the inner pores of the sorbents on storage and need to be washed from the plate. Last, there are the monomeric/polymeric binders in the hard layer plates that might not have cross-linked as much as possible.

Prewashing a plate is accomplished by allowing a solvent (methanol, the mobile phase, or the extraction solvent mixture—whichever is the strongest to ensure nothing but the components will elute from the sample band) to migrate up the TLC plate in a developing chamber. Dipping in some solvent as a prewashing step is not as effective and uses considerably more solvent which then presents a disposal problem.

After this prewashing is complete (overnight or after the solvent has traveled up the plate to some predetermined height), a slight colored band of impurities is often seen at the top of the plate. These impurities can be removed by scraping the plate or scoring below it to stop the final developing solvent from moving into this area. Had these impurities remained throughout the sorbent, they would have interfered with the final MS work that was done.

The final step in preparing the TLC or HPTLC plate is to activate any silica gel layer to remove moisture that may have been absorbed onto the layer during storage or after the prewash. This is done in a forced air oven at 95–100°C for 30 min.

Although bonded thin layers usually are not activated before use, if developing in a higher water content mobile phase (>50%) then also heating these thin layer plates (95°C for 30 min) might strengthen the binder in a hard layer plate to prevent swelling or lifting of the layer.

If using a new HPTLC plate made to higher purity standards (for MS work or if so stated, premium purity), then a prewashing step is probably not necessary, as long as the package had not been opened or has been properly stored.

## 2.8   SAMPLE LOCATION IN THE SORBENT LAYER

When a sample is placed on a thin layer, where in the sorbent matrix are the separated bands during and after their movement? This had always intrigued the chromatographer from the time optical quantitation began because any reflectance densitometry that was done at the time is only able to detect compounds in the top of the layer. Likewise, if doing desorption TLC–MS, the majority of the compound being near the surface for impact would be desired. Can this be controlled and is it reproducible?

One can imagine that depending on the sample solubility, the developing solvent composition and its component's volatility, the layer thickness and chemistry, the temperature, especially if force drying of some kind is used, that any one sample band might be almost anywhere in the sorbent matrix as shown in Figure 2.2.

An initial inquiry into this question was simply accomplished by scrapping small layer after small layer of silica gel at the sample band, extracting and weighing [7]. Some years later, investigations began by using photoacoustic spectroscopy (PAS), which sends sound waves into the layer [8]. Both gave identical results, the majority of the compound is found in the top 25% of the 250-μm layer, or a version of the band at the asterick in Figure 2.2.

But continued PAS work found concentration differences of samples located across a single plate, and it seemed to be related to the way the layer was dried after development [9]. The different drying routines investigated were those most commonly used by all chromatographers: (1) simple air drying (in the hood), (2) with a stream of warm air (hair dryer or similar), and (3) in a forced air oven at 50°C. The most reproducible was the latter. This is certainly because the layer is heated more evenly than by the other drying techniques, a point to be remembered for inclusion in any new protocol. Continued work by Prosek et al. [10] on this topic allowed the

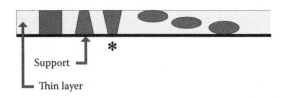

**FIGURE 2.2**   Possible configurations for a sample band in a sorbent matrix. The asterisk is under the closest representation of sample band concentrations found from the experimental data outlined in Section 2.8.

development of an efficient TLC plate drying oven. From experience, if drying a flexible layer in an oven, place it on a metal or glass plate so it heats evenly. If placed on a metal grid of some designs, the flexible support will heat unevenly, will warp, and the layer will flake off.

If a surface is to be bombarded directly from an MS source (MALDI, SALDI, or other desorption techniques), then the best possibility of getting sufficient sensitivity is if the sample molecules are near the surface to be ionized and pulled into the MS. Those compounds deeper within the thin layer are essentially unchanged. The study with different layer thicknesses [6] was discussed previously showing that the thinner layer gave improved results for that MALDI-TOF study of lipids. The disadvantage of the thicker layer gave more matrix background. Obviously, this is something to be concerned with when trying to get the best results from the TLC–MS work.

If elution TLC–MS is being done, then the sample mass location is not important as long as the correct eluting solvent is chosen for dissolution and compatibility with the MS mode being used.

## 2.9 SORBENTS USED IN THIN-LAYER CHROMATOGRAPHY

### 2.9.1 SILICA GEL

Because column chromatography using silica gels preceded their use for TLC layers, most of the major manufacturers either made their own silica gel or had a reliable source from which to purchase it. Only the specification of particle size had to be modified. Classically, the thin-layer plates manufactured have been made with irregular silica gels with average 60 A pores, surface areas about 500 $m^2g^{-1}$, a particle distribution of 5–20 μm, with an average particle size of 15 μm. Other properties of these silica gels include silanol content of about 8 $m^2g^{-1}$ onto which the polar moieties of sample components are attracted to various degrees to give a separation in the presence of the correct mobile phase. These silanols also play an important role in the bonding of silica gels discussed next.

A few manufacturers also supplied silica gel prepared plates with irregular silica gels with 150 A pores, surface areas of about 300 $m^2g^{-1}$, which in effect gave some variety of selectivity and mobility to the layers. With fewer silanols on the smaller surface area, silica gel generally gives faster moving solutes. Other properties regarding particle size range and average particle size are as for the 60-A pore silica.

Around 1975, thin layers of particles with a distribution of 4–8 μm were made from the same irregular 60-A silica gel, with an average particle size of 5–7 μm, hence leading to the high-performance plates preferred by many for their advantages.

In 1990, Merck (EMD) Millipore introduced a line of HPTLC prepared plates made from 3 to 5-μm spherical LiChrospher silica gel 60 and an RP18-bonded version. These also had the advantage of even faster chromatography. Also among their offering were HPTLC plates made with both silica gel 60 and LiChrospher with thinner layers, 100 μm, for use with the CAMAG AMD device. Since thinner layers seem to give improved results in many TLC–MS procedures, these are other available layers that might be tried during method development because all layer formulations differ.

Merck (EMD) Millipore also introduced a UTLC plate composed of monolithic silica gel, which promised even better speed and lower limits of detection, but this has been discontinued.

In general, as newer detection techniques and sensitivities are developed in the analytical laboratory, the demands are more stringent regarding the purity of the new products whether they are solvents or thin-layer plates. This is particularly true for the silica gels, bonded phases, or binders used in HPTLC plates to be used in TLC–MS work. If doing elution-based TLC–MS or desorption-based TLC–MS, the requirements are the same.

Recently, Merck (EMD) Millipore began to offer HPTLC plates specifically for the MS market. Promoting higher purity and less background as shown in Figure 2.3, comparing the standard HPTLC plate with the MS-grade plate, both eluted with a combination of acetonitrile/water (95:5). On their website, applications for a number of TLC–MS applications are shown both with elution MS and MALDI. Presently, they are offering four different prepared TLC–MS plates, three with silica gel (both standard TLC and HPTLC) layers, and one bonded HPTLC RP-18 layer. These are shown in Table 2.4 together with other offerings that might be of interest because of their packaging or thinner layers. The final step to ensure the purity of the MS grade layers is the special packaging to prevent contamination.

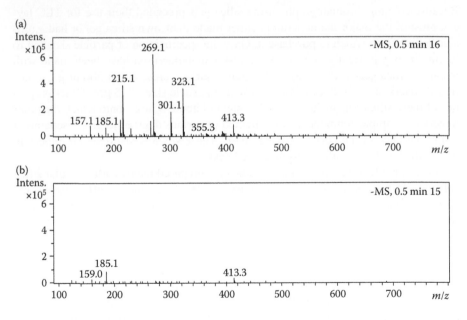

**FIGURE 2.3** Comparison of background noise of a standard HPTLC silica gel 60 $F_{254}$ plate compared to an HPTLC silica gel 60 F MS grade plate. (a) LC–MS background signal measurement on an HPTLC silica gel 60 $F_{254}$ standard plate, 20 × 10 cm (1.05642.0001) with mobile phase ACN/water (95/5). (b) LC–MS background measurement on an HPTLC silica gel 60 $F_{254}$ MS-grade plate, 20 × 10 cm (1.00934.0001) with mobile phase ACN/water (95/5). (Courtesy of Merck Millipore, a division of Merck KGaA, Darmstadt, Germany. With permission.)

**TABLE 2.4**

**Merck (EMD) Millipore TLC/HPTLC MS Plus Offerings**

| Catalog # | Description | Layer Thickness (μm) | Size (cm) | Plates/ Box | Support |
|---|---|---|---|---|---|
| 1.00933.0001 | TLC silica gel 60 $F_{254}$ MS-grade | 200 | $20 \times 20$ | 25 | Glass |
| 1.51160.0001 | HPTLC silica gel 60 $F_{254}$ MS-grade for MALDI | 100 | $5 \times 7.5$ | 20 | Alum |
| 1.00934.0001 | HPLC silica gel 60 $F_{254}$ MS-grade | 100 | $20 \times 10$ | 25 | Glass |
| 1.51161.0001 | HPTLC silica gel 60 RP-18 $F_{254s}$ | 100 | $20 \times 10$ | 25 | Glass |
| 1.05648.0001 | HPTLC silica gel 60 F254 premium purity* | 200 | $20 \times 10$ | 50 | Glass |
| 1.05650.0001 | ProteoChrom HPTLC silica gel 60 $F_{254s}$ | 100 | $20 \times 10$ | 25 | Glass |
| 1.15445.0001 | HPTLC LiChrospher silica gel 60$_{254s}$ | 200 | $20 \times 10$ | 25 | Glass |
| 1.05586.0001 | HPTLC LiChrospher silica gel 60F$_{254s}$ | 200 | $20 \times 20$ | 25 | Alum |
| 1.05646.0001 | HPTLC LiChrospher silica gel 60 RP-18 W $F_{254s}$ | 200 | $20 \times 10$ | 25 | Glass |
| 1.11764.0001 | HPTLC silica gel 60 AMD extra thin layer | 100 | $20 \times 10$ | 25 | Glass |
| 1.12363.0001 | HPTLC silica gel 60 AMD WR $F_{254s}$ extra thin layer | 100 | $20 \times 10$ | 25 | Glass |
| 1.05647.0001 | HPTLC LiChrospher silica gel 60 AMD WR $F_{254s}$ | 100 | $20 \times 10$ | 25 | Glass |

*Note:* Particle size for both HPTLC silica gel 60 and LiChrospher 60 are 5–7 μm.

The HPTLC premium purity plate and the HPTLC–MS plates are wrapped in a special, plastic-coated aluminum foil. This prevents plasticizers (such as phthalates) from leaving deposits.

*Codes:* W—water tolerant and R—specially purified.

At present, no other company is offering an MS-grade plate. It might be possible to use any other prepared plates if they are pretreated as described next. The other TLC plate manufacturers do make HPTLC plates that are for special applications or are made with thinner layers and their websites or catalogs can be consulted.

## 2.9.2 Bonded Phase Silica Gels

The availability of many silanol (Si–O–H) sites on the silica gel surface allows for relatively easy bonding with organosilyl reagents with one or more leaving groups such as a halide or a hydroxyl. The bonding reaction is done most often under anhydrous or moisture-controlled conditions to control the carbon loading. In general, the longer the chain length of the silyl reagent (C-2, C-8, C-18), the more carbon is bonded to the silica gel, so that a stronger mobile phase (usually methanol/water, so more methanol) is needed to move the samples through the thin layer.

Whatever steps in the manufacturing process, the final product has to be reproducible as mentioned. When bonded silica gel layers started to be produced, more variables become important during their manufacture. There was also the consideration of scale of the manufacturing process. If making a bonded phase sorbent for HPLC columns, the batch size need be only 1–2 kg to fill a few hundred HPLC columns; the batch size for bonded sorbents for coating thin layers may be 10 or 20 times this amount.

The purity and reproducibility of the final bonded product starts with the reproducibility of the silica gel. It must have the correct physical properties (particle size and range, pore size, surface area, surface pH, and silanol content). Then, various steps might be involved to make the bonded phase. These include treating or washing the silica gel, type of bonding reagent and conditions, batch size, etc. Each is developed and monitored to ensure reproducibility. It should be remembered that the final bonded phase thin layer is going to be vastly different from one manufacture to another. The upside of this is a variety of thin layers that exist and could be tried during the method development for their different properties and selectivities. The downside is the time involved in testing this large number of plates, if given the incentive to do so.

Normally, few problems will be encountered with the use of the TLC or HPTLC products, but the chromatographer should routinely record any batch numbers on the packing of that product to allow back tracking with the manufacturer should this be necessary.

### 2.9.2.1  Reversed Phase Bonded Silica Gels

The usual RP sorbents manufactured for TLC and HPTLC use are those with various chain lengths, such as dimethyl (RP-2/C-2), octyl (RP-8/C-8), and octadecyl (RP-18/C-18) phases. The bonded CN might also be considered a slightly polar butyl (RP-4/C-4) phase. Macherey-Nagel states that they bond only C-18 (with the exception of their C-2 dimethyl bonded product), but control the amount of carbon to produce their various RP bonded layers. The carbon loading or silanol coverage, often given for HPLC column sorbents, is proprietary for bonded-phase TLC plates generally.

Although a second reaction step to bond more silanols with a smaller "endcapping" reagent to HPLC sorbents is routine today, only one stage of bonding is done with the sorbents for TLC, which saves cost and time in making the bonded sorbent.

Another factor to consider with bonded RP layers is their usual use in water-rich mobile phases that can cause lifting of the layer. To solve this potential problem, some RP layers are available with water-tolerant (the W-type of plate) binders. This, too, is a variable in their resulting selectivity that should be noted.

RP thin layers are available for TLC and HPTLC applications. For routine work, perhaps a quick test of purity, then the standard TLC bonded RP plate is suitable. For other more demanding or quantitative work, then the HPTLC bonded prepared plates are recommended. Other bonded phases are made only on the HPTLC silica gel because the advantages of these are a vast improvement over TLC versions, especially development times and lower limits of detection. The C18-bonded phase is also available bonded to a spherical silica gel.

An interesting paper by Klingselhoffer and Morlock [11] pointed out that it took four decades to discover RP thin layers as a solution to overcome a problem with bioautography on silica gel layers. With this technique, after separation on the silica gel TLC plate, the plate undergoes a few immersions and incubation periods resulted in extreme diffusion of the detected components. Of course, these aqueous immersion solutions were causing the problem with their great affinity for the silica gel. Switching to the separation on a bonded RP plate where water is repelled through all of these operations allowed for sharper bounded zones. Therefore, thinking about problems and possible solutions constantly may lead to a breakthrough in a long-standing problem.

### 2.9.2.2 Hydrophilic-Bonded Silica Gels

Sales of prepared TLC and HPTLC plates are dominated by (1) silica gel and then (2) bonded RP plates. However, because of the ease of bonding to silica gel, the manufacturers have had hydrophilic/polar phases on HPTLC available for many years, but have not found wide use. These are amino, cyano, and diol phases described next. These allow different modes of chromatography to be accomplished depending on the mobile phase chosen for development. These can be used in developing orthogonal methods to ensure complete separation of unknown mixtures. Even if finding a separation that nearly works on a silica gel layer, utilizing any one or all of these during method development, using even the same nonpolar mobile phase as on the silica gel plate, a different elution order and resolution can be found. Another uniqueness of these hydrophilic-bonded layers is their ability to be used in both the normal phase (NP) and the RP mode. This opens up the potential to use any or all of them for 2D TLC during method development.

#### 2.9.2.2.1 Amino-Bonded Layers

The amino group is bonded to the silanols of silica gel with an organosilane with a trimethylene ($-(CH_2)_3-$) between the silicon atom (with its three leaving groups for bonding) and an amino group. It is one of the most versatile thin layers because it can perform as an NP partition with nonpolar solvent, RP with polar solvents, and finally as a weak anion exchanger with suitable buffers. Caution is necessary optimizing these latter two modes as high water content will lift the layer unless the correct binder is incorporated into the layer or with the use of the 1M sodium chloride as mentioned previously. Demand is generally small for this bonded phase, and hence, a water-tolerant prepared plate has not been developed by the manufacturers.

One special mode of chromatography that is gaining wider use in HPLC and can also be applied to both silica gel and bonded amino phase plates is the hydrophilic interaction chromatography (HILIC). It is, in fact, a version of NP. With this mode, very polar solutes that elute too rapidly in the RP mode, even with water as the mobile phase, are retained on these two layers with mobile phases with a high percentage of acetonitrile in water. This mode might be tried if appropriate during method development to investigate its potential. Amino thin layers with acetonitrile/water combinations are well known for separating carbohydrate mixtures [12].

One other unique property of the amino thin layer is its ability to be another detection tool. Separated mixtures of carbohydrates, catecholamines, and fruit acids

[13] are detected as stable fluorescent zones by simply heating the plate between 105°C and 220°C to effect thermochemical activation.

Often other detection techniques are first done before any MS work. This is especially true when large numbers of samples have to be looked at as in numerous batches of animal feeds. First separating the extracted samples onto HPTLC, then using bioautography with a bioluminescent bacteria (*Alivibrio ficheri*) gives a yes/no pass on whether MS work is needed. Chen and Schwack [14] started their investigation using HPTLC silica gel plates, but looked at other bonded phases (RP2, RP18W, CN, DIOL, NH2) to see any obvious advantages. As it turned out, RP2, RP18, CN, and DIOL layers actually made the bioluminescence almost useless. However, the NH2 layer gave enhanced bioluminescence after 3 h of incubation, better than what had been observed on the silica gel layers, a completely unexpected but welcome finding.

### 2.9.2.2.2   Cyano-Bonded Layers

As with the amino-bonded phase, the organosilane reagent used for bonding the CN phase has a trimethylene ($-(CH_2)_3-$) between the silicon atom (with its three leaving groups for bonding) and a cyano group. This thin layer can be used in the RP mode with polar mobile phases or in the NP mode with nonpolar mobile phases. As mentioned, it has less activity compared to a silica gel layer and also a less nonpolar character than C18- or C8-bonded phases.

### 2.9.2.2.3   Diol-Bonded Layers

The organosilane used for bonding this phase is derived from glycerol, where one of its hydroxyl groups is attached to the silicon atom with the three leaving groups. In nonpolar mobile phases, acting in the NP mode, attraction is on the remaining silanols with the possibility of hydrogen bonding or dipole interactions of the diol groups. In the RP mode with organic/water mobile phases, this bonded phase generally retains compounds to a smaller degree than amino-bonded phases.

## 2.9.3   Nonsilica Sorbents

Other nonsilica sorbent thin layers are available, but almost all are only available as standard TLC prepared plates. This is a limiting factor to some, but if sample sizes are reduced, there could be a special application found or sorbent layer that aids in its selectivity or detection.

### 2.9.3.1   Alumina (Aluminum Oxide)

Of the sorbents available on prepared layers, alumina is one of the most unique. It can be made into different forms so that it not only has the basic character, but also neutral and acidic versions. This allows a great versatility for selectivity where the acid, neutral, or basic character need not be controlled with buffers in the mobile phase, certainly a disadvantage if doing TLC–MS work lest a buffer interfere in some manner. It also is a complex sorbent with hydroxyl groups, partial positive and negative surface charges, onto which water is also attracted. Only TLC precoated layers are available. Check with the manufacturers as to the pH character of the alumina prepared layers they offer.

### 2.9.3.2 Cellulose

Cellulose thin layers are derived from natural sources and are mainly used in NP partition separation where water is bound to the hydroxyl groups and compounds move between the mobile phase and the water bound to the cellulose surface. The prepared layers can be fibrous or "microcrystalline" depending on the manufacturer. Recently, ProteoChrom® HPTLC cellulose plates, 10 × 10 cm (Merck [EMD] Millipore) have been introduced. Other cellulose prepared plates on the market are standard TLC-sorbent layers. Cellulose sorbents bond extremely well to all supports and no binder is required in their formulations.

### 2.9.3.3 Other Less Used Thin-Layer Chromatography Plates/Layers

Cellulose can be bonded easily and versions of PEI (polyethyleneimine), DEAE (diethylaminoethyl), and AC (acetylated) bonded cellulose standard layers are available. Polyamide 6 (ε-aminopolycaprolactam) prepared layers have been used for separations of compounds in which hydrogen bonding aids in the separation. Ion exchange (strong anion and cation) sorbents can be combined with cellulose to make prepared plates.

Diatomaceous earth is a nonsorbent silica gel formed under the oceans from the skeletons of diatoms millennia ago. Its main use is on preadsorbent zone plates described previously. Prepared TLC layers of this material are available to hold impregnated reagents for special applications.

### 2.9.4 MISCELLANEOUS LAYERS

#### 2.9.4.1 Impregnated Layers

There are a number of prepared thin layers into which various chemicals have been added to the slurry during manufacture. These have been found to enhance or make possible a separation, usually on a certain class of compounds. Among these are layers from Analtech containing silver nitrate (for aiding in the separation of compounds containing C=C bonds), sodium hydroxide (for aiding in the separation of organometallics and some acidic classes), Carbomer®, a generic term for a series of polymers primarily made from acrylic acid (for aiding the separation of mannitol and sorbitol), magnesium acetate (for aiding the separation of phospholipids), potassium oxalate (for aiding the separation of polyphosphoinositides), and ammonium sulfate (this reagent allows for self-charring of compounds with simple heating at 150–200°C). They also make silica gel prepared plates with sodium borate, potassium phosphate, ammonium sulfate, sodium carbonate, and sodium dihydrogen phosphate. Many of these layers are available with different concentrations of these reagents. Last, Analtech also makes both a TLC and HPTLC plate impregnated with 5% hydrocarbon for RP separations, the precursor to bonded RP phases. Because of their limited use and stability, they are often custom made. Macherey-Nagel makes a couple of impregnated layers. They are SIL G-25 Tenside (silica gel with ammonium sulfate for separating surfactants), Nano-SIL PAH (HPTLC silica gel with electron acceptors), and CHIRALPLATE (with a chiral selector and Cu(II) ions). Unless noted otherwise in their descriptions, these impregnated layers are only available in standard TLC sorbents.

Obviously, if used for a separation and elution is to be done, those impregnated layers with inorganic salts would generally not present a problem. However, those with some organic additives would require special extraction or workup. No further details will be given but the reader can contact the manufacturers.

An alternative before purchasing these and for initial investigation would be to dip a prepared hard layer plate into reagent solutions. For a review of these and other possibilities of impregnations, see References 15 and 16.

### 2.9.4.2  Mixed-Phase Layers

Some prepared layers are available that are mixed sorbent plates. Sometimes, the mixture is to allow multiple modes of chromatography to be used at once or in sequence. Other times, the mixture has been chosen to improve the separation characteristics or to aid in holding the active sorbent onto the support. This latter is often the reason cellulose is part of the layer formulation.

The majority of the mixed-phase layers are manufactured by Macherey-Nagel. These include CEL 300 DEAE/HR (cellulose and DEAE cellulose), Ionex-25 SA-Na (silica and a strong acidic cation exchanger), Ionex-25 SB-AC (silica and a strong basic anion exchanger), ALOX/CEL-AC-Mix (aluminum oxide and acetylated cellulose), SILCEL-Mix (silica and cellulose), and GURSIL-Mix (silica and kieselguhr). Merck (EMD) Millipore makes only a plate of silica gel and kieselguhr. They can be contacted for further information and possible applications performed on them.

### 2.9.5  Noncommercial Thin Layers Used with MS Detection

A few researchers have developed their own thin layers for MS work because those available commercially have not been suitable for their applications or they were curious to see if any advantages could be found on these new layers. Since silica gel TLC use began, many other inorganic oxides, silicates, etc., have been cast as thin layers to investigate their properties as sorbents [17]. More recently, with newer techniques for making UTLC layers, some of these have been revisited.

Morlock [18] has looked at a number of inorganic oxides that could be made in ultrathin layers using glancing angle deposition (GLAD). Of these, $TiO_2$ and $ZrO_2$ proved to work well for the separation of food dyes. Of greater interest is the ability to modify the sorptive nature of these layers with UV light or oxidation heat treatment. Much of this work was also accomplished with commonly used devices such as inkjet printers for streaking samples to ease researchers into the field of UTLC–MS.

Clark and Olesik [19] have made ULTC layers of various compositions by electrospinning to form nanofibrous stationary phases.

Song et al. [20] first formed patterned carbon nanotubes (CNT) as templates onto which they deposited silica giving layers that surpassed HPTLC in performance and speed.

Returning to one of the oldest synthetic routes for making a sorbent, Zhang et al. [21] used smaller particles of silica gel (350, 700, and 900 nm) to coat with polyacrylamide from which 15-μm layers were made.

Lv et al. [22] are another research group who also used an organic polymer, those being styrenic chemistries, to form 50-μm monomeric layers on which they were able to separate proteins, peptides, and dyes.

Whether any of these UTLC layers can be made commercially at a reasonable cost remains to be seen. Still, such research is invaluable because everyone in the community can learn and perhaps be stimulated to think in another direction that would benefit all.

## 2.10 CHOOSING THE PRECOATED PLATES AND SOURCES

With the variety of TLC prepared plates now available from numerous manufacturers, what plate should be purchased when doing TLC–MS work? First, the tendency might be to use what is at hand, already on the shelves of your company. If developing a method, it is better to use fresh stock, nothing that may have been on the shelves for a long time, which may have become contaminated.

Also, consider what has been used or recommended by recent papers dealing with the new protocol being developed. The time spent searching the literature can save time, energy, and contribute to the longevity of a method. It is better to spend the time in preparation of any method development than having to return later when some problems arise because some thin layer might have been available but not considered.

Obviously, the most important consideration is what thin layer plate will give the speed, resolution, and limits of detection required. However, from the examples given above, even years after their introduction, some of the classic bonded phases have found new applications and offered solutions to problems.

## 2.11 COMMENTS

In the United States and Canada, the company is EMD Millipore Corporation, 290 Concord Road, Billerica, Massachusetts, a division of Merck KGaA, Darmstadt, Germany. In the rest of the world, the company is Merck Millipore, a division of Merck KGaA, Darmstadt, Germany. Throughout the chapter, Merck (EMD) Millipore was used, trying to accommodate both versions of this international company.

## REFERENCES

1. Chen, Y.C., Shiea, J., and Sunner, J. Thin-layer chromatography–mass spectrometry using activated carbon, surface-assisted laser desorption/ionization, *J. Chromatogr. A*, 826, 77–86, 1998.
2. Guittare, J., Hronowski, X.L., and Costello, C.E. Direct matrix-assisted laser desorption/ionization mass spectrometric analysis of glycosphingolipids on thin layer chromatographic plates and transfer membranes, *Rapid Commun. Mass Spectrom.*, 13, 1838–1849, 1999.
3. Himmelsbach, M., Waser, M., and Klampfl, C.W. Thin layer chromatography—spray mass spectrometry: A method for easy identification of synthesis products and UV filters from TLC aluminum foils, *Anal. Biomed. Chem.*, 406, 3647–3656, 2014.

4. Rabel, F.M. Sorbents and precoated layers in thin-layer chromatography, in Sherma, J. and Fried, B. (Eds.), *Handbook of Thin-Layer Chromatograph*, 3rd edition, CRC Press/Taylor & Francis Group, Boca Raton, FL, p. 123, 2003.

5. Morlock, G. and Kovar, K.A. Detection, identification, and documentation, in Sherma, J. and Fried, B. (Eds.), *Handbook of Thin-Layer Chromatograph*, 3rd edition, CRC Press/Taylor & Francis Group, Boca Raton, FL, pp. 211–212, 2003.

6. Griesinger, H., Fuchs, B., Süß, R., Matheis, K., Schultz, M., and Schiller, J. Stationary phase thickness determines the quality of thin-layer chromatography/matrix-assisted laser desorption and ionization mass spectra of lipids, *Anal. Biochem.*, 451, 45–47, 2014.

7. Rimmer, J.G. Sample distribution in the TLC layer, *Chromatographia*, 1, 219–220, 1968.

8. Vovk, I., Franko, M., Gibkes, J., Prosek, M., and Bicanic, D. Photoacoustic investigation of secondary chromatographic effects on TLC plates, *Anal. Sci.*, 13, 191–194, 1997.

9. Prosek, M. and Vovk, I. Basic principles of optical quantification in TLC, in Sherma, J. and Fried, B. (Eds.), *Handbook of Thin-Layer Chromatograph*, 3rd edition, CRC Press/Taylor & Francis Group, Boca Raton, FL, pp. 289–291, 2003.

10. Prosek, M., Golc-Wondra, A., Vovk, I., and Zmitek, J. The importance of controlled drying in quantitative TLC, *J. Planar Chromatogr.*, 18, 408–414, 2005.

11. Klingelhofer I. and Morlock, G.E. Sharp-bounded zones link to the effect in planar chromatography–bioassay–mass spectrometry, *J. Chromatogr. A*, 1360, 288–295, 2014.

12. Maloney, M.D. Carbohydrates, in Sherma, J. and Fried, B. (Eds.), *Handbook of Thin-Layer Chromatograph*, 3rd edition, CRC Press/Taylor & Francis Group, Boca Raton, FL, 2003.

13. Klaus, R., Fischer, W., and Hauck, H.E. Application of a thermal *in situ* reaction for fluorometric detection of carbohydrates on $-NH_2$ layers, *Chromaographia*, 29, 467–472, 1990.

14. Chen, Y. and Schwack, W. High performance thin-layer chromatography screening of multi class antibiotics in animal food by bioluminescent bioautography and electrospray ionization mass spectrometry, *J. Chromatogr. A*, 1356, 249–257, 2014.

15. Gasaric, J. Chromatography on thin layers impregnated with organic stationary phases, *Adv. Chromatogr.* 31, 153–252, 1992.

16. Nikolova-Damhanova, B. and Sv. Momchilova, Sy. Silver ion thin-layer chromatography of fatty acids: A Survey, *J. Liq. Chromatogr. Related Technol.*, 24, 1447–1466, 2001.

17. Stahl, E. (Ed.), *Thin Layer Chromatography, A Laboratory Handbook*, Springer-Verlag, New York., 1969.

18. Wannenmacher, J., Jim, S.R., Taschuk, M.T., Brett, M.J., and Morlock, G.E. Ultrathin-layer chromatography on $SiO_2$, $Al_2O_3$, $TiO_2$, and $ZrO_2$ nanostructured thin films, *J. Chromatogr. A*, 1318, 234–243, 2013.

19. Clark, J.E. and Olesik, S.V. Technique for ultrathin layer chromatography using an electrospun, nanofibrous stationary phase, *Anal. Chem.*, 81, 4121–4129, 2009.

20. Song, J., Jensen, D.S., Hutchison, D.H., Turner, B., Wood, T., Dadson, A., Vail, M.A., Linford, M.R., Vanfleet, R.R., and Davis, R.C. Carbon-nonotube-templated microfabrication of porous silicon-carbon materials with application to chemical separations, *Adv. Funct. Mater.*, 21, 1132–1139, 2011.

21. Zhang, Z., Ratnayaka, S.N., and Wirth, M.J. Protein UTLC-MALDI-MS using thin films of submicrometer silica particles, *J. Chromatogr. A*, 1218, 7196–7202, 2011.

22. Lv, Y., Lin, Z., Tan, T., and Svec, F. Preparation of porous styrenic-based monolithic layers for thin layer chromatography coupled with matrix-assisted laser-desorption/ionization time of flight mass spectrometric detection, *J. Chromatogr. A*, 1316, 154–159, 2013.

# 3 The CAMAG TLC–MS Interface

*Joseph Sherma and Jacob Strock*

## CONTENTS

## 3.1 HISTORY AND DEVELOPMENT

Direct coupling of thin-layer chromatography (TLC) and mass spectrometry (MS) was reported by Issaq et al. as early as 1977 using benz(a)pyrene and pyrene as model compounds [1]. The zones were detected under ultraviolet (UV) light on a silica gel 60 TLC plate, and a circle perimeter of 2.5 cm diameter was scored through the layer around each zone using a milling device provided as an accessory with the Eluchrom Automatic Elution System available from CAMAG until 1992. The elution head was placed over each scored adsorbent-free circle and tightly clamped on the plate forming a Teflon (elution head)-glass plate seal. Quantitative elution of each zone was carried out with 0.15 mL of methanol at a 0.1 mL/min flow rate. The eluents were introduced into a Finnigan Model 3300 mass spectrometer through a specially built heated Pyrex inlet probe forming a tight seal between the Eluchrom outlet and mass spectrometer ion source.

In 2004, the elution-based ChromeXtractor interface was reported by Dr. Heinrich Luftmann of the University of Muenster, Germany [2] and commercialized by the ChromAn Company. This TLC–MS interface, pictured in an earlier article [3], was designed to remove a zone or spot completely from flexible plastic or aluminum TLC plates (foils) using a miniaturized elution head similar to the Eluchrom that was first pressed tightly on the layer to form a tight seal around the desired zone via its hard cutting ring edge. Then, a solvent flow was forced through the enclosed spot and extracted it quantitatively and directly with 50–100 µL of solvent into a mass spectrometer in the online approach [4]. It could also be used in the offline approach where the eluate is collected in a vial or other container followed by subsequent transfer into the MS instrument [5]. No tedious and time-consuming scraping off the plate, elution into a tube, and subsequent transfer into the mass spectrometer was needed. TLC–MS aids substance identification or structure elucidation. An advantage of elution-based TLC–MS is that all of the analyte in the entire zone is transferred to the mass spectrometer and not only that in the surface region as with desorption-based techniques.

Prosek et al. also in 2004 [6] described construction of a new online computer-controlled TLC–MS approach for collection of sample and programmed loop injection into an LCQ $MS^n$ ion trap mass spectrometer with an atmospheric pressure chemical ionization (APCI) source. The elution head was positioned manually, and knives on the bottom cut around the zone of interest. One pump applied eluent onto the plate and a second pump removed it. Morlock and Schwack [4] stated that this interface was more laborious and less sensitive than the ChromeXtractor because the recovery rate was less than 10%, and its use was not reported further in the literature.

The current CAMAG TLC–MS interface evolved from the ChromeXtractor after modifications (see the next paragraph), and it became commercially available in mid-2009 [7] for rapid, contamination-free elution of zones from usually high-performance TLC (HPTLC) layers with online transfer to a mass spectrometer, and it has proven to be one of the most reliable and versatile interfaces for TLC/HPTLC–MS coupling [8]. It can be connected to any HPLC/MS instrument without modification and can accommodate plates up to $20 \times 20$ cm on its positioning table. It is designated as semiautomatic because the only automatic steps are pneumatic operation (lifting/lowering) for sealing the zone and cleaning of the elution head between elutions (purging of silica gel particles) [9]. An integrated laser light cross-hairs gives exact positioning of the elution head (also termed the piston or plunger) onto the zone to be eluted, or positioning can be based on coordinates determined earlier by a CAMAG TLC scanner or TLC visualizer. It works with both glass plates and flexible aluminum of plastic-backed layers. Zones can be efficiently extracted from layers ranging from polar to nonpolar. The regular elution head has a cutting edge of 0.2 mm useful for HPTLC plates, while 0.5 mm edge height is used for thicker preparative layers and 0.1 mm for ultrathin-layer chromatography (UTLC) layers. The interface has thus far been used with electrospray ionization (ESI) mass spectrometers and is the main ESI-based TLC-coupling method, but it can also be directly coupled with instruments having APCI, atmospheric pressure photoionization (APPI), and inductively coupled plasma (ICP) sources [10]. Use with direct inlet electron impact (EI) MS, matrix-assisted laser desorption ionization (MALDI) MS, static nanospray, nuclear magnetic resonance (NMR) spectrometry, and infrared (IR) spectrometry requires intermediate collection in a vial (offline approach) [11]. The mechanism of the ESI process in MS was described by Sherma [12].

Many papers were published reporting modifications and applications of the original ChromeXtractor before it was commercialized by CAMAG as the TLC–MS interface. These included ability to use glass plates rather than just flexible aluminum or plastic plate foils by introducing buffering of the plunger to reduce leakage, use of a torque screwdriver for fixation to give reproducible contact pressure and avoid plate breakage, and extension of use with plates having 100 μm layer thickness by reducing the height of the plunger's cutting edge [13]. Values of HPTLC/ESI–MS for limit of detection (LOD) with a single quadrupole (40 pg) and limit of quantification

(LOQ) with MS/MS (20 pg) were found to be similar to HPLC/MS for the first time in the analysis of the heterocyclic aromatic amine harman (harmane) [14].

Morlock and Jautz [15] published a comparison of circular or ring-shaped (4 mm) and oval-shaped (4 × 2 mm) extraction heads for TLC–MS or HPTLC–MS coupling with harman and Glu-P-1 analytes. The performance of both extraction heads was similar with regard to the delay time between switching the valve and recording the signal, the system pressure, the short negative baseline amplitude at the signal start of the elution peak, the time for complete extraction (peak width), and blank plate signals. The plunger with oval geometry, especially designed for the more common band-shaped zones resulting from application of samples and standards with automated applicators such as the widely used CAMAG Linomat or ATS4 in quantitative HPTLC, was better for exact positioning on the substance band of interest and for avoiding the codetection of adjacent zones. The oval plunger was demonstrated to be more selective than the circular plunger was and produced more intense signals for adjacent zones. The circular plunger was easier to position on a zone and for nonadjacent zones resulted in generally higher signal intensity because of its larger cross section. There is also a round elution head with 5 mm diameter available from CAMAG for layer thickness up to 500 μm (preparative layer chromatography) [16].

## 3.2 INSTALLATION AND PERFORMANCE

Detailed information on the installation and performance of the TLC–MS interface was discussed in detail in a handbook chapter [10] based on first-hand experience by the person who has published the most papers on its use, Professor Dr. Gerda Morlock. "Plug and play" installation on a given HPLC/MS system by connecting the interface by PEEK tubing (fitting) with the pump of the HPLC system and another with the inlet of the ion source of the mass spectrometer was described, as well as change of the elution heads with different sized cutting edges by two valve fittings within 5 min.

Morlock [10] reported that in instrumental HPTLC, ionization occurs comparably on plates compared to HPLC/MS and that amounts detected are similar, in the 1–500 ng range. The MS recording sequence of the interface was described: placing the plate on the positioning table and exact positioning of the head on the colored or outlined zone of interest; pneumatically lowering the elution head so the cutting edge was tightly around the zone to be eluted; pumping the elution solvent through the inlet capillary to dissolve the analyte from the layer and continuously introducing the eluent through the outlet capillary containing a Teflon frit; and automated cleaning of the elution head using pressurized air. Figure 3.1 is a photograph of the CAMAG TLC–MS interface, Figure 3.2 is a close-up image of the plate under the head, and Figure 3.3 is a schematic diagram showing the flow path of the solvent through the elution head.

The handbook chapter [10] section on the TLC–MS interface ends with subsections on characteristics of ESI mass spectra for identification of various compounds in different matrices, capability of detection (LOQ values), capability for quantification (relative standard deviation [RSD] and determination coefficient [$r^2$] values), and automated operation of the elution head. In the latter section, a paper is cited

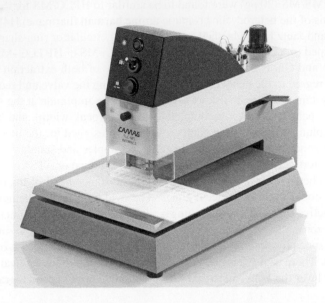

**FIGURE 3.1** CAMAG TLC–MS interface. The three controls on the top front panel are laser on/off button (upper), plunger up/down button (middle), and cleaning switch (lower). The moving lever on the right side is the on/off connection valve used to start the solvent flow into the MS instrument. (From Advion, Inc., Ithaca, New York. With permission.)

[17] in which it was shown that full automation of manual plate positioning and valve switching in an advanced version of the interface (R3D3) gave RSD ($\leq$5.6%) and $r^2$ (0.9973) values for the quantification of caffeine in energy drinks and pharmaceutical tablets without an internal standard that were a match for other automated systems even with use of an internal standard for correction of results, as well as

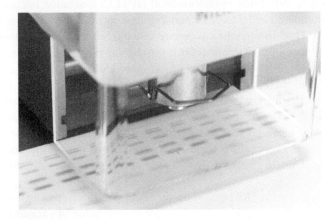

**FIGURE 3.2** Close-up view of a plate under the raised elution head. The laser light on the left is the source of the crosshairs image formed on the plate for correct positioning of the zone under the head. (From CAMAG, Muttenz, Switzerland. With permission.)

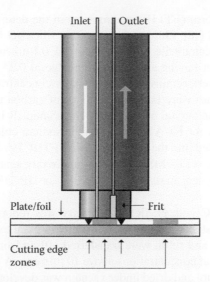

**FIGURE 3.3** Schematic diagram of solvent flow through the extraction head (piston) to elute a zone directly into a mass spectrometer. The extraction head is lowered onto the layer with a force of approximately 20 kg to completely seal the zone to be extracted. The cutting edges on either side of the zone are shown. Typical flow rates of the HPLC pump are 0.05–5 mL/min, with a solvent such as methanol or methanol–ammonium formate buffer, 10 mM, pH 4(95:5). The frit prevents contamination of the mass spectrometer with washed out layer particles [7]. (From Advion, Inc., Ithaca, New York. With permission.)

pg/band LOD. Manual positioning error was found to be responsible for up to 6% of total random error, calculated by correction with an isotopically labeled internal standard, in another study [9]. Full automation of the CAMAG TLC–MS interface seems to be advantageous and feasible, although it has not yet been offered in the current commercial version [9].

Morlock [9] discussed background signals in TLC/HPTLC–ESI–MS using the CAMAG interface with a circular elution head connected by one PEEK tube to an Agilent 1100 HPLC pump and by another containing an inline filter to the source inlet of a single quadrupole mass spectrometer. Use of acidic solvents in mobile phases caused intense background signals and ion suppression in analyte mass spectra. Plate prewashing with methanol–water (3:1) reduced background mass signals to a minimum. Different Merck silica gel 60 plates with and without manganese activated zinc silicate fluorescence indicator did not show significant differences. Extent of the formation of sodium adducts was different with different plate types. Practical recommendations were provided for optimum plate handling, integration of the inline filter, pressure increases, and leakage using the interface.

## 3.3 OFFLINE USE WITH IR AND NMR SPECTROMETRY

Extraction of zones on TLC plates into vials using the TLC–MS interface was reported for offline HPTLC-attenuated total reflectance (ATR)-IR spectrometry and

HPTLC-Fourier transform (FT) IR spectrometry in the determination of lubricant additives in mineral oil [18]. Elution of zones from silica gel $60F_{254}$ plates (0.2 mm thickness) was with acetonitrile at a flow rate of 0.1 mL/min via the interface equipped with a plunger having a round cutting edge of 0.25 or 0.5 mm into glass vials with a 300-$\mu$L insert, requiring 5–7 min. After concentration to dryness under nitrogen gas, the residues were taken up in 10 $\mu$L of carbon tetrachloride that was dropped on the diamond crystal of a SMART DuraSamplIR installed on an Avatar 320 FTIR spectrometer for FT-ATR-IR, or on the sodium chloride carrier with the applied sample assembled into the spectrometer for FTIR. For HPTLC/MS, the acetonitrile eluent from the TLC–MS interface was directly sent to the ESI source of a single quadrupole Agilent mass spectrometer by an HP 1100 pump operating at 0.1 mL/min [7].

Combination of TLC with NMR spectrometry was reported by Gaugler et al. [19]. Three natural substances occurring frequently in plant extracts, that is, caffeic acid, chlorogenic acid, and rutin, were transferred offline from an HPTLC plate to an NMR spectrometer at concentrations above 10 $\mu$g/zone. A silica gel $60F_{254}$ plate prewashed with methanol and dried under vacuum was developed with formic acid–ethyl acetate–water–methyl ethyl ketone (5:30:6:18) in a CAMAG twin trough chamber (TTC). After 5 min drying, elution of zones into respective vials was performed using the TLC–MS interface with the round elution head and methanol eluent at a flow rate of 0.3 mL/min for 6 min. The NMR instrument used was a 400-MHz Bruker Advance I with 5 mm BBO sample head under TOPSPIN 2.1.

A later publication by Gossi et al. [20] described utilization of the TLC–MS interface to characterize zones of interest by NMR spectrometry with a focus on quantification of active pharmaceutical ingredients in formulations and identification of active principles in plant extracts. A CAMAG Automatic Sampler 4 was used for initial zone application, and silica gel $F_{254}$ DC plates were developed with different mobile phase in a CAMAG automatic developing chamber (ADC 2). Zones of interest were eluted with methanol into vials. Solvent was removed by a stream of nitrogen, and the sample was finally collected in 600 $\mu$L of methanol-$d_4$ for subsequent NMR spectrometry measurement with the same 400-MHz Bruker instrument mentioned previously. The compounds quantified were rutin, caffeic acid, chlorogenic acid, amiodarone, and aminodarone from Aminodarone Mepa 200 tablet.

## 3.4 ALLIANCE BETWEEN CAMAG AND ADVION INC.

It was announced on February 26, 2013, that Advion, Inc. and CAMAG joined in an exclusive original equipment manufacturing (OEM) and distribution agreement to commercialize an integrated system including the CAMAG TLC–MS interface and Advion's single quadrupole expression compact mass spectrometer (CMS) offering unit resolution (Figure 3.4). The CMS mass detector can be operated in full-scan mode to provide mass assignment of eluted compounds within 1 min, and in the selected ion monitoring (SIM) mode for concentration-dependent detection (quantitative analysis) [21]. Cretu et al. [22] reported use of this commercial system for the determination of anthocyanins in powdered extracts by TLC linked with bioassay.

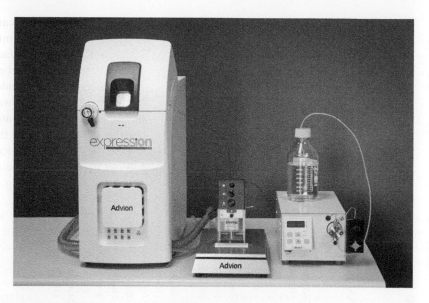

**FIGURE 3.4** CAMAG-Advion TLC–MS/CMS system. Left to right: expression compact mass spectrometer (CMS), TLC–MS interface, and pump for elution solvent. (From Advion, Inc., Ithaca, New York. With permission.)

## 3.5 SURFACE ANALYSIS WITHOUT THIN-LAYER CHROMATOGRAPHY

The TLC–MS interface was assessed as a tool for direct determination of drugs from dried blood spot (DBS) samples on Ahlstrom grade 237 paper using an MS detector with and without HPLC separation. The HPLC–MS system consisted of an Agilent 1100 binary pump with integrated column oven. MS detection was by a Sciex API-3000 instrument equipped with a Turbo Ion Spray source. Acceptable sensitivity, linearity, accuracy, and precision date were achieved with and without the inclusion of HPLC separation, and sensitivity was increased compared to conventional extraction methods (punching of the DBS and elution prior to HPLC/MS analysis). Parameter optimization was carried out, and it was shown that the TLC–MS interface has the potential to be superior to manual practices in terms of simplicity, cost, and greater sensitivity, allowing determination of additional analytes [23]. This type of surface analysis could probably be extended to other types of samples such as clinical, forensic, and food packaging (migration studies) [10].

## 3.6 APPLICATIONS

Table 3.1 contains a list of some of the published applications given in Sections 3.1 and 3.2 for the ChromeXtractor and CAMAG interfaces arranged chronologically. The analyte, sample, layer, mobile phase, elution solvent, MS instrument, and reference are given in the table. The full methodology in each case typically includes sample preparation; sample application, most likely bandwise using an automated

**TABLE 3.1**
**Previous Usage of HPTLC–MS**

| Analyte | Sample Matrix | Plate | Mobile Phase | Eluent | Mass Spectrometer | References |
|---|---|---|---|---|---|---|
| Heterocyclic aromatic amines | NA[a] | Silica gel 60WRF$_{254}$s[b] HPTLC | Diethyl ether–methanol–chloroform, with alkaline conditioning via gas phase | NA | NA | 28 |
| Heterocyclic aromatic amines | NA | Silica gel 60F$_{254}$ HPTLC preconditioned with aqueous ammonia (pH 10.4) | Diethyl ether–methanol (98:2) | Methanol–formate buffer (10 mM, pH 4.0) (95:5) | 4000 Q Trap (Applied Biosystems/MDS Sciex) with an ESI source | 14 |
| Isopropylthioxanthone | Milk, yogurt, fat | Silica gel 60 HPTLC, RP-18 HPTLC | Toluene–*n*-hexane (4:1) for silica gel 60, acetonitrile–water (9:1) for RP-18 | Methanol–ammonium formate buffer (10 mM, pH 4) (95:5) | VG Platform II quadrupole (micromass) with an ESI source | 29 |
| Riboflavin, pyridoxine, nicotinamide, caffeine, taurine | Energy drinks | Silica gel 60F$_{254}$ HPTLC | Chloroform–ethanol–acetic acid–acetone water (54:27:10:2:2) | Methanol–formate buffer (10 mM, pH 4.0) (95:5) for pyridoxine, nicotinamide, caffeine, taurine; acetic acid–water (1:9) for riboflavin | VG Platform II quadrupole (micromass) with an ESI source | 30 |
| Heterocyclic aromatic amines | Beef patties | LiChrospher[c] silica gel 60WRF$_{254}$s preconditioned with ammonia vapor | Methanol–chloroform (1:9) | Methanol–formate buffer (10 mM, pH 4.0) (95:5) | VG Platform II quadrupole (micromass) with an ESI source | 31 |

*(Continued)*

**TABLE 3.1 (*Continued*)**
**Previous Usage of HPTLC–MS**

| Analyte | Sample Matrix | Plate | Mobile Phase | Eluent | Mass Spectrometer | References |
|---|---|---|---|---|---|---|
| Isopropylthi-oxanthone, caffeine | NA | Silica gel 60F$_{254}$ HPTLC | Toluene–*n*-hexane (4:1) for isopropylthioxanthone; acetonitrile–aqueous ammonium hydroxide 2.5% (400:1) for caffeine | Methanol–ammonium formate buffer (10 mM, pH 4) (95:5) | VG Platform II quadrupole (micromass) with an ESI source | 32 |
| Caffeine, ergotamine, metamizol | Pharmaceutical products | Silica gel 60F$_{254}$ HPTLC | Ethyl acetate–methanol–ammonia (90:15:1) | Methanol–formate buffer (10 mM, pH 4.0) (19:1) | VG Platform II single quadrupole (micromass) with an ESI source | 33 |
| Caffeine | Energy drinks, pharmaceutical products | Silica gel 60F$_{254}$ HPTLC | Chloroform–ethanol–acetic acid–acetone–water (54:27:10:2:2) for energy drinks; ethyl acetate–methanol–ammonia 25% (90:15:1) for pharmaceutical products | Methanol–formate buffer (10 mM, pH 4.0) (19:1) | VG Platform II single quadrupole (micromass) with an ESI source | 34 |
| Caffeine | Energy drinks, pharmaceutical products | Silica gel 60F$_{254}$ HPTLC | Chloroform–ethanol–acetic acid–acetone–water (54:27:10 2:2) for energy drinks; ethyl acetate–methanol–ammonia (25%) (90:15:1) for pharmaceutical products | Methanol–ammonium formate buffer (10 mM, pH 4) (19:1) | Z-Spray ESI Quattro LCZ triple quadrupole (micromass) | 17 |

*(Continued)*

**TABLE 3.1 (*Continued*)**

**Previous Usage of HPTLC–MS**

| Analyte | Sample Matrix | Plate | Mobile Phase | Eluent | Mass Spectrometer | References |
|---|---|---|---|---|---|---|
| Zinc bis(*O,O'*-diisobutyl dithiophosphate), zinc bis(*O,O'*-didodecyl dithiophosphate), Anglamol 99® | Mineral oil lubricants | Silica gel 60F$_{254}$ HPTLC, RP2 F$_{254}$S HPTLC | Methanol–water–acetic acid (6:3:2) (45 mm), acetonitrile–water (11:9) (60 mm), acetonitrile–water (9:11) for RP2; 14 step gradient based on toluene, methanol, *n*-hexane for silica gel 60F$_{254}$S HPTLC | Acetonitrile | Single quadrupole (Agilent) | 18 |
| Acrylamide | Drinking water | Silica gel 60F$_{254}$ HPTLC | Ethyl acetate, postchromatographic derivatization with 25% polypropylene glycol in *n*-hexane | Methanol–ammonium formate buffer (10 mM, pH 4) (95:5) | VG Platform II quadrupole (micromass) with an ESI source | 35 |
| Sudan I, Sudan II, Sudan Red B, Sudan Orange G Sudan III, Sudan IV, Sudan Red 7B, Para Red) | Spices | NANO-SIL-PAH[d] HPTLC | Isohexane–methyl ethyl ketone (5:1) | Methanol–formic acid (1%) (95:5) | 1100 LC/MSD (Agilent) with an ESI source | 36 |
| Water-soluble food dyes | Energy drinks, bakery inks | Silica gel 60F$_{254}$ HPTLC | Ethyl acetate–methanol–water–acetic acid (65:23:11:1) | Methanol | Single quadrupole mass spectrometer (Agilent) with an ESI source | 37 |

*(Continued)*

**TABLE 3.1 (Continued)**
**Previous Usage of HPTLC–MS**

| Analyte | Sample Matrix | Plate | Mobile Phase | Eluent | Mass Spectrometer | References |
|---|---|---|---|---|---|---|
| Plasticizers, other plastic additives | Polyvinyl chloride plastic foils | Silica gel 60F$_{254}$ HPTLC | Isooctane–toluene–diethyl ether–ethyl acetate (8:7:4:1) | Ethanol (95%) | 1100 LC/MSD (Agilent) with an ESI source | 38 |
| Pyritinol | Pharmaceutical tablet | Silica gel 60F$_{254}$ HPTLC | Dichloromethane–methanol–formic acid (9:1:1) | Methanol–ammonium formate (10 mM, pH 4.0) (19:1) | VG Platform II single quadrupole (micromass) with an ESI source | 39 |
| Single peptides of angiotensin-converting enzyme inhibitors | Pharmaceutical compounds | Silica gel 60 TLC, and UTLC$^e$ | Ethyl acetate–acetone–acetic acid–water (4:1:0.25:0.5) | Methanol, 0.2% acetic acid in methanol for UTLC plates | LCQ (Thermo Finnigan) with an ESI source | 25 |
| 5-Hydroxymethyl-furfural | Honey | Silica gel 60 TLC, and silica gel 60F$_{254}$ HPTLC | Ethyl acetate | Methanol | G1956B MSD single quadrupole (Agilent) | 40 |
| Sucralose | Sewage effluent, surface water, and drinking water | Silica gel 60F$_{254}$ HPTLC | Isopropyl acetate–methanol–water (15:3:1), acetonitrile–water (5:1) for focusing up to 11 mm, methanol–water (4:1) for cleaning | Methanol–ammonium formate buffer (10 mM, pH 4) (19:1) | MSD single quadrupole (Agilent) with an ESI source | 41 |

(Continued)

**TABLE 3.1 (Continued)**
**Previous Usage of HPTLC–MS**

| Analyte | Sample Matrix | Plate | Mobile Phase | Eluent | Mass Spectrometer | References |
|---|---|---|---|---|---|---|
| Pesticides | Apples, cucumbers, red grapes, tomatoes | Silica gel 60 NH$_2$ F$_{254}$s | Acetonitrile, in reverse direction with acetone, postchromatographic derivatization with 0.05% primuline in acetone–water (4:1) | Acetonitrile–ammonium formate buffer (10 mM) (1:1) | G1956B MSD single quadrupole (Agilent) with an ESI source | 42 |
| Phenolic acids, flavonoids | Salvia lavendulifolia | Silica gel F$_{254}$ | Ethyl acetate–toluene–formic acid (7:3:1) for phenolic acids, acetate–toluene–formic acid (5:5:0.1) for flavonoids | Methanol, methanol–acetic acid (95.5:0.5) | 100-MS (Varian) | 43 |
| Phenolic acids | Salvia lavendulifolia | RP-18 F$_{254}$s | Methanol–water–acetic acid (5:5:0.1) | Methanol, methanol–acetic acid (95.5:0.5) | 500-MS (Varian) with an ESI source | 44 |
| Spinochrome pigments | Sea urchin shells | Kieselgel 60F$_{254}$ treated with oxalic acid | Chloroform–methanol–acetic acid–water (5:1.1:0.5:0.2) | Methanol | micrOTOF-Q (Bruker Daltonics) | 45 |
| Acetamiprid, penconazole, azoxystrobin, chlorpyrifos, pirimicarb, fenarimol, mepanipyrim | Green and black teas | Silica gel F$_{254}$ TLC | Acetonitrile–ultrapure water (95:5) | Acetonitrile–ammonium formate buffer (10 mM) (1:1) | G1956B MSD single quadrupole (Agilent) with an ESI source | 46 |

(Continued)

**TABLE 3.1 (*Continued*)**
**Previous Usage of HPTLC–MS**

| Analyte | Sample Matrix | Plate | Mobile Phase | Eluent | Mass Spectrometer | References |
|---|---|---|---|---|---|---|
| NA | Food dyes, carotenoids | Silicon dioxide, aluminum oxide, titanium dioxide, zirconium dioxide GLAD[g] UTLC | Ethyl acetate–methanol–water (65:23:5) | Methanol | Single quadrupole MSD (Agilent) | 27 |
| Lactose, sucrose, fructose | Chocolate | GLAD-UTLC | Ethyl acetate–methanol–formic acid–dionized water (8:2:1:0.5) | Methanol | MSD (Agilent) with ESI source | 26 |
| Preservatives | Nonalcoholic beverage | Polyacrylonitrile microfiber with manganese-activated zinc silicate and UV$_{254}$ photoluminescent indicator | Water–acetonitrile (13:7) containing 0.1 M tetra-*n*-butyl–ammonium phosphate | Methanol | G1956B MSD single quadrupole (Agilent) with an ESI source | 47 |
| Anthocyanes | Pomace, animal feed, juice, wine | Silica gel 60F$_{254}$ HPTLC | Ethyl acetate–2-butanone–formic acid–water (7:3:1.2:0.3) for anthocyanins, ethyl acetate–toluene–formic acid–water (10:3:0.8:1.2) for anthocyanidin development in automatic developing chamber 2 (CAMAG) | Methanol | Single quadrupole (Agilent) with an ESI source | 48 |

(*Continued*)

**TABLE 3.1 (Continued)**
**Previous Usage of HPTLC–MS**

| Analyte | Sample Matrix | Plate | Mobile Phase | Eluent | Mass Spectrometer | References |
|---|---|---|---|---|---|---|
| Difloxacin, difloxacin photodegradation products | NA | Silica gel $F_{254}$ TLC | Methylene chloride–methanol–2-propanol–ammonia (25%) (4:4:5:2) | Methanol | TQD (waters) with an ESI source | 49 |
| Flavonols | Extracts from Juniper seeds *Juniperus communis* L. and pomegranate fruit *Punica granatum* L. | Silica gel 60 HPTLC and cellulose HPTLC | n-Propanol–water–acetic acid (4:2:1) and pure water for cellulose plates, acetone–toluene–acetic acid (6:3:1) for silica plates | 1% formic acid in methanol, methanol–acetonitrile (1:1) for silica gel 60 | Unknown manufacturer, used with an ESI source | 50 |
| Tetracycline, flouroquinolone antibiotics | Milk | Silica gel 60 HPTLC | Chloroform–methanol–ammonium hydroxide (25%) (60:35:5) | Acetonitrile–ammonium formate (10 mM + 2% methanol) (9:1) | G1956B MSD single quadrupole (Agilent) | 51 |
| Acetylcholinesterase | Galbanum, gum resin from *Ferula gummosa* | Silica gel 60F$_{254}$ HPTLC | Chloroform–ethylacetate–methanol (100:10:2) | Acetonitrile–water (80:20) with 0.1% formic acid | Single quadrupole 6120 (Agilent) with an ESI source | 52 |
| Desamido insulin, human insulin | NA | Silica gel 60F$_{254}$ HPTLC MS-grade | 2-Butanol–pyridine–ammonia (25%)–water (39-34-10-26) | Acetonitrile–water (19:1) | NA | 53 |
| Antibiotics | Bovine milk, porcine kidney | Silica gel 60 NH$_2$ F$_{254}$S | Methanol–acetonitrile (4:6) | Acetonitrile–aqueous ammonium formate (10 mM) (70:30), acetonitrile–aqueous formic acid (0.03%) (70:30) depending specific analyte | G1956B MSD single quadrupole (Agilent) with an ESI source | 54 |

*(Continued)*

**TABLE 3.1 (Continued)**
**Previous Usage of HPTLC–MS**

| Analyte | Sample Matrix | Plate | Mobile Phase | Eluent | Mass Spectrometer | References |
|---|---|---|---|---|---|---|
| Anthocyanes | Bilberry, blueberry, chokeberry, açai berry, and cranberry powdered extracts | Silica gel 60F$_{254}$ HPTLC | Ethyl acetate–2-butanone–wate–formic acid (7:3:0.8:1.2) | Methanol | Expression CMS single quadrupole (Advion) | 22 |
| Colorants, isoflavones, caffeine | Urine, rum-watermelon beverage, soy drink, energy drinks, pharmaceutical products | Silica gel 60F$_{254}$ HPTLC MS-grade | NA | Acetonitrile–water (95:5) | Expression CMS (Advion) with an ESI source | 55 |
| Estrogen-effective compounds | Spices | RP-18 W HPTLC | n-hexane–toluene–ethyl acetate (4:1.5:1) | Methanol–ammonium formate (10 mM, pH 4.0) (98:2) | Single quadrupole (Advion) with an ESI source | 56 |
| Endocrine disrupting compounds | Food samples, beer | RP-18 W HPTLC | n-hexane–toluene–ethyl acetate (4:1.5:1) with postchromatographic derivatization with 20 mg 4-methylumbelliferyl-β-D-galactopyranoside in dimethyl sulfoxide-reaction buffer (citric acid 6 g/L, disodium hydrogen phosphate 10g/L, pH 12) (1:39) | Methanol–ammonium formate (10 mM, pH 4) (98:2) | Single quadrupole (Advion) with an ESI source | 57 |

*(Continued)*

**TABLE 3.1 (Continued)**
**Previous Usage of HPTLC–MS**

| Analyte | Sample Matrix | Plate | Mobile Phase | Eluent | Mass Spectrometer | References |
|---|---|---|---|---|---|---|
| Sibutramine | Herbal slimming supplements | Silica gel 60 F$_{254}$ HPTLC preconditioned with a saturated solution of MgCl$_2$ | Toluene–methanol (9:1) | Methanol–ammonium formate (1:1) | 3200 Q-trap hybrid (AB SCIEX) with an ESI source | 58 |
| Neutral sphingolipids | Human plasma | Primuline-postimpregnated silica gel | 2-Step AMD[h] with undefined solvents | NA | NA | 59 |
| Monoacylglycerides | Fatty acid methyl esters (biodiesels) | HPTLC | t-Butyl methyl ether–dichloromethane–n-heptane | NA | NA | 60 |
| Sulfonamide antibiotics | Bovine milk, porcine kidney and liver | Silica gel 60F$_{254}$ HPTLC | Ethyl acetate–methanol–ammonium hydroxide (28%) (8:2:0.1), postchromatographic derivatization with fluram solution (10 mg in 100 mL acetone) | Acetonitrile–ammonium formate buffer (20 mM) (7:3), and methanol–ammonium formate (20 mM) (7:3) for derivatized plates | G1956B MSD single quadrupole with an ESI source (Agilent) | 61 |
| Insulin, UV filters, steroids, caffeine, peptides, protein | Food, beverage, pharmaceutical ingredients, cosmetic additives, sun cream, energy drinks | NA | NA | Acetonitrile–water (95:5) | Unknown manufacturer, used with an ESI source | 62 |

*(Continued)*

**TABLE 3.1 (Continued)**
**Previous Usage of HPTLC–MS**

| Analyte | Sample Matrix | Plate | Mobile Phase | Eluent | Mass Spectrometer | References |
|---|---|---|---|---|---|---|
| Antioxidant isoflavone aglycones, glycosides | *Genista saharae* Coss. & Dur. | NA | NA | Dichloromethane–methanol (95:5) | Qtrap 2000 triple quadruple (AB SCIEX) with an ESI source | 63 |
| Antibacterial products, antioxidant products | Plants | NA | NA | NA | NA | 64 |
| Lecithins | Chocolate, soybean, and sunflower extracts | NA | NA | NA | Single quadrupole | 65 |
| Coumarin | Cinnamon samples, and cinnamon-containing foods | Silica gel 60 HPTLC | *n*-hexane–ethyl acetate–ammonia, and postchromatographic derivatization with ethanolic KOH solution | NA | NA | 66 |
| Steviol glycosides | *Stevia* formulations and sugar-free food products | Silica gel 60 HPTLC and silica gel 60F$_{254}$ HPTLC | Ethyl acetate–methanol–acetic acid (3:1:1), in two stage at (7:2:2) then (6:1:1) for candy samples | Methanol | Expression CMS single quadrupole (Advion) with an ESI source | 67 |
| Pesticides | Apples, cucumbers, red grapes, tomatoes | Silica gel 60 NH$_2$ F$_{254}$s | Acetonitrile, acetone in the reverse direction | Acetonitrile–ammonium formate (10 mM) (1:10) | Unique HT TOFMS (LECO) with an ESI source | 68 |

*(Continued)*

**TABLE 3.1 (*Continued*)**
**Previous Usage of HPTLC–MS**

| Analyte | Sample Matrix | Plate | Mobile Phase | Eluent | Mass Spectrometer | References |
|---|---|---|---|---|---|---|
| Gangliosides, sulfatides | Bovine brain | Silica gel TLC | Chloroform–methanol–aqueous calcium chloride (0.2%) (55:45:10), chloroform–methanol–water–acetic acid (90:50:5:2) for total lipid extract in bovine brain | Isopropyl alcohol–methanol–water (9:1:1) | QSTAR Pulsar *i* quadrupole-orthogonal TOF (AB SCIEX) with an ESI source | 69 |
| Potential cosmetic compounds | Plant extracts | HPTLC | NA | NA | Polaris Q (Finnigan) | 70 |
| Saponin glycosides | Plant materials | Silica gel 60F$_{254}$ HPTLC | Chloroform–methanol–water (6:4:0.9), and chloroform–acetic acid–methanol–water (6.4:3.2:1.2:0.8) | Aqueous formic acid (0.1%), and acetonitrile–water (40:60) | (Bruker Daltonic) | 71 |
| Anthocyanes | Plants | NA | NA | NA | NA | 72 |
| Melamine | Milk | Silica gel 60F$_{254}$S HPTLC | Iso-propanol–dichloromethane–water (5:2:5:3) | Acetonitrile | Single quadrupole | 73 |
| Triterpenoids, carotenoids, proanthocyanidins, flavanols | Food derived from plants | NA | NA | NA | NA | 74 |

(*Continued*)

**TABLE 3.1 (Continued)**
**Previous Usage of HPTLC–MS**

| Analyte | Sample Matrix | Plate | Mobile Phase | Eluent | Mass Spectrometer | References |
|---|---|---|---|---|---|---|
| Antidiabetic polysaccharides | Ocimum basilicum seeds | Silica gel 60 HPTLC | Isopropyl acetate–ethyl acetate–methanol–water (5:4:1:0.1) and derivatization with aniline diphenylamine o-phosphoric acid reagent | Methanol | Expression CMS single quadrupole (Advion) with an ESI source | 75 |
| Dibenzyl cyclooctadiene lignans | Schisandra grandiflora | Silica gel 60F$_{254}$ HPTLC | Toluene–ethyl acetate–methanol (6:1:1) | Methanol | NA | 76 |

a  NA = Information not available in the cited reference.
b  WR = Water resistant and purified; s = acid stable indicator.
c  LiChropher = Spherical particles.
d  NANO-SIL-PAH = Macherey–Nagel, impregnated with caffeine.
e  UTLC = Ultrathin-layer chromatography.
f  NH2 = Amino-bonded silica gel.
g  GLAD UTLC = Glancing angle deposition ultrathin-layer chromatography.
h  AMD = Automated multiple development.

instrument; plate development in a TTC, horizontal chamber, or CAMAG Automatic Developing Chamber (ADC 2) [22]; zone detection under UV light or with a derivatization spray or dip reagent; chromatogram documentation with a camera or scanner; and densitometry if the method involved quantification. These details can be found by consulting the cited references. The applications are all based on one-dimensional ascending linear chromatograms, but a paper has been published on application of the CAMAG TLC–MS interface to different variations of TLC including circular and two-dimensional developments [24]. The large number of papers published in 2014 cited in Table 3.1 clearly demonstrates the current high level of use of the CAMAG interface.

In almost all cases, commercial HPTLC plates have been used with the TLC–MS interface. A few papers (e.g., Reference 25) were published involving its use with commercial Merck ultrathin layers (UTLC) (introduced in 2001 and now discontinued), and, more recently, laboratory-made UTLC plates such as those produced by glancing angle deposition (GLAD) [26,27]. Layers for TLC–MS are covered in detail by Rabel in Chapter 5, and Table 3.1 lists layers used with the TLC–MS interface.

## ACKNOWLEDGMENT

We thank Dr. Gerd Battermann, head of Instrumental Analytics, Merck KGaA, Darmstadt, Germany, for financial support of Jacob Strock within the Lafayette College EXCEL Scholars Program.

## REFERENCES

1. Issaq, J.H., Schroer, J.A., and Barr, E.W. 2008, A direct on-line thin layer chromatography/mass spectrometry coupling system, *Instrum. Sci. Technol.*, 8: 51–53.
2. Luftmann, H. 2003, A simple device for the extraction of TLC spots: Direct coupling with an electrospray mass spectrometer, *Anal. Bioanal. Chem.*, 378: 964–968.
3. Sherma, J. 2008, A field guide to instrumentation: Instrumentation for modern thin-layer chromatography, *J. AOAC Int.*, 91: 55A–58A.
4. Morlock, G. and Schwack, W. 2010, Coupling of planar chromatography to mass spectrometry, *Trends Anal. Chem.*, 29: 1157–1171.
5. Luftman, H. 2011, Thin layer chromatography (TLC): Online and offline coupling with mass spectrometry, *GIT Lab. J.*, 5–6: 37–39.
6. Prosek, M., Milivojevic, M., Krizman, M., and Fir, M. 2004, On-line TLC–MS, *J. Planar Chromatogr.-Mod. TLC*, 17: 420–423.
7. Loppacher, M. and Rolli, R. 2009, The new TLC–MS interface, *CAMAG Bibliography Service (CBS)*, 102: 2–3.
8. Tuzimski, T. 2011, Application of different modes of thin-layer chromatography and mass spectrometry for the separation and detection of large and small biomolecules, *J. Chromatogr. A*, 1218: 8799–8812.
9. Morlock, G.E. 2014, Background mass signals in TLC/HPTLC–ESI–MS and practical advices for use of the TLC–MS interface, *J. Liq. Chromatogr. Relat. Technol.*, 37: 2892–2914.
10. Morlock, G.E. 2012, High-performance thin-layer chromatography-mass spectrometry for analysis of small molecules, in *Handbook of Mass Spectrometry*, Lee, M., Ed., John Wiley & Sons, New York, pp. 1181–1206.

11. Tuzimski, T. 2011, Basic principles of planar chromatography, in *High-Performance Thin-Layer Chromatography (HPTLC)*, Srivastava, M., Ed., Springer, New York, pp. 277–310.

12. Sherma, J. 2002, High performance liquid chromatography/mass spectrometry (LC/MS), *Inside Lab. Manage.*, 6(4): 24–29.

13. Alpmann, A. and Morlock, G.E. 2006, Improved online coupling of planar chromatography with electrospray mass spectrometry: Extraction of zones from glass plates, *Anal. Bioanal. Chem.*, 386: 1543–1551.

14. Jautz, U. and Morlock, G. 2006, Efficacy of planar chromatography coupled to (tandem) mass spectrometry for employment in trace analysis, *J. Chromatogr. A*, 1128: 244–250.

15. Morlock, G.E. and Jautz, U. 2008, Comparison of two different plunger geometries for HPTLC–MS coupling via an extractor-based interface, *J. Planar Chromatogr.-Mod. TLC*, 21: 367–371.

16. About TLC–MS interface, CAMAG Web Site, http://www.camag.com/printpage.cfm?nav=43&content=100, accessed March 30, 2014.

17. Luftman, H., Aranda, M., and Morlock, G.E. 2007, Automated interface for hyphenation of planar chromatography with mass spectrometry, *Rapid Commun. Mass Spectrom.*, 21: 3772–3776.

18. Dytkiewitz, E. and Morlock, G.E. 2008, Analytical strategy for rapid identification and quantification of lubricant additives in mineral oil by high-performance thin-layer chromatography with UV absorption and fluorescence detection combined with mass spectrometry and infrared spectroscopy, *J. AOAC Int.*, 91: 1237–1243.

19. Gaugler, S., Scherer, U., Gössi, A., Schlotterbeck, G., Wyss, S., Büttler A., Hettich, T., and Baron, A. 2013, Rapid structure confirmation and quantitation by HPTLC-NMR, *CAMAG Bibliography Service (CBS)*, 110: 2–4.

20. Gössi, A., Uta, S., and Götz, S. 2012, Thin-layer chromatography-nuclear magnetic resonance spectroscopy—A versatile tool for pharmaceutical and natural products analysis, *CHIMIA*, 66: 347–349.

21. Advion and CAMAG form exclusive alliance to commercialize unique TLC/CMS assay system for synthetic organic and peptide chemists, Advion website, http://www.advion.com/advion-camag-form-exclusive-alliance-commercialize-unique-tlccms-assay-system-synthetic-organic-peptide-chemists/, accessed May 1, 2014.

22. Cretu, G.C. and Morlock, G.E. 2014, Analysis of anthocyanins in powdered berry extracts by planar chromatography linked with bioassay and mass spectrometry, *Food Chem.*, 146: 104–112.

23. Abu-Rabie, P. and Spooner, N. 2009, Direct quantitative bioanalysis of drugs in dried blood spot samples using a thin-layer chromatography mass spectrometer interface, *Anal. Chem.*, 81: 10275–10284.

24. Chausov, A.V., Khrebtova, S.S., Borisov, R.S., Dizdo, T., Berezkin, V.G., and Zaikin, V.G. 2013, The application of CAMAG TLC–MS interface in two dimensional TLC TLC-capillary GC, *Sorbtsionnye i Khromatograficheskie Protsessy*, 12: 248–260.

25. Vovk, I., Popovic, G., Simonovska, B., Albreht, A., and Agbaba, D. 2011, Ultra-thin-layer chromatography mass spectrometry and thin-layer chromatography mass spectrometry of single peptides of angiotensin-converting enzyme inhibitors, *J. Chromatogr. A*, 1218: 3089–3094.

26. Krchert, S., Wang, Z., Taschuk, M.T., Jim, S.R., Brett, M.J., and Morlock, G.E. 2013, Inkjet application, chromatography, and mass spectrometry of sugars on nanostructured thin films, *Anal. Bioanal. Chem.*, 405: 7195–7203.

27. Wannenmacher, J., Jim, S.R., Taschuk, M.T., Brett, M.J., and Morlock, G.E. 2013, Ultrathin-layer chromatography on $SiO_2$, $Al_2O_3$, $TiO_2$, and $ZrO_2$ nanostructured thin films, *J. Chromatogr. A*, 1318: 234–243.

28. Schwack, W., Häberle, S., Jautz, U., and Morlock, G. 2004, New HPTLC–MS method for determination of heterocyclic aromatic amines, *Camag Bibliography Services (CBS)*, 93: 14–15.

29. Morlock, G. and Schwack, W. 2006, Determination of isopropylthioxanthone (ITX) in milk, yoghurt and fat by HPTLC-FLD, HPTLC–ESI/MS and HPTLC-DART/MS, *Anal. Bioanal. Chem.*, 385: 586–595.

30. Morlock, G. and Aranda, M. 2006, Simultaneous determination of riboflavin, pyridoxine, nicotinamide, caffeine and taurine in energy drinks by planar chromatography-multiple detection with confirmation by electrospray ionization mass spectrometry, *J. Chromatogr. A*, 1131: 253–260.

31. Morlock, G. and Jautz, U. 2007, Validation of a new planar chromatographic method for quantification of the heterocyclic aromatic amines most frequently found in meat, *Anal. Bioanal. Chem.*, 387: 1083–1093.

32. Morlock, G. and Ueda, Y. 2007, New coupling of planar chromatography with direct analysis in real time mass spectrometry, *J. Chromatogr. A,* 1143: 243–251.

33. Aranda, M. and Morlock, G. 2007, Simultaneous determination of caffeine, ergotamine, and metamizol in solid pharmaceutical formulation by HPTLC-UV-FLD with mass confirmation by online HPTLC–ESI–MS, *J. Chromatogr. Sci.*, 45: 251–255.

34. Aranda, M. and Morlock, G. 2007, New method for caffeine quantification by planar chromatography coupled with electrospray ionization mass spectrometry using stable isotope dilution analysis, *Rapid Commun. Mass Spectrom.*, 21: 1297–1303.

35. Alpman, A. and Morlock, G. 2008, Rapid and sensitive determination of acrylamide in drinking water by planar chromatography and fluorescence detection after derivatization with dansulfinic acid, *J. Sep. Sci.*, 31: 71–77.

36. Schwack, W. and Elodie, P. 2009, Determination of unauthorized fat-soluble azo dyes in spices by HPTLC, *CAMAG Bibliography Service*, 103: 13–15.

37. Morlock, G. and Oellig, C. 2009, Rapid planar chromatographic analysis of 25 water-soluble dyes used as food additives, *J. AOAC Int.*, 92: 745–756.

38. Dytkiewitz, E. and Wolfgange, S. 2010, Determination of additives in plastics foils, *CAMAG Bibliography Service*, 105: 13–15.

39. Arando, M. and Morlock, G. 2010, Quantification of pyritinol in solid pharmaceutical formulation by high-performance thin-layer chromatography-ultraviolet detection and selectivity evaluation by mass spectrometry, *J. Liq. Chromatogr. Relat. Technol.*, 33: 957–971.

40. Chernetsova, E., Revelksy, I, and Morlock, G. 2011, Fast quantitation of 5-hydroxymethylfurfural in honey using planar chromatography, *Anal. Bioanal. Chem.*, 401: 325–332.

41. Morlock, G., Scuele, L., and Sebastian, G. 2011, Development of a quantitative high-performance thin-layer chromatographic method for sucralose in sewage effluent, surface water, and drinking water, *J. Chromatogr. A*, 1218: 2745–2753.

42. Oellig, C. and Schwack, W. 2011, Planar solid phase extraction-a new clean-up concept in multi-residue analysis of pesticides by liquid chromatography–mass spectrometry, *J. Chromatogr. A*, 1218: 6540–6547.

43. Sajewicz, M., Staszek, D., Natić, M., Wojtal, Ł., Waksmudzka-Hajnos, M., and Kowalska, T. 2011, TLC–MS versus TLC–LC–MS fingerprints of herbal extracts. Part II. Phenolic acids and flavonoids. *J. Liq. Chromatogr. Relat. Technol.,* 34: 864–887.

44. Sajewicz, M., Staszek, D., Natic, M., Waksmundzka-Hajnos, M., and Kowalska, T. 2011, TLC-MS versus TLC–LC–MS fingerprints of herbal extracts. Part III. Application of the reversed-phase liquid chromatography systems with chromatography systems with $C_{18}$ stationary phase, *J. Chromatogr. Sci.*, 49: 560–567.

45. Shikov, A., Ossipov, V., Martiskainen, O., Pozharitskaya, O., Ivanova, S., and Makarov, V. 2011, The offline combination of thin-layer chromatography and high-performance liquid chromatography with diode array detection and micrOTOF-Q mass

spectrometry for the separation and identification of spinochromes from sea urchin (*Strongylocentrotus droebachiensis*) shells, *J. Chromatogr. A*, 1218: 9111–9114.

46. Oellig, C. and Schwack, W. 2012, Planar solid phase extraction clean-up for pesticide residue analysis in tea by liquid chromatography–mass spectrometry, *J. Chromatogr. A*, 1260: 42–53.

47. Kampalanonwat, P., Supaphol, P., and Morlock, G. 2013, Electrospun nonofiber layers with incorporated photoluminescence indicator for chromatography and detection of ultraviolet-active compounds, *J. Chromatogr. A*, 1299: 110–117.

48. Krüger, S., Urmann, O., and Morlock, G. 2013, Development of planar chromatographic method for quantitation of anthocyanes in pomace, feed, juice and wine, *J. Chromatogr. A*, 1289: 105–118.

49. Hubicka, U., Żuromska-Witek, B., Żmudzki, P., Matwiej, B., and Krzek, J. 2013, Thin-layer chromatography with densitometry for the determination of difloxacin and its photodegradation products. Kinetic evaluation of the degradation process and identification of photoproducts by mass spectrometry, *J. Liq. Chromatogr. Relat. Technol.*, 36: 2431–2445.

50. Smrke, S. and Vovk, I. 2013, Comprehensive thin-layer chromatography mass spectrometry of flavanols from *Juniperus cummunis* L. and *Punica granatum* L., *J. Chromatogr. A*, 1289: 119–126.

51. Chen, Y. and Schwack, W. 2013, Planar chromatography mediated screening of tetracycline and fluoroquinolone antibiotics in milk by fluorescence and mass selective detection, *J. Chromatogr. A*, 1312: 143–151.

52. Adhami, H., Scherer, U., Kaehlig H., Hettich, T., Schlotterbeck, G., Reich, E., and Krenn, L. 2013, Combination of bioautography with HPTLC–MS/NMR: A fast identification of acetylcholinesterase inhibitors from galbanum, *Phytochem. Anal.*, 24: 395–400.

53. Schulz, M., Schubach, B., Minarik, S., and Griesinger, H. 2013, Introduction of special HPTLC and TLC plates for coupling with mass spectrometry, *CAMAG Bibliography Service (CBS)*, 110: 10–11.

54. Chen, Y. and Schwack, W. 2014, High-performance thin-layer chromatography screening of multi class antibiotics in animal food by bioluminescent bioautography and electrospray ionization mass spectrometry, *J. Chromatogr. A*, 1356: 249–257.

55. Altmaier, S. and Schulz, M. 2014, Fast analysis of "dirty" samples with monolithic silica LC and silica gel TLC stationary phases, *LCGC N. America*, 32: 504–512.

56. Morlock, G. and Klingelhöfer, I. 2014, Liquid chromatography–bioassay–mass spectrometry for profiling of physiologically active food, *Anal. Chem.*, 86: 8289–8295.

57. Klingelhöfer, I. and Morlock, G. 2014, Sharp-bounded zones link to the effect in planar chromatography–bioassay–mass spectrometry, *J. Chromatogr. A*, 1360: 288–295.

58. Mathon, C., Ankli, A., Reich, E., Bieri, S., and Christen, P. 2014, Screening and determination of sibutramine in adulterated herbal slimming supplements by HPTLC–UV densitometry, *Food Addit. Contam. A: Chem. Anal. Control Expo Risk Assess*, 31: 15–20.

59. Cebolla, V., Dominguez, A., Jarne, C., Membrado, L., Saviron, M., Orduna, J., Galban, J., and Lapieza, M. July 2–4, 2014, A hyphenated technique based on AMD–FDIC–MS for separating and determining biomarkers of lysosomal storage diseases in human fluids, *HPTLC 2014*, Lyon, France, abstract O-3.

60. Cebolla, V., Jarne, C., Membrado, L., Saviron, M., and Orduna, J. July 2–4, 2014, Separation, quantitative determination, and fatty acid profiling of monoacylgliceraides in fatty-acid methyl esters (FAME) using an on-line, hyphenated technique based on AMD–FDIC–ESI–MS, *HPTLC 2014*, Lyon, France, abstract P-29.

61. Chen, Y. and Schwack, W. 2014, Rapid and selective determination of multi-sulfonamides by high-performance thin layer chromatography coupled to fluorescent densitometry and electrospray ionization mass detection, *J. Chromatogr. A*, 1331: 108–116.

62. Griesinger, H., Oberle, M., Matheis, K., and Schulz, M. July 2–4, 2014, HPTLC–MS using an elution based TLC–MS interface, *HPTLC 2014*, Lyon, France, abstract P-30.

63. Mariane, D., Genta-Jouve, G., Kaabeche, M., Michele, S., and Boutefnouchet, S. 2014, Rapid identification of antioxidant compounds of *Genista saharae* Coss. & Dur. by combination of DPPH scavenging assay and HPTLC–MS, *Molecules*, 19: 4369–4379.

64. Móricz, A., Ott, P., and Morlock, G. July 2–4, 2014, HPTLC-bioassay-MS, a rapid tool to search and analyse bioactive plant products, *HPTLC 2014*, Lyon, France, abstract O-16.

65. Morlock, G., Krüger, S., Bürmann, L., and Lochnit, G. July 2–4, 2014, HPTLC–FLD–ESI–MS and HPTLC–MALDI-TOF/TOF MS analysis of lecithins used in the production of chocolate, *HPTLC 2014*, Lyon, France, abstract P-8.

66. Morlock, G., Winheim, L., and Krüger, S. July 2–4, 2014, Quantitation of coumarin in food, confirmed by mass spectrometry, *HPTLC 2014*, Lyon, France, abstract P-6.

67. Morlock, G., Meyer, S., Zimmermann, B., and Roussel, J. 2014, High-performance thin-layer chromatography analysis of steviol glycosides in *Stevia* formulations and sugar-free products, and benchmarking with (ultra) high-performance liquid chromatography, *J. Chromatogr. A*, 1350: 102–111.

68. Oellig, C. and Schwack, W. 2014, Planar solid phase extraction clean-up and microliter-flow injection analysis-time-of-flight mass spectrometry for multi-residue screening of pesticides in food, *J. Chromatogr. A*, 1351: 1–11.

69. Park, H., Zhou, Y., and Costello, C. 2014, Direct analysis of sialylated or sulfated glycosphingolipids and other polar and neutral lipids using TLC–MS interfaces, *J. Lipid Res.*, 55: 773–781.

70. Pasquier, L., Blanchot, L., and Tranchant, J. July 2–4, 2014, Development of an off-line HPTLC–MS technique for plant extracts, *HPTLC 2014*, Lyon, France, abstract P-43.

71. Reim, V. and Rohn, S. July 2–4, 2014, Hyphenation of HPTLC with ESI–MS for characterization of saponins in different plant matrices, *HPTLC 2014*, Lyon, France, abstract P-33.

72. Spina, R., Héma, A., Palé, E., Dupire, F., Lachaud, F., Nacro, M., and Laurain-mattar, D. July 2–4, 2014, A rapid identification of anthocyanins in various plants from Burkina Faso by HPTLC/MS, *HPTLC 2014*, Lyon, France, abstract O-14.

73. Srivastava, M., Rani, R., and Medhe, S. July 2–4, 2014, Development and validation of HPTLC–MS determination of melamine in milk, *HPTLC 2014*, Lyon, France, abstract O-31.

74. Vovk, I., Glavnik, V., Albreht, A., Naumoska, K., Simonovska, B., and Smrke, S. July 2–4, 2014, Planar chromatography and mass spectrometry in analysis of phytonutrients in the extracts of edible plants, *HPTLC 2014*, Lyon, France, abstract O-29.

75. Yili, A., Yimamu, H., Ghulameden, S., Quing, Z., Aisa, H., and Morlock, G. 2014, Determination of antidiabetic polysaccharides of *Ocimum basilicum* seeds indigenous to Xinjiang of China by high-performance thin-layer chromatography–UV/vis–mass spectrometry, *J. Planar Chromatogr. Mod. TLC,* 27: 11–18.

76. Kumar, K., Ramesh, B., Rao, V., Poornima, B., Sarma, V., Nissankararao, S., Rao, M., and Babu, S. 2014, Validated high-performance thin-layer chromatographic method for the determination of dibenzyl cyclooctadiene lignans from *Schisandra grandiflora, J. Planar Chromatogr. Mod. TLC*, 27: 460–465.

# 4 Principles of Mass Spectrometry Imaging Applicable to Thin-Layer Chromatography

*Przemysław Mielczarek, Anna Bodzoń-Kułakowska, Jerzy Silberring, and Piotr Suder*

## CONTENTS

## 4.1 INTRODUCTION

Mass spectrometry, as an analytical technique, has been known since the first years of the twentieth century, when Sir Joseph John Thompson observed the isotopes of helium ions traveling in the tube through the magnetic field. Since 1911, a fast development of the mass spectrometry-based techniques has been observed. One of the most promising branches of this analytical method, the so-called imaging mass spectrometry (IMS), dynamically developed during the last few years. Not only does IMS allow for $m/z$ ratio determination of the ionized molecules, but also what is more important, it can show the spatial distribution of the molecules on the two-dimensional surface. It allows for mapping of a variety of components that can be ionized and sputtered from the surface, like tissue sections [1], cell cultures [2], skin, or even thin layer chromatography (TLC) plates [3]. For some cases, there is also a possibility to build three-dimensional maps of the compounds, but such analysis is more complex [4]. In the latter case, usually the sample must be cut into slices prior to IMS analyses and then every section should undergo imaging analysis, which consumes much more time to complete analysis.

Currently, there are at least three ionization techniques routinely used in IMS: (1) secondary ion mass spectrometry (SIMS), (2) matrix-assisted laser desorption ionization (MALDI), and (3) desorption electrospray ionization (DESI). Each of these ion sources has their own advantages and drawbacks; thus, they are usually selected in the context of the imaged sample. In the following text, we provide a concise description of these devices.

### 4.1.1 SECONDARY ION MASS SPECTROMETRY

This source utilizes an ion gun emitting beam of ions (e.g., $Bi^+$, $Ga^+$, and $Au^+$) or ion clusters (e.g., $C_{60}^+$ and $Bi_3^+$) toward the analyzed surface. Ions, treated with the ion gun, and desorbed from the surface are traveling to the time-of-flight (TOF) analyzer, where their $m/z$ are determined [5,6]. The main advantage of this ion source is its high spatial resolution. For routine analyses, the pixel resolution of the final image is usually better than $10 \times 10$ μm, sometimes reaching the value of $1 \times 1$ μm or less, providing the ion beam can be precisely focused on the area of interest [7]. This parameter corresponds to the image resolution in a range from 2500 to 25,000 dpi. However, the ion beam carries a high quantity of energy, which results in the pronounced and unwanted fragmentation of the molecules in the source, especially those of higher MW. In conclusion, SIMS is mainly used for imaging of small objects (e.g., single cells, internal parts of the electronic components, metal ions, catalysts, pollutants, and others) where high resolution of the image is the most important factor. Additionally, MW range of the ionized molecules usually does not exceed 1000 Da, which significantly limits the nature of the samples successfully undergoing analysis performed by this method.

### 4.1.2 MATRIX-ASSISTED LASER DESORPTION IONIZATION–IMAGING MASS SPECTROMETRY

This technique is based on the principles of a typical MALDI ionization, where the liquid sample is deposited on the stainless steel or silicone dioxide target and then covered or mixed with the low MW organic acid capable of absorption of the energy from the UV laser, followed by desorption and ionization.

In the case of MALDI imaging, the sample is also placed on the MALDI target, but this time the sample is represented by the thin section of the material, mounted on the plate by the hydro- or lipophilic interactions with the target surface [8,9]. In the next step, the sample is covered by the matrix with the aid of, for example, an automatic spotter, depositing the appropriate matrix, left under ambient conditions to evaporate solvent, and introduced into the ionization chamber. It is important to cover the sample equally with tiny drops of dissolved matrix, while maintaining no contact between them. If the sample would have been covered with the evenly deposited matrix, this would lead to the exchange and mixing of the compounds from various surface regions. Dot after dot, the laser beam ionizes the sample surface in both $x$ and $y$ dimensions. Resolution of the reconstructed image depends on the density of the dots hit by the laser beam [10]. Usually, a single dot has dimensions of approximately $10 \times 10$ μm, which allows for achieving the image resolution of approximately 2500 dpi. This ion source is mainly used for examination of biological and medical samples (tissues or cross sections of the whole animals) as it is capable of effectively ionizing high MW substances, such as proteins, peptides, lipids, polysaccharides, or oligonucleotides. The effective MW determination varies from around 100 Da to even 100 kDa. This soft ionization technique is often utilized in the MS/MS mode, which substantially increases a quality of structural information gained from the experiments.

### 4.1.3 DESORPTION ELECTROSPRAY IONIZATION

In contrast to both techniques described above, desorption electrospray ionization occurs at ambient conditions (atmospheric pressure and room temperature), and thus seems to be the most convenient ion source among those used in IMS methodology. The ionization process is similar to that appearing in the typical electrospray source. Briefly, spraying capillary (ID: 20–50 µm, fused silica) delivers solvent to the DESI source at the flow rate from 1 to 5 µL/min. The spraying process is supported by the nitrogen delivered from the nozzle surrounding the spraying needle. Nitrogen pressure is usually set to 10–15 bar. Solvent is sprayed on the imaged material, which causes desorption of the ions from the surface [11]. Desorbed ions travel toward the MS inlet. Movement of the sample is realized by the moving $x$–$y$ stage, while both capillaries remain at the same positions. Composition of the sprayed solvent depends on the type of the analyzed sample but, in most cases, it consists of water, methanol, acetonitrile, dimethylformamide (DMF), and small quantities of additives (e.g., formic acid and $NH_{3aq}$) in various proportions. Because of the nature of the ionization process, spatial resolution of the DESI system is the worst among the IMS ionization sources, due to the solvent spraying on the scanned surface. A sample is wetted on the wide area (in comparison to the focused ion, or laser beams); therefore, the achievable spatial resolution is usually not better than 300–600 dpi. To enhance resolution, the so-called nanoDESI, which was introduced by Laskin et al. [12], is a methodology where spraying capillary is bent, forming a liquid bridge directly on the scanned surface. In this solution, a small amount of the solvent extracts substances from the sample surface and then nebulizes them like in a typical nanoelectrospray source. Despite the low spatial resolution of the DESI system, its advantages, such as versatility, simple construction, and operation under ambient conditions, make this source very popular (Figure 4.1).

## 4.2 DESORPTION ELECTROSPRAY IONIZATION–THIN-LAYER CHROMATOGRAPHY PRINCIPLES

Thin-layer chromatography (TLC) is a simple separation technique that is usually applied in the pharmaceutical industry, organic chemistry, and environmental laboratories for fast, basic analyses of sample purity, detection of the reaction products, or verification of the presence or absence of some compounds in the mixtures. TLC methodology and equipment are simple and cost-effective, and such separations may also be performed outside the laboratory, for example, wherever the sample has been taken from the source localized hundreds of miles from the nearest facility. One of the weakest points of TLC separation is visualization of the obtained chromatogram.

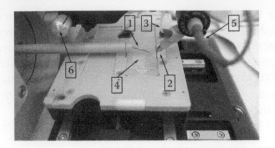

**FIGURE 4.1** DESI ion source (OMNIspray, Prosolia Inc., Indianapolis, IN). 1—MS inlet capillary; 2—Spraying capillary; 3—Tubing delivering nitrogen; 4—$x$–$y$ moving stage with the mounted sample (on the glass microscopic slide); 5—High-voltage cable; 6—Micromanipulator knob positioning spraying capillary (2). (Photo courtesy of Piotr Suder.)

If all separated compounds absorb visible light, it is usually sufficient to estimate quantity of the compounds using optical supervision. For other cases, it is necessary to use a detection system, compatible with the nature of the separated substances. The most often used are UV light emitters, allowing for the observation of the light emission. Sometimes, the more specific methodologies are applied, like chemical staining directly on the TLC plate (e.g., ninhydrin). For TLC chromatograms, quantitative analysis is also possible. In such cases, various densitometers are utilized to provide quantitative results from chromatograms.

Mass spectrometry brings a powerful detection system to TLC, being able to identify almost every compound present on the TLC plate. Moreover, fragmentation procedure (MS/MS or MS$^n$) can be done to fully identify components present on the chromatogram.

Formerly, connection between MS and TLC was more complicated. Keeping in mind that earlier mass spectrometers were the instruments unable to sample the surface point after point, it was necessary to scrape a small amount of the TLC layer containing the compound of interest. Then the sample was desorbed from the beads, dissolved in a solvent compatible with the MS source, and introduced into the mass spectrometer [13]. Such a procedure was laborious, inaccurate, and definitely not quantitative. Those disadvantages prevented the dissemination of the mass spectrometers as effective detectors in TLC. Additionally, it should be noted that mass spectrometers were (and still are) expensive analytical tools, but they are becoming more popular in various laboratories nowadays.

The modern approach, linking mass spectrometry to TLC, is much more convenient and reliable. Progress in mass spectrometry imaging allows for fast and simple TLC plate mounting in the system and visualization of the compounds by ionizing them directly on the surface. In contrast to the previously applied "off-line" techniques, the novel approach is easy to apply, gives repeatable results, and allows for unambiguous compounds' identification and quantitation independently from their separation effectivity. In the case of the DESI-TLC connection, the methodology of the measurements is simple but still the quality of the results is mainly dependent on the DESI source settings and DESI solvent selection. Technically, using desorption electrospray ionization source, it is sufficient to immobilize the dried TLC plate on the moving $x$–$y$ stage to find the chromatographic traces on the plate. Then, DESI head moves over the entire chromatogram, desorbing the molecules from the TLC plate, ionizing them, and directing into the MS inlet. Although the analytical procedure does not seem to be complicated, there are at least a few variables, which should be appropriately set before a TLC-DESI-MS experiment. One of the most important is selection of the proper solvent composition for DESI spraying. The selected solvent must be able to effectively destroy physical interactions between matrix (silica gel, aluminum oxide, cellulose, etc.) and the separated sample compounds. Solvent must also be compatible with the DESI source and serve as an environment for the effective ionization process. Solvents used for DESI-TLC analyses are similar to those applied in electrospray (ESI) and nanoelectrospray (nanoESI). Their optimal composition depends on the TLC matrix, a nature of separated compounds, and is adjusted empirically. Another important step is optimization of the geometrical settings of the DESI source. Such process consumes significant amount of time, as there are at least a few important parameters to be optimized like distances between capillaries, height of the spraying capillary over the surface of TLC plate, angle of the spraying capillary, voltage between capillaries, speed of the moving stage, and other settings of the mass spectrometer. It is worth mentioning that careful optimization is absolutely crucial for the successful DESI-TLC analysis. Although all MS-based methods need to be adjusted at the preparation step, it seems that DESI-based techniques and final quality of results are extremely sensitive to proper optimization.

During TLC-DESI-MS analysis, the spraying capillary moves over the chromatographic trace on the TLC plate, while the MS inlet collects ions desorbed from the surface and ionized. The speed of a moving stage is precisely controlled in a range from 50 to 200 µm/s. Moving speed, along with MS scanning speed, allows for adjustment of the resolution of the final MS chromatogram or image. A decrease of the moving speed with simultaneous increase of the MS scanning speed allows for an increase of resolution, as the mass spectrometer acquires more spectra from the smaller distance. After scanning, spectra acquired from the TLC trace can be transformed into a mass chromatogram. Then every $m/z$ identified from the surface of the TLC plate can be visualized in various modes. Direct observation of MS spectra allows for $m/z$ identification of the compounds, while extracted ion chromatograms (EIC) carry semi-quantitative information about compounds' concentrations. In case of uncertainties about the structure of the observed ion, it is possible to find an area where the compound is located and perform MS/MS experiment. Even if the compounds are poorly or not separated, a mass spectrometer can distinguish between them, based on the $m/z$ of the ions. Similarly, for the fragmentation process, identification of overlapping molecules present on the same area of the plate is not challenging.

In the case of typical TLC plates, DESI seems to be a very useful technique of visualization due to its ambient working conditions. The limited spatial resolution of this source is not important for a majority of the TLC plates, including high-performance TLC (HP-TLC). However, for some applications, it is recommended to apply another ion source providing better imaging capabilities, such as MALDI–IMS.

## 4.3   MATRIX-ASSISTED LASER DESORPTION IONIZATION–THIN-LAYER CHROMATOGRAPHY PRINCIPLES

Since MALDI was developed in the 1980s, many efforts were done for over 30 years to combine TLC with MALDI–MS. The biggest advantage of this type of analyses is a possibility to obtain a detailed "image" of the TLC plate, without compromising TLC spatial resolution. MALDI–MS seems to be more demanding for sample preparation in comparison to DESI–MS. However, the major benefit of this type of ionization is its high versatility, higher spatial resolution than for DESI-TLC–MS, and a possibility to identify and quantify compounds that belong to many different chemical types. TLC–MALDI–MS has already been used for analyses of compounds such as pesticides, drugs [14], and dyes [15]. The biggest achievement, as compared to other MS-based techniques linked to TLC analyses, is the possibility to apply this technique for high-MW compounds such as polymers, proteins, peptides, nucleotides, and lipids [16,17]. As it was described earlier, MALDI requires application of a matrix to produce efficient ionization of the analyte. Application of the matrix on the TLC plate is the key to successful analysis, as this is the most important step of sample pretreatment. The most commonly used matrices are listed in Table 4.1.

In general, there are five techniques for spreading the matrix over the TLC plate. The first one, and the simplest, is to place a small droplet of the matrix solution on the TLC plate directly from the pipette tip. Unfortunately, this methodology does not allow for continuous scanning of the entire surface of the plate. This type of analysis is usually performed to measure masses of the compounds present in various spots that have been *a priori* marked on the plate. This approach can be improved by using matrix solution of a relatively high surface tension. This can consist of a mixture of water and organic solvent, instead of a pure organic solution of the matrix. As a result, formation of small spots on the plate covered with the matrix is observed, which significantly increases spatial resolution. Nowadays, the most popular way to prepare samples for analysis is to spray the TLC plate with the matrix solution, as such spraying instruments are currently commercially available. The spray may be produced in different ways, for example, by electrospray equipment or nebulizers using compressed gases. The most sophisticated way is to use piezoelectric nozzles (similar to those used in ink jet printers). This technique offers the smallest droplets

---

**TABLE 4.1**
**Popular Matrices in MALDI–MS**

| Sinapinic Acid<br>SA | α-Cyano-4-hydroxycinnamic Acid<br>CHCA | 2,5-Dihydroxybenzoic Acid<br>DHB |
|---|---|---|

on the TLC surface, their regular shapes, and, finally, each spot is separated from the others, which allows avoiding mixing of the compounds present in distinct TLC spots. Two other techniques of matrix deposition should also be mentioned; however, they are rarely used. One is based on brushing the TLC plate with a supersaturated solution of the matrix, and the other utilizes pressing the matrix crystals on the TLC surface usually by a stainless-steel block.

Additionally, the most important advantage that should be added to all benefits mentioned above is the simplicity of coupling TLC with MALDI–MS. Basically, it is sufficient to mount the TLC plate directly on the stainless-steel MALDI target. The only limitation is that the surface has to be conductive, and the TLC plate with glass support needs to be replaced with a TLC plate with stationary phase immobilized on the aluminum foil. Care must also be taken to keep the overall dimension of the MALDI target with the TLC plate to maintain its smooth insertion into the ion source.

Some limitations should be pointed out here. The obstacle is that commercially available lasers used in MALDI sources are based on UV light that do not deeply penetrate into the stationary phase. This significantly reduces signal intensity. To overcome this problem, the analyte can be brought onto the plate surface using organic solvents; however, this procedure reduces spatial resolution of the image because the sample can be spread over a larger surface. The other way to solve this problem is usage of IR lasers with glycerol as a matrix. Not all commercially available instruments can be equipped with IR lasers, and glycerol cannot be used to ionize all chemical classes of compounds. The next problem is irregularity of the TLC surface that reduce mass accuracy obtained on the mass spectra. In the MALDI method, even small inequality of the surface may result in the affected flying time of ions having identical $m/z$. This problem may be partially eliminated by using an internal standard placed on the TLC plate or by performing the experiment in MALDI-TOF(/TOF) instruments.

## 4.4 CONCLUSIONS

The discussed mass spectrometry-based imaging techniques can be easily implemented for visualization and identification of the compounds separated by TLC. MS-based methods need to be appropriately arranged and optimized before the experiment, which costs a significant amount of time and additional reagents. However, their advantages, such as unambiguous identification of the compounds separated on the plate and visualization of every spot, independently from the quality of the separation itself, make them the perfect choice for detection in combination with the very simple TLC separation technology.

## REFERENCES

1. Eberlin, L.S., Liu, X., Ferreira, C.R., Santagata, S., Agar, N.Y., and Cooks, R.G. 2011, Desorption electrospray ionization then MALDI mass spectrometry imaging of lipid and protein distributions in single tissue sections, *Anal. Chem.*, 15: 8366–8371.
2. Bodzon-Kulakowska, A., Drabik, A., Marszalek, M., Kotlinska, J.H., and Suder, P. 2014, DESI analysis of mammalian cell cultures—Preparation and method optimisation, *J. Mass Spectrom.*, 49: 613–621.

3. Van Berkel, G.J., Ford, M.J., and Deibel, M.A. 2005, Thin-layer chromatography and mass spectrometry coupled using desorption electrospray ionization. *Anal. Chem.*, 1: 1207–1215.
4. de Rijke, E., Hooijerink, D., Sterk, S.S., and Nielen, M.W. 2013, Confirmation and 3D profiling of anabolic steroid esters in injection sites using imaging desorption electrospray ionisation (DESI) mass spectrometry. *Food Addit. Contam. A: Chem. Anal. Control Expo Risk Assess.*, 30: 1012–1019.
5. Pacholski, M.L. and Winograd, N. 1999, Imaging with mass spectrometry, *Chem. Rev.*, 99: 2977–3006.
6. Todd, P.J., Schaaff, T.G., Chaurand, P., and Caprioli, R.M. 2001, Organic ion imaging of biological tissue with secondary ion mass spectrometry and matrix-assisted laser desorption/ionization, *J. Mass Spectrom.*, 36: 355–369.
7. Winograd, N. 2005, Imaging mass spectrometry on the nanoscale with cluster ion beams, *Anal. Chem.*, 6: 328–333.
8. Spengler, B., Hubert, M., and Kaufmann, R. 1994, MALDI ion imaging and biological ion imaging with a new scanning UV-laser microprobe, *Proc. 42nd Annual Conf. Mass Spectrom. Allied Topics*, Chicago, Illinois, 1041.
9. Caprioli, R.M., Farmer, T.B., and Gile, J. 1997, Molecular imaging of biological samples: Localization of peptides and proteins using MALDI-TOF MS, *Anal. Chem.,* 69: 4751–4760.
10. Martin-Lorenzo, M., Balluff, B., Sanz-Maroto, A., van Zeijl, R.J., Vivanco, F., Alvarez-Llamas, G., and McDonnell, L.A. 2014, 30 µm spatial resolution protein MALDI MSI: In-depth comparison of five sample preparation protocols applied to human healthy and atherosclerotic arteries, *J. Proteomics*, 28: 465–468.
11. Bodzon-Kulakowska, A., Drabik, A., Ner, J., Kotlinska, J.H., and Suder, P. 2014, Desorption electrospray ionisation (DESI) for beginners—How to adjust settings for tissue imaging, *Rapid Commun. Mass Spectrom.*, 15: 1–9.
12. Laskin, J., Heath, B.S., Roach, P.J., Cazares, L., and Semmes, O.J. 2012, Tissue imaging using nanospray desorption electrospray ionization mass spectrometry, *Anal. Chem.*, 84: 141–148.
13. Chen, Y. and Schwack, W. 2014, High-performance thin-layer chromatography screening of multi class antibiotics in animal food by bioluminescent bioautography and electrospray ionization mass spectrometry, *J. Chromatogr. A*, 22: 249–257.
14. Kuwayama, K., Tsujikawa, K., Miyaguchi, H., Kanamori, T., Iwata, Y.T., and Inoue, H. 2012, Rapid, simple, and highly sensitive analysis of drugs in biological samples using thin-layer chromatography coupled with matrix-assisted laser desorption/ionization mass spectrometry, *Anal. Bioanal. Chem.*, 402: 1257–1267.
15. de Oliveira, D.N., Siqueira, M., Sartor, S., and Catharino, R. 2013, Direct analysis of lipsticks by Sorptive tape-like extraction laser desorption/ionization mass spectrometry imaging, *Int. J. Cosmet. Sci.*, 35: 467–471.
16. Yang, J. and Caprioli, R.M. 2014, Matrix pre-coated targets for high throughput MALDI imaging of proteins, *J. Mass Spectrom.*, 49: 417–422.
17. Mainini, V., Lalowski, M., Gotsopoulos, A., Bitsika, V., Baumann, M., and Magni, F. 2014, MALDI-imaging mass spectrometry on tissues, *Methods Mol. Biol.*, 1243: 139–164.

# 5 Mass Spectrometry Applicable to Electrophoretic Techniques

*Anna Drabik, Joanna Ner, Przemysław Mielczarek,*
*Piotr Suder, and Jerzy Silberring*

## CONTENTS

## 5.1 INTRODUCTION

Studies of complex samples are the most demanding tasks in analytical methods and therefore must combine high-resolution separation systems with an equally advanced, selective detector. During the last decades, planar forms of electrophoresis, such as polyacrylamide gel electrophoresis (PAGE) and agarose gel electrophoresis, additionally supported with imaging documentation systems, are very useful tools for separation and identification of the complex biological samples.

## 5.2   PREPARATION OF BIOLOGICAL SAMPLES

Sample preparation for electrophoretic separations is crucial and the quality of this step decides on the final results of an experiment. Unwanted precipitation of proteins during the isolation process is one of the most common causes of sample loss. Addition of small amounts of detergents helps to protect against this phenomenon. In addition, the presence of high salt concentration causes unstable voltage conditions during electrophoresis, which results in smudges and heterogeneous bands. It is also important to note that, during blood sample analysis or tissue samples containing blood, the immunodepletion of albumin and immunoglobulins is recommended. Otherwise, those highly abundant proteins (approximately 95% of blood content) will obscure information regarding substances present in very low concentrations. It is necessary to establish protein content before electrophoretic separation. Too large amount of the sample will result in poor resolution of the gel image, and large bands will overlay the neighboring protein signals (Figure 5.1). Too low protein concentration will lead to the very poor signal, and therefore, information about low-abundant proteins will be lost.

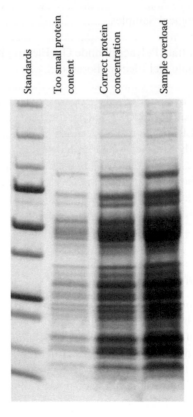

**FIGURE 5.1**   Optimization of the protein content applied on the polyacrylamide gel. Staining performed with Coomassie Brilliant Blue (CBB).

Electrophoresis can be performed either under denaturing or nondenaturing conditions. In the case when the biological activity of proteins or protein complexes should be retained, addition of nonionic detergent (e.g., Triton X-100) or Coomassie Brilliant Blue (CBB) to the sample in order to create anion complexes with proteins might be necessary. The most common type of electrophoretic separation is performed under denaturing conditions with addition of sodium dodecyl sulfate (SDS), due to the higher resolution of protein bands.

## 5.3  SEPARATION MECHANISM

During the electrophoresis process, the molecules migrate in the gel under the influence of an applied electric field. The distance the compounds can travel in the gel depends on several factors, which are as follows:

1. Pore size
2. Molecular weight
3. Total charge
4. Shape

Electrophoretic mobility can be described by the following equation:

$$\mu = \frac{V}{E} = \frac{Z}{f}$$

$$f = 6\pi\eta nr$$

where
  $\mu$—electrophoretic mobility
  $E$—strength of the electric filed
  $V$—velocity of the ion
  $Z$—total molecular charge
  $f$—coefficient of friction
  $\eta$—viscosity
  $r$—hydrodynamic radius

Depending on the type of material being separated and on the applied conditions, several types of electrophoretic separations can be taken into account, as shown in Figure 5.2.

One of the popular options for the separation of proteins under native or denaturing conditions is polyacrylamide gel. The gel results from the polymerization of acrylamide with $N,N$-methylenebisacrylamide (bisacrylamide) in the presence of additives that accelerate the polymerization process (Table 5.1).

The separation process depends on the size of pores present in the gel. The pore size is defined by two parameters as presented below:

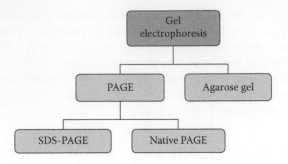

**FIGURE 5.2**    Types of electrophoretic separation.

**TABLE 5.1**
**Polyacrylamide Gel Components**

| Compound | Function |
|---|---|
| Acrylamide (toxic) | Main component of the gel |
| N, N-methylenebisacrylamide (toxic) | Cross-linking agent |
| Ammonium persulfate (APS) | Polymerization starter |
| β-Dimethylaminoproprionitril (DMAP) | Reaction catalyst |
| N,N,N,N-tetramethylethylenediamine | Reaction catalyst |

The total amount of acrylamide: $\%T = (\text{acrylamide} + \text{bisacrylamide})\ [\text{g}]$

The amount of cross-linker: $\%C = \dfrac{(\text{bisacrylamide})\ [\text{g}] \times 100}{(\text{acrylamide} + \text{bisacrylamide})\ [\text{g}]}$

The resulting pore size is determined by the percentage of the following two reagents: acrylamide and bisacrylamide. If the parameter $\%C$ is constant, and $\%T$ increases, gel pores are reduced. If $\%C$ increases, gel pores will be altered, according to a parabolic function [1]. Different types of gels used for the separation of proteins, depending on the range of their size, are commercially available or can be prepared in the laboratory. In the latter case, care should be taken, as components of the gel are toxic and cancerogenous.

## 5.4 SODIUM DODECYL SULFATE POLYACRYLAMIDE GEL ELECTROPHORESIS

Sodium dodecyl sulfate polyacrylamide gel electrophoresis (SDS-PAGE) is one of the most important separation techniques for proteins. The addition of an anionic detergent, SDS, to the sample causes denaturation of proteins. Detergent donates the negative charge to the protein, which is proportional to the polypeptide chain length. SDS specifically binds to proteins in a mass ratio of 1.4:1. In this type of separation, migration rate of proteins exclusively depends on their molecular masses and not on other factors, listed previously. Such a system allows for the separation of molecules

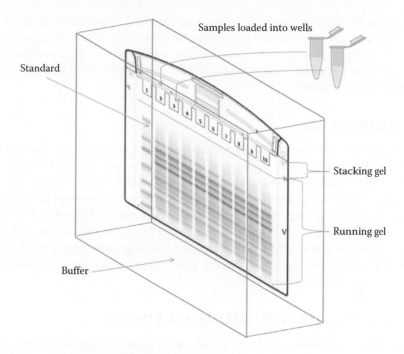

**FIGURE 5.3** System for the SDS-PAGE separation.

in a wide range of molecular masses (0.5–300 kDa). A mixture of proteins migrates through the polyacrylamide gel creating lanes of protein bands. Larger proteins progress slower than the smaller ones do (Figure 5.3). High salt concentration causes high electrical current and makes effective separation impossible [2].

## 5.5 NATIVE POLYACRYLAMIDE GEL ELECTROPHORESIS

This type of gel electrophoresis is used for the separation of native proteins, multi-protein complexes, and enzymes. Separation takes place under nondenaturing conditions. In this approach, migration rate depends on the negative charge of molecules. The higher the charge, the faster protein migration is. In the native polyacrylamide gel electrophoresis (PAGE), it is important to minimize denaturation and proteolysis by keeping the device cooled.

Blue native electrophoresis (BN-PAGE) and clear native electrophoresis (CN-PAGE) are variants of the native PAGE. BN-PAGE, first described in 1991, is a separation method very often used for the analysis and identification of multiprotein complexes [3]. Proteins are separated according to their size and shape. Addition of CBB results in assigning a negative charge for molecules. Moreover, BN-PAGE can be connected with SDS-PAGE as a two-dimensional blue native separation method to enhance resolution.

In the CN-PAGE technique, the proteins are separated according to their iso-electric points (pI). Proteins do not gain additional charge, and their migration in the gel depends on their native charges. Therefore, only proteins characterized by pI below the pH value of the electrophoresis buffer (pH ~ 7) can be resolved, for the reason that they are able to obtain proper electric charge and move to the appropriate electrode. Basic proteins can be separated in an additional run, after switching the positions of the electrodes. In comparison to SDS-PAGE, BN-PAGE is characterized by a much lower resolution.

## 5.6    AGAROSE GEL

An additional option among electrophoretic techniques is agarose gel, first applied in 1964 for DNA separations. Agarose is a copolymer, consisting of 1,3-linked β-*D*-galactose and 1,4-linked 3,6-anhydro-α-*L*-galactose, which is in the liquid state at a temperature above 40°C. The solution forms a gel after cooling to room temperature. Crosslinking of the gel depends on the type of sample and can be modified by varying the concentration of polysaccharide. Agarose electrophoresis is a method used for the separation of both small DNA fragments and large molecules (1 million Da). Various proportions of agarose-acrylamide gels are applied for the determination of gene maps (e.g., HUGO project) [4].

## 5.7    STAINING AND VISUALIZATION METHODS

Visualization of proteins and nucleic acids is an important aspect of electrophoretic separation techniques. Actually, there are several commercially available staining reagents. Selection of the appropriate detection method and types of reagents depend on various factors.

CBB is a well-known reagent used for the detection of proteins (8–10 ng) in the PAGE method. It visualizes proteins as blue bands on the transparent background. There are two types of this reagent: G-250 greenish and R-250 reddish (Figure 5.4); however, reddish (Figure 5.5) has lower sensitivity

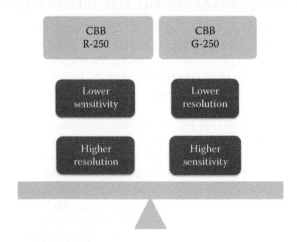

**FIGURE 5.4**   Comparison of two types of Coomassie Brilliant Blue.

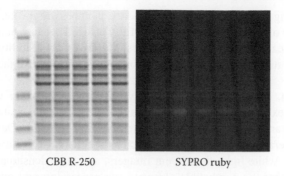

CBB R-250                SYPRO ruby

**FIGURE 5.5** Examples of stained gels.

than greenish. CBB can be used for densitometric measurements (quantitative) because it binds stechiometrically to the proteins. This stain is characterized by a good reproducibility, low cost, and MS compatibility.

Silver staining has high sensitivity—below 1 ng of protein per spot. The principle of operation using the reagent is based on silver precipitation in the gel. Silver staining has good reproducibility and enables quantitative analysis. Proteins can be analyzed using MS, after destaining with $K_3[Fe(CN)_6]$ and $Na_2S_2O_3$, followed by standard in-gel digestion protocol.

Zinc stain is a negative staining method. This is because the reagent has no effect on proteins but on the background only. This detection method is used in qualitative analysis only, and no destaining protocol is required prior to MS analysis.

Copper stain—This detection method cannot be used in quantitative analysis because it is a negative staining method. Like the zinc labeling method, copper stain does not require any additional dye removal. However, this technique is compatible with SDS-PAGE only, and therefore, it is not suitable for native separations.

Fluorescence staining (Figure 5.5)—This kind of visualization is very popular, and there are many commercial reagents that might be selected, depending on the sample type; the basic SYPRO Ruby (ruthenium chelate) binds to basic amino acids in proteins. The more specific reagents allow for detection of selected posttranslational modifications. For instance, Pro-Q-Emerald should be chosen for glycoproteins identification and Pro-Q-Diamond for detection of phosphoproteins. All of the mentioned dyes are easily removable and compatible with MS, and proteins can be identified using a basic, in-gel digestion method.

Ethidium bromide (3,8-diamino-5-ethyl-6-phenylphenanthridinium bromide) is an organic compound often applied for visualization of nucleic acid upon illumination with UV light.

Isotope labeling—Although radioactive isotope labeling has been used for 2D-electrophoresis, it is not a popular method because of the exceptional safety requirements. There is a need for a separate laboratory room, advanced equipment (radioactivity counters), and conditions designed for the staining protocol, when the radioactive isotopes are involved. The high sensitivity of this technique cannot be fully utilized because none of the MS methods reach that low detection limits. Moreover, a possibility of radioactive contamination of the mass spectrometer is a prohibitive factor.

Visualization, documentation, and analysis of the results are very important aspects of each experiment. Commercially available gel documentation systems are equipped with various types of detection methods and software. Depending on the type of dye, several devices can be used, such as scanners, CCD cameras, illuminators with UV or white light, fluorescent imagers, and laser densitometers. For each image system, there is compatible software for processing and evaluation of the results and for data documentation.

## 5.8   ISOLATION OF PEPTIDES PRIOR TO MS ANALYSIS

There are several protocols for sample preparation after separation of proteins on the gel, prior to MS analysis. An exemplary scheme is presented in Figure 5.6.

Proteins can be visualized by various detection and imaging methods, which allow selecting interesting lanes and bands. Bands are excised from the gel. The use of CBB enforces destaining of this blue dye as the first step. If the bands are intensely colored, this procedure should be repeated a few times, until a completely transparent gel will be obtained. Application of fluorescent dyes allows skipping this routine.

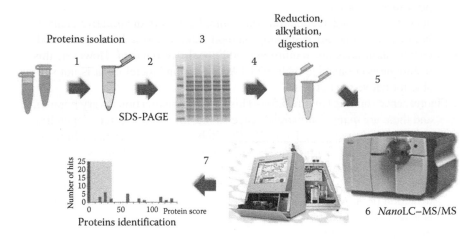

1   Proteins isolation
2   SDS-PAGE
3   CBBstain bands are excised from the gel
4   Reduction of disulfide bonds,
    blocking by alkylation,
    Digestion directly in the gel

5   Extraction peptides from the gel
6   NanoLC–MS/MS
7   Proteins identification

**FIGURE 5.6**   Sample preparation strategy.

The next step in sample preparation for MS analysis is reduction of intramolecular disulfide bonds by using reducing agents, such as dithiothreitol (DTT), dithioerythritol (DTE), tributylphosphine (TBP), tris(2-carboxyethyl)phosphine (TCEP), or β-mercaptoethanol (BME). The reduced disulfide bonds should be blocked by alkylation to prevent refolding. For this type of reaction, the typical procedures involve carbamidomethylation of cysteines with iodoacetamide or pyridylethylation.

The proteins are digested directly in the gel by applying various enzymes, depending on the sample type. Most frequently, trypsin is used due to the release of peptides of the length, appropriate for MS analysis and efficient sequencing. For thorough sequence analysis, several (at least two) enzymes of various specificities should be applied to cover the entire protein sequence and to assign proper position of peptides in the protein. After protein digestion, the peptides are extracted from the gel and analyzed by LC–MS/MS.

## 5.9 TWO-DIMENSIONAL ELECTROPHORESIS

For the very complex samples, the use of two-dimensional electrophoresis (2DE) is suggested. During the first step, the proteins are resolved, according to their isoelectric points. This part of the experiment can be processed in solution (with the application of semiconducting membranes) or performed using immobilized pH gel immobilized pH gradient (IPG) strips. Incorporation of ampholytes into the polyacrylamide gel results in the higher resolving power, and therefore, posttranslational modifications can be observed using 2DE. The isoelectrofocusing (IEF) step requires the presence of chaotropic substances (e.g., urea and thiourea) that denaturate protein structure as well as surfactants (e.g., 3-[(3-cholamidopropyl) dimethylammonio]-1-propanesulfonate CHAPS), which improve protein solubility. Also dithiothreitol (DTT), a reducing agent, is routinely added to abolish disulfide bond formation and to destabilize protein structure. During IEF, the substances are focused, according to their isoelectric points. This means that the molecules migrate to the corresponding pH regions where they became zwitterions and therefore do not possess net charge, and cannot move any further. After focusing is completed (the voltage gains constant value), an IPG strip is placed on the top of the SDS-PAGE system, and separation in the second dimension is performed, following the similar protocol as in 1DE (Figure 5.7).

The next challenging task is the gel image analysis. The high-resolution image is crucial for further gel analysis. The image warping is necessary to overlap all gel repeats, so that the corresponding bands can be analyzed both qualitatively and quantitatively to compare proteomes (protein profiles). Although often ignored, software analysis of gel images might be the source of abnormalities, associated with the postexperimental examination and manipulation of the software parameters. In particular, cropping the gel images prior to quantitative analysis has been shown to contribute to a significant inaccuracy through image analysis. There are various methods describing determination of spot areas, including computer-based approaches and fitting algorithms, and different image analysis software proposed by manufacturers of the gel documentation systems are available on the market.

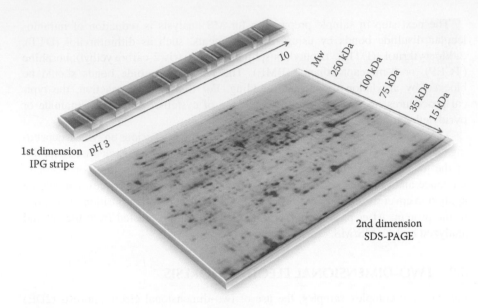

**FIGURE 5.7**   Two-dimensional gel electrophoresis.

However, none of them is capable of automatic functioning [5]. Each method has some drawbacks, particularly when addressing a wide variety of images. On the other hand, extensive manipulation of the software variables by the operators may lead to poor reproduction of the results, and also to some "improvements" of the data to, for example, clean up for outliers to obscure bad separations.

For the reliable protein identification and quantitation, it is important to minimize the variability associated with 2DE image analysis obtained from different gels/samples. Since this step of image examination might be the reason of the divergence, the difference gel electrophoresis (DIGE) method was developed (Figure 5.8). This technique enables separating up to three different samples during one experiment, and avoiding the increased precision error. Three fluorescent dyes are used to label each individual sample, Cy2, Cy3, and Cy5. There is, however, one limitation of this method. It cannot be applied to the proteins that do not contain cysteines or lysines.

## 5.10   DIRECT ANALYSIS OF THE GEL-SEPARATED PROTEINS

Nevertheless, planar electrophoretic techniques are very popular in biotechnological and biochemical laboratories. There is still no online interface, directly linking such techniques with mass spectrometric detectors. A handful of experiments were described, regarding the identification of proteins transferred onto the membrane after immunoblotting [6,7]. Secondary ion mass spectrometry (SIMS) and matrix-assisted laser desorption/ionization (MALDI) techniques were used for the direct analysis of intact proteins or after sputtering blots with trypsin solution for digestion

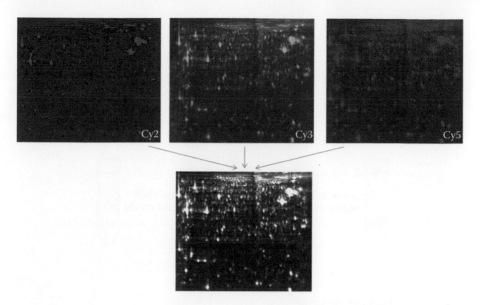

**FIGURE 5.8** Differential gel electrophoresis (DIGE).

into shorter peptides [8]. In addition, ambient ionization methods, including desorption electrospray ionization (DESI) and dielectric barrier discharge ionization (DBDI) have been applied for the rapid and direct analysis of complex mixtures with slight sample modifications [8]. However, there is still no report on the routine use of mass spectrometry for the direct analysis of proteins present in the gel.

## 5.11 ROBOTICS

To overcome disadvantages of the time-consuming sample preparation step, prior to the MS analysis, robots are applied for the excision of the bands, proteins in gel digestion, and spotting sample on the MALDI plate. Moreover, application of autosamplers is commonly applied in the high-throughput facilities. These robotic systems are often interfaced with the image analysis software and with MS instrumentation. The use of spot picking and protein handling machines not only shortens the time of analysis, but also decreases a possibility of contamination of the samples with keratins that interfere with protein identification. This offline approach is only used in the high-throughput analyses. Usually, the sample is manually extracted from a single band and further processed.

## 5.12 CAPILLARY ELECTROPHORESIS

Only capillary electrophoresis offers the possibility for online coupling with the mass spectrometer. The most popular combination is based on the direct connection of capillary zone electrophoresis (CZE) outlet with ESI ion source. The CZE technique is based on the movement of ions inside the fused silica capillary filled

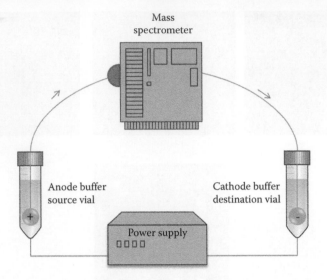

**FIGURE 5.9**   Capillary electrophoresis.

with buffer, where one end of the capillary is a cathode and the other one is an anode (Figure 5.9). Small, highly charged ions, travel to the electrode faster than the bigger components with minor charge. Only volatile buffers can be used for the online coupling, such as formates, acetates, or ammonium salts. Capillary gel electrophoresis is very similar to CZE; however, the fused silica is filled with the gel that results in a better resolution but it is also more prone to clogging.

## 5.13   CONCLUSIONS

Proteomics aims at development and application of techniques for the global and rapid analysis of proteins. This strategy is very useful for identification of the functions of biomolecules, discovery of disease state biomarkers, and revelation of potential therapeutic targets. In the traditional bottom-up approach, gel electrophoresis is the most widely used technique for separation of the complex protein mixtures. On the other hand, the procedures involving in-gel digestion, chemical extraction of the separated proteins, are time-consuming and often lead to the sample loss. Application of robots for the excision of protein spots from 2D gels, and modules for automated protein digestion have been developed to expedite the identification of proteins in proteomics. Their drawback is that they are mostly suitable for the high-throughput facilities and, in the case of a low number of samples, there is a substantial waste of all reagents.

The planar electrophoretic techniques are frequently used in biochemical and biotechnological laboratories as a good alternative for the separation of biological samples; however, there is no online interface with mass spectrometers for their direct connection. Further technical improvements are needed to enable detection and characterization of the low-abundance proteins, to improve protein quantitation using planar electrophoresis, and to increase the high-throughput of the methodology. The weakest point to date seems to be a lack of efficient imaging software, capable of identifying proteins present in the spots and obtained during multiple, parallel experiments.

## ACKNOWLEDGMENTS

The research was supported by The Polish National Science Center 2013/09/B/NZ4/02531, and EuroNanoMed "META" 05/EuroNanoMed/2012.

## REFERENCES

1. Hawcroft D.M. (Ed.). 1997. *Electrophoresis the Basics*, IRL Press at Oxford University Press, Oxford, England, Chapter 1.
2. Gallagher S.R. 2001. One-dimensional SDS gel electrophoresis of proteins, *Curr. Protoc. Protein Sci.*, Chapter 10, Unit 10.1.
3. Wittig I. and Schägger H. 2009. Native electrophoretic techniques to identify protein–protein interactions, *Proteomics*, 23: 5214–5223.
4. Voytas D. 2001. Agarose gel electrophoresis. *Curr. Protoc. Immunol.*, Chapter 10, pp. 1–9, Unit 10.4. http://www.ncbi.nlm.nih.gov/pubmed/18432695.
5. Brauner J.M., Groemer T.W., Stroebel A., Grosse-Holz S., Oberstein T., Wiltfang J., Kornhuber J., and Maler J.M. 2014. Spot quantification in two dimensional gel electrophoresis image analysis: Comparison of different approaches and presentation of a novel compound-fitting algorithm, *BMC Bioinform.*, 15: 181.
6. Aebersold R.H., Teplow D.B., Hood L.E., and Kent S.B. 1986. Electroblotting onto activated glass. High efficiency preparation of proteins from analytical sodium dodecyl sulfate-polyacrylamide gels for direct sequence analysis, *J. Biol. Chem.*, 261: 4229–4238.
7. Vestling M.M. and Fenselau C. 2015. Polyvinylidene difluoride (PVDF): An interface for gel electrophoresis and matrix-assisted laser desorption/ionization mass spectrometry, *Biochem. Soc. Trans.*, 22: 547–551.
8. Han F., Yang Y., Ouyang J., and Na N. 2015. Direct analysis of in-gel proteins by carbon nanotubes-modified paper spray ambient mass spectrometry, *Analyst*, 140: 710–715.

# 6 Selection of Ionization Methods of Analytes in the TLC–MS Techniques

*Michał Cegłowski and Grzegorz Schroeder*

## CONTENTS

## 6.1   INTRODUCTION

Thin-layer chromatography (TLC) is probably one of the most frequently used and by far the simplest chromatographic techniques used to separate or purify compound mixtures. Commercially available TLC plates that are used in laboratories allow resolution of compounds on many types of stationary phases such as thin-layer silica, reversed phase (RP) modified silica, cellulose, or aluminum oxide. TLC technique is widely used because it has many important advantages such as low cost, low solvent consumption, simultaneous elution of many different samples on one TLC plate, and no "memory" effects [1–2].

To improve the separation efficiency in TLC, many different modifications of this chromatographic technique have been developed [3]. The most important is high-performance thin-layer chromatography (HPTLC), which has increased precision by one order of magnitude, lowered analysis time, reduced development distances on the layer, and lowered solvent consumption [4]. These benefits were mainly achieved by using sorbent with smaller and more uniform particle sizes (usually between 4 and 8 μm) and thinner layers of the sorbent in comparison with conventional TLC. HPTLC has been turned into a semiautomated chromatographic technique, which provides accuracy comparable to high-performance liquid chromatography (HPLC) [4].

One of the biggest issues of TLC is the visualization and characterization of compounds resolved on the TLC plate. Although there is no problem with visualization of naturally colored or fluorescent compounds, these compounds are rare in the laboratory. Other compounds can be visualized with UV light or by using appropriate TLC-visualization reagents. These methods, however, provide only little information about the nature of the compounds resolved on the TLC plate. For this reason, coupling of TLC with other techniques permitting better detection and characterization of compounds has become a subject of many research projects and scientific papers [5–6].

The coupling of TLC and mass spectrometry (MS) allows mass spectrometric characterization of compounds resolved on TLC plates. Many setups connecting TLC and MS have been developed, but generally they can be divided into "indirect sampling TLC–MS" and "direct sampling TLC–MS" [6]. To date, many reviews considering TLC–MS [3,5–10], TLC–MS analysis of particular groups of compounds [11–15], or TLC–MS using particular ionization methods have been published [1,16–17].

Indirect sampling TLC–MS setups are the least state-of-the-art techniques used. They rely on extraction of the analyte from TLC spots using appropriate solvents, purification of solutions obtained, and the obtainment of mass spectra (sometimes after concentration of the analyte solution or even isolation of the pure analyte). The extraction is usually preceded by scraping the gel containing the analyte from the TLC surface. These techniques are technically undemanding and effective, but overall are time-consuming and tedious due to the steps that must be carried out to obtain a mass spectrum. Because the end analyte is in solution or pure form, however, the choice of mass spectrometer is straightforward and is determined solely by the availability and the type of the analyte.

Direct sampling TLC–MS setups are usually more sophisticated than indirect sampling setups, but allow for more rapid analysis; they are sometimes partially or fully automated. Generally, direct sampling techniques rely on desorption of the analyte from the TLC surface followed by its ionization, or the use of a special sampling probe that extracts the analyte and transfers it directly to the ion source. Some of these setups are now available commercially and can be attached to different types of mass spectrometers.

TLC–MS techniques will be reviewed first based on the ion source and second by the analyte type. Chromatographic and mass spectrometric procedures will be described in detail to inform the reader of the possibilities and limitations of a particular technique. The selection of ion source is determined by the analyte type that has been resolved on a TLC plate. Appropriate combinations of ionization methods and analyte types allow one to easily obtain and interpret high quality mass spectra. Therefore, the choice of mass spectrometric instrument is a key step in the process of characterization of compounds using TLC–MS techniques.

## 6.2 THIN-LAYER CHROMATOGRAPHY–SECONDARY ION MASS SPECTROMETRY

### 6.2.1 ALKALOIDS

TLC spots obtained after resolving ethanolic extracts of Inocybe napipes have been investigated using secondary ion mass spectrometry (SIMS). Concentrated extracts containing 2.0 µg/µL muscarine were applied (75 µL) onto aluminum-backed cellulose sheets and were developed with a solution of n-butanol, methanol, and water (58:25:17). The scan of the whole TLC plate was performed by SIMS, by placing the plate into a vacuum chamber on a hemispherical holder attached to the sample manipulator, or mass spectra of particular TLC spots were obtained after their visualization with iodine vapors. The second procedure was preferred due to the lower analysis time in comparison with the first procedure. SIMS spectra were obtained by argon ion bombardment, whereas the positive surface charge of chromatographic support was neutralized by flooding the surface with low-energy electrons. Muscarine cations at $m/z$ 174 were observed along with many background ions from the decomposition of the cellulose support. It has been observed that using alumina or silica thin-layer plates substantially reduced the lower mass background. Moreover, it has been suggested that the thickness of the adsorbent layer is responsible for spectral quality, and therefore, HPTLC plates have been recommended for direct analysis. For calculation of the detection limits, a solutions containing 10 µg each of choline and muscarine was chromatographed and analyzed directly. The spectra obtained showed signals at $m/z$ 104 and 174 for choline and muscarine, respectively [18].

### 6.2.2 TERPENES

A mixture of two diterpenes (abietic acid and gibberellic acid) was separated on three different TLC plates and then analyzed using SIMS technique. The selected three different TLC plates were as follows: a monolithic ultrathin-layer chromatography (UTLC) plate, an aluminum-backed TLC plate with modified silica gel, and a commercially available Raman spectrometric thin-layer plate. The plates were cleaned with methanol, dried, and after application of analyte mixture were developed with ethanol/water (4:6). For SIMS measurements, an electron impact ion gun was used that generated $Ar^+$ ions with energy of 10 keV. Macroscanning with SIMS was used to identify the analytes after chromatographic separation. The most applicable analytical signal response for positive-ion macroscans was obtained on the UTLC plate [19].

## 6.3 THIN-LAYER CHROMATOGRAPHY–LIQUID SECONDARY ION MASS SPECTROMETRY

### 6.3.1 GLYCOLIPIDS

Neoglycolipid products derived from mucin oligosaccharide alditols after periodate oxidation and coupling by reductive amination to the aminolipid dipalmitoyl–glycero–phosphoethanoloamine have been resolved on HPTLC plates. After resolving, the neoglycolipid bands were cut out as strips and placed on a standard stainless steel liquid secondary ion mass spectrometry (LSIMS) target probe. A matrix of tetramethylurea/triethanolamine/$m$-nitrobenzyl alcohol (2:2:1) and chloroform/methanol/water (25:25:8) was placed onto the TLC strip, and the sample was ionized using a cesium ion gun. The sequence data derived by LSIMS analysis of the neoglycolipid derivatives were in excellent agreement with the assignments that had been made previously by MS and NMR analysis of the free oligosaccharide alditols. The TLC–LSIMS characterization of neoglycolipids obtained allowed structural assignment of several oligosaccharide fractions [20].

### 6.3.2 Phenothiazine-Derived Drugs

Phenothiazine drugs have been resolved on silica gel TLC using methanol/ammonia (100:1.5) as a developing solvent. Glycerol and threitol have been used as matrices in LSIMS experiments using cesium ions to obtain positive secondary ion spectra. After developing, the plate was attached to a direct insertion probe and the appropriate matrix was applied to the plate. The plate was spatially resolved using a sample manipulator. For all but one of the compounds investigated, the [M+H]+ ion was the base peak in the spectrum [21].

## 6.4 THIN-LAYER CHROMATOGRAPHY–FAST ATOM BOMBARDMENT

### 6.4.1 Glycolipids

Native neoglycolipids, derived from oxidative cleavage of the C4–C5 bond in the terminal glycan alditols, have been characterized by thin-layer chromatography–fast atom bombardment (TLC–FAB) technique. Oligosaccharide alditols were treated with sodium periodate. After incubation, the oxidation was stopped by the addition of an excess of butan-2,3-diol and via prolongation of the reaction time. Schiff base formation of oxidized alditols with dipalmitoyl-glycero-phosphoethanolamine was followed by reduction with sodium cyanoborohydride. The reaction mixture was applied onto HPTLC plates, which were developed with chloroform/methanol (1:1) and chloroform/methanol/water (130:50:9). To perform the TLC/FAB experiment, the HPTLC plates were cut into strips and placed on a standard stainless steel target. A matrix of thioglycerol was used and solubilization of the neoglycolipids was aided by methanol. The target was than analyzed using xenon atoms having a kinetic energy equivalent to 8.5–9.5 kV. Data obtained using TLC–FAB technique allowed assignment of the structures of neoglycolipids [22].

### 6.4.2 Polyether Antibiotics

A mixture of antibiotics (lasalocid, septamycin, and monensin) was applied to TLC silica gel plates that were subsequently developed with ethyl acetate/dichloromethane (70:30). Xenon was used as a gas for the FAB gun and thioglycerol as the FAB matrix liquid. The FAB probe tip was made of copper, and the sample surface was beveled at an angle of 70° to the probe axis. Lasalocid and monensin gave [M+Na]+ ions at $m/z$ 613 and 693, respectively. Septamycin also produced an [M+Na]+ ions peak at $m/z$ 937, but additionally an intense fragment ion at $m/z$ 875 was observed. With monensin spotted on a TLC plate, the sensitivity of detection was established to be below 0.1 µg [23].

## 6.5    THIN-LAYER CHROMATOGRAPHY–MATRIX-ASSISTED LASER DESORPTION/IONIZATION

### 6.5.1 PEPTIDES

The thin-layer chromatography–matrix-assisted laser desorption/ionization (TLC–MALDI) method was found to be suitable for direct TLC imaging of bradykinin, angiotensin, and enkephalin derivatives. This method was found to be suitable for larger peptides and small proteins like bovine insulin chain B, insulin, horse heart cytochrome $c$, and myoglobin. However, to produce a signal, analytes from inside the sorbent must be transferred onto the surface of the TLC plate following matrix deposition and crystallization, because after TLC development the analyte is presumably located 100–500 µm inside the bulk of the adsorbent. Therefore, to extract an analyte onto the plate surface and to improve the sensitivity of TLC–MALDI, an extraction solvent was applied before matrix deposition. Due to the concentration gradient, diffusion moved the analyte toward the plate surface and into the extraction solvent. The matrix was added to the extraction solvent in small increments after the extraction was finished. The time of crystallization was less than 10–15 min, after which the TLC plate was introduced into the mass spectrometer and analyzed. This method was successful for all analytes examined. The absolute detection limit was in the 2–4 ng range for a spot area of $7 \times 7$ mm [24].

Bradykinin was used as an analyte in the investigation and optimization of the TLC–MALDI coupling protocol. In this protocol, a matrix solution (α-cyano-4-hydroxycinnamic acid) was deposited onto a stainless steel or polyester plate. The resolved TLC plate was sprayed with extraction solvent and placed into a solvent-saturated atmosphere. Afterward, the stainless steel or polyester plate was placed face-to-face with the dampened TLC plate and pressed. The pressing step puts pressure on the stationary phase, forcing solvent toward the top surface of the TLC plate and the matrix layer and also transfers the matrix to the top of the TLC plate. After removal of the stainless steel or polyester plate, the matrix remains on the TLC plate cocrystallized with analyte. The TLC plate is then analyzed in a MALDI mass spectrometer. According to the discussed paper, the parameters of the TLC–MALDI coupling protocol, particularly for the extraction solvent selection, extraction time and pressure have been investigated and optimized [25].

### 6.5.2 LIPIDS

A mixture of 1-palmitoyl-2-linoleoyl-$sn$-phosphatidylcholine (PLPC) and 1-palmitoyl-2-linoleoyl-$sn$-phosphatidylethanolamine (PLPE) was oxidized under the influence of atmospheric oxygen and characterized by TLC–MALDI. TLC separation was performed using TLC plates with an aluminum back, which were developed using chloroform/ethanol/water/triethylamine (30:35:7:35). After visualization, the matrix solution was manually applied onto the center of each spot of interest. After drying, the TLC plate was mounted onto a TLC–MALDI adapter target and loaded into the MALDI mass spectrometer. Mass spectra of oxidation products of substrates used, and in particular carboxylic acid, aldehyde, epoxide, and hydroperoxide derivatives, have been obtained [26].

IR–MALDI in combination with TLC has been used for structural analysis of glycosphingolipids in crude lipid extracts. Total lipids were first extracted from THP-1 cells using methanol and chloroform/methanol mixtures. Next, phospholipids were enzymatically digested using phospholipase C, an enzyme that cleaves the polar head groups from phospholipids. Glycosphingolipids were detected on a TLC plate with the use of a mixture of various anti-GSL antibodies during the same TLC run. To perform MS measurements, a TLC plate was placed into a commercially available MALDI–MS–TLC holder. Structural analysis of glycosphingolipids was achieved with direct IR–MALDI analysis using a 2.94 µm Er/YAG pulse laser in combination with collision-induced dissociation. This merged approach delivers data on the glycosphingolipids' composition and specific structural information about individual glycosphingolipids in complex mixtures, with limited investment in sample preparation [27].

### 6.5.3 Psychoactive Drugs

TLC–MALDI has been used to analyze drugs in pure solutions and biological samples such as urine, plasma, and organs. The samples were spotted onto the TLC plate and developed using acetone/28% aqueous ammonium (99:1). Then, a matrix solution (α-cyano-4-hydroxycinnamic acid) was sprayed onto a TLC plate and the plate was fixed in a TLC plate holder. A MALDI laser (Nd/YAG) was used to scan a plate in a straight line from the spotted sample position to the front line of the developing solvent, using a 150-µm laser step-size. In total, 11 psychotropic compounds were tested (3,4-methylenedioxymethamphetamine, 4-hydroxy-3-methoxymethamphetamine, 3,4-methylenedioxyamphetamine, methamphetamine, p-hydroxymethamphetamine, amphetamine, ketamine, caffeine, chlorpromazine, triazolam, and morphine) on a TLC plate. When the urine containing 3,4-methylenedioxymethamphetamine (MDMA) without sample dilution was spotted onto a TLC plate and was analyzed by TLC–MALDI, the detection limit of the MDMA spot was estimated to be 0.05 ng/spot. The value was the same as that seen in an aqueous solution spotted on a stainless steel plate [28].

### 6.5.4 Reaction Monitoring

A nanomaterial-assisted method that combines TLC and MALDI has been developed to directly monitor a simple esterification reaction. To obtain appropriate functional nanomaterials, $Fe_3O_4$ magnetic nanoparticles (MNP) have been functionalized first with tetraethyl orthosilicate and subsequently with 2,5-dihydrobenzoic acid (DHB), yielding DHB-coated MNP (DHB@MNP) [29]. The esterification reaction monitored was a reaction between triethylene glycol monomethyl ether and 2-chloro-2-phenylacetyl chloride. After the reaction was started, the sample reaction mixture was spotted onto a TLC plate and was developed using ethyl acetate/hexane (1:1). The DHB@MNP solution was then deposited onto the spots of interest and dried. The MALDI mass spectra were acquired using a pulsed 337-nm nitrogen laser. Strong signals from sodium adducts with substrate and product were observed, accompanied by potassium adducts. The use of DHB@MNP almost eliminated the background level of DHB fragmentation and considerably enhanced the signal intensity of both substrate and product. In comparison, when the pure DHB was used as a matrix, multiple peaks derived from DHB fragments were observed, leading to suppression of the signals of compounds of interest [30].

### 6.5.5 DENDRIMERS

The potential of TLC–MALDI for analyzing dendrimers was investigated using three different samples of polyamidoamine (PAMAM) dendrimers: the first-generation ammonia-cored PAMAM, the completely glycine-modified first-generation ammonia-cored PAMAM, and the N-(tert-butoxycarbonyl)phenylalanine-modified first-generation ammonia-cored PAMAM. All compounds were developed on HPTLC silica gel 60 aluminum-backed plates using triethylamine/water/methanol (10:45:45), or, in the case of N-(tert-butoxycarbonyl)phenylalanine modified first-generation ammonia-cored PAMAM, by using a water/methanol (10:90) solvent mixture. After drying, the TLC plate was inserted into a commercially available TLC target adapter. The TLC plate was raster scanned with the Nd/YAG 355-nm laser in an automated manner to collect a data set. The combination of TLC and MALDI appeared to be particularly powerful in monitoring the synthesis and chemical modification of PAMAM dendrimers. Comparisons with MALDI experiments performed using dried droplet deposit on the MALDI stainless steel target plate have been performed. It was noted that the analyte was randomly detected, depending on the position of the laser shot on the MALDI target. Moreover, many ions present in the MALDI spectrum were difficult to attribute, as they did not correspond to expected dendrimers or defective structures. Thus, the coupling of TLC and MALDI seemed to allow for the reduction in discrimination effects and ensured detection of all species present in the sample, in comparison with conventional analysis on MALDI stainless-steel target plates [31].

## 6.6 THIN-LAYER CHROMATOGRAPHY–ATMOSPHERIC PRESSURE MATRIX-ASSISTED LASER DESORPTION/IONIZATION

### 6.6.1 DRUGS

Midazolam, verapamil, and metoprolol were resolved using ethyl acetate containing 0.5% ammonium hydroxide on monolithic UTLC glass-backed plates. The plates were prewashed once with acetonitrile before sample application. The UTLC plates were attached to the face of an in-house-modified AP–MALDI target plate with double-sided conductive tape after cutting the plate to match the target probe.

A nitrogen laser at 337 nm was focused on the sample zone on the plate and the ions formed in the laser pulses were directed to the ion trap via an extended capillary of the ion trap instrument. The applicability of UTLC–AP–MALDI has been shown to be good enough for the identification of small drug molecules in relatively simple samples in MS mode. The limits of detection were in the picomolar range. Because of the thinner adsorbent layer, the UTLC plates provided 10–100 times better sensitivity than conventional HPTLC plates [32].

### 6.6.2 BENZODIAZEPINES

The feasibility of a combination of UTLC and AP–MALDI for bioanalysis was studied with benzodiazepines, and in particular with midazolam, triazolam, diazepam, oxazepam, *N*-desalkylflurazepam, nitrazepam, and lorazepam. These seven compounds were used in the development of the 2D UTLC method using monolithic glass-backed UTLC plates. The 1D separation was performed with dichloromethane/acetone and the 2D separation with toluene/acetone/ethanol/25% ammonia solution. After separation, the α-cyano-4-hydroxycinnamic acid matrix was sprayed over the separated sample zone, and the UTLC plate was cut to match the face of an in-house-modified AP–MALDI target plate to which it was attached using double-sided conductive tape. A nitrogen laser at 337 nm was focused on the sample zone of the plate. The size of the laser spot was 0.5 mm. The ions that formed were directed to the ion trap via an extended capillary. All MS spectra of benzodiazepines showed an abundant protonated molecule with minimal fragmentation. Moreover, the applicability of the 2D UTLC–AP–MALDI was demonstrated in a qualitative screening analysis of an authentic urine sample after intake of a single dose of diazepam [33].

## 6.7 THIN-LAYER CHROMATOGRAPHY–ELECTROSPRAY IONIZATION

### 6.7.1 DYES

A combined surface sampling probe/electrospray emitter was used for the direct analysis of TLC plates by electrospray ionization (ESI) MS. The plates used for the TLC/ESI coupling were glass-backed HPTLC RP plates. A three-dye mixture composed of methylene blue, crystal violet, and rhodamine 6G was developed with methanol/tetrahydrofuran (60:40) containing NH4OAc, and analyzed in positive ion mode. A mixture of fluorescein, naphthol blue black, and fast green FCF was developed with methanol/water (70:30) and was analyzed in negative ion mode. The sampling probe consisted of the stainless steel tee and the metal sampling/sprayer tube. The sampling end of the sampling tube was positioned laterally, relative to the TLC plate. During the experiment, the TLC plate was pulled back slightly to eliminate direct physical contact of the probe and the surface. The soluble components present in the developed TLC plate were dissolved in the eluting solvent and taken into the sampling capillary, which allowed the authors to obtain a mass spectrum. The presented method proved to be effective, and detection levels measured were shown to be in the low nanogram range [34].

An automation system was developed to control surface sampling probe-to-surface distance during the operation of a surface-sampling electrospray system. It allowed for hands-free reoptimization of the microjunction thickness during surface scanning, which resulted in a fully automated surface sampling system. The effectiveness of this system was tested during the analysis of a mixture of rhodamine dyes (rhodamine 6G, B, and 123) developed on RP C8 plates using methanol/water (80:20) containing ammonium acetate. After drying, developed TLC plates were attached to the *XYZ* stage and their position relative to the stationary sampling probe and the liquid microjunction thickness was monitored with a closed-circuit camera. The aspiration rate of the probe/emitter was matched to the pumped flow rate by adjustment of the nebulizing gas flow rate. The data obtained were sufficient to produce a 3D map of the TLC plate, where the *X* and *Y* axes corresponded to the horizontal and vertical range of the scanned surface, and the *Z* axis represented the corresponding mass spectral signal intensities, respectively [35].

### 6.7.2 PEPTIDES

Separation, detection, and identification of structurally related angiotensin-converting enzyme inhibitors (lisinopril, cilazapril, ramipril, and quinapril) and their corresponding active diacid forms was performed on conventional TLC silica gel plates and monolithic UTLC plates. Plates were developed in a modified horizontal developing chamber using ethyl acetate/acetone/acetic acid/water (4:1:0.25:0.5). Mass spectra of resolved compounds were obtained using a commercially available CAMAG TLC–MS interface allowing online extraction from plates, combined with ESI. All analyzed compounds showed a substantial affinity for alkali metal ions, which could be seen as a high relative abundance of sodium adduct ions in the MS spectra. UTLC appeared to be more efficient than conventional TLC for the separation of the compounds examined. UTLC was faster, cheaper, and produced less waste but its coupling to MS is necessary for full compound identification [36].

### 6.7.3 OLIGOSACCHARIDES

Hyaluronan oligosaccharides were resolved on an aluminum-backed TLC plate using 1-butanol/formic acid/water (3:5:2). These oligosaccharides were produced in-house by digestion and subsequent purification of hyaluronan from *Streptococcus zooepidemicus*. Spots of interest were then extracted using a CAMAG TLC–MS interface. High-resolution ESI spectra were recorded in negative ion mode, revealing [M–H]⁻ and [M–2H]²⁻ ions as characteristic peaks. The purity of the analytes was confirmed because no odd-number sugars were detected [37].

### 6.7.4 TETRACYCLINES

Four tetracyclines (tetracycline, chlortetracycline, oxytetracycline, and doxycycline) and three fluoroquinolones (enrofloxacin, ciprofloxacin, and marbofloxacin) were analyzed by HPTLC–ESI technique. HPTLC silica gel 60 glass plates were functionalized to obtain ethylenediaminetetraacetic acid-modified silica gel plates.

After application of analytes, the plates were developed with chloroform/methanol/ammonium hydroxide solution (25%) (60:35:5). A CAMAG TLC–MS interface coupled to a single quadrupole mass spectrometer equipped with an ESI source was used to extract and characterize spots of interest. Full-scan mass spectra recorded in the ESI positive mode generally provided the protonated molecules (partly accompanied by sodium adducts) with the highest abundancies for both tetracyclines and fluoroquinolones. In the ESI-negative mode, tetracyclines produced the deprotonated molecules, but only with low intensities, whereas fluoroquinolones noticeably showed strong signals for formate adducts. Despite these differences, the characteristic signals from both mass polarities are seemingly of value for qualitative confirmations [38].

### 6.7.5 Preservatives

Manganese-activated zinc silicate was directly mixed into polyacrylonitrile solution, which was further fabricated into a fibrous substrate by the electrospinning process. The electrospun polyacrylonitrile nanofibrous phase, incorporating a photoluminescent indicator was employed to study the separation of seven preservatives (sorbic acid, benzoic acid, 4-hydroxybenozic acid, methyl 4-hydroxybenzoate, ethyl 4-hydroxybenzoate, propyl 4-hydroxybenzoate, and butyl 4-hydroxybenzoate). To obtain chromatographic plates, the polyacrylonitrile solution with photoluminescent indicator was electrospun on a rotating collector covered with clean aluminum foil. After the process, the foil was cut from the middle into rectangular pieces. Analyte solutions were then applied to the plates, which were subsequently developed with water/acetonitrile (13:7) containing 0.1 M tetra-*n*-butyl-ammonium phosphate. For recording mass spectra, the electrospun polyacrylonitrile nanofiber phase was coupled online using a CAMAG TLC–MS interfaced to the ESI source of the single-quadrupole mass spectrometer. For all preservatives, the deprotonated molecule $[M-H]^-$ was the characteristic base peak except for the deprotonated dimer for sorbic acid $[2M-H]^-$. In some mass spectra, for example, for methyl and ethyl 4-hydroxybenzoate, the electrospun polyacrylonitrile nanofiber background was visible. It has been estimated that elution of relatively small analyte amounts (20 ng/zone for all preservatives except benzoic acid, which was 600 ng/zone) is sufficient for obtaining strong mass signals and strong total ion current elution profiles visible in the chronogram and its respective mass spectra [39].

### 6.7.6 Flavanols

TLC coupled to ESI was used for the analysis of monomeric flavanols and proanthocyanidins from standard stock solutions and from extracts of natural samples. Specifically, standard solutions of (−)-epicatechin, (+)-catechin, procyanidin B2, (−)-epigallocatechin, and extracts of pomegranate peel and juniper seeds were developed on HPTLC cellulose plates and HPTLC silica gel 60 plates. Effects of eluent flow, sorbent material, and developing solvent on TLC–ESI mass spectra were studied. A CAMAG TLC–MS interface was used for the elution of compounds from HPTLC plates into the ESI source. For silica plates, it was necessary to use an HILIC guard column mounted between the CAMAG TLC–MS interface and ion source. This need was caused by the presence of stationary phase impurities in the extracts, which in turn caused suppression of the ionization of compounds of interest. Ultimately, the most effective method for the analysis of flavanols by TLC–ESI was via separation on a cellulose sorbent, development with $n$-propanol/water/acetic acid (4:2:1) or pure water, and elution with methanol using a CAMAG TLC–MS interface without an HILIC column, directly to the ESI source [40].

### 6.7.7 ANTHOCYANINS

Pomace, animal feed, and various food samples, along with 11 anthocyanin standards, were developed on HPTLC silica gel 60 plates. The plates were developed using ethyl acetate/2-butanon/water/formic acid (5:3:1:1). Zones of interest were directly eluted using a CAMAG TLC–MS interface using pure methanol. The mass spectrometer used was a single-quadrupole mass spectrometer with an ESI interface as an ion source. The zones of interest were those from the sample tracks that did not match any of the 11 anthocyanin standards developed. The detection sensitivity for anthocyanidins was much better compared to the anthocyanins. Nevertheless, the anthocyanin mass spectra showed the molecular ion $[M]^+$, and in the case of diglycosides, the loss of one sugar moiety and the parent aglycone was also observed [41].

### 6.7.8 SULFONAMIDES

Twelve representative sulfonamides were developed on HPTLC silica gel 60 plates using ethyl acetate/methanol/28% ammonium hydroxide solution (8:2:0.1). Additionally, some plates were derivatized by immersion of the plate into a solution of fluram, which fluorescently labels $p$-aminobenzene sulfonamide group of the sulfonamides. Zones of interest were eluted using CAMAG TLC–MS interfaced to a single-quadrupole mass spectrometer equipped with an ESI source. For nonderivatized plates, the eluent consisted of acetonitrile/20-mM ammonium formate buffer (7:3), and for derivatized plates, the eluent was methanol/20-mM ammonium formate buffer (7:3). From the nonderivatized plates, protonated molecules $[M+H]^+$ and sodium ion adducts $[M+Na]^+$ were the most pronounced signals in the ESI-positive mode, while in the negative mode, deprotonated molecules were generally produced. On derivatized plates, a mass increase of 278 amu was expected, resulting from the reaction of the sulfonamides with fluram. However, in both ESI-positive and ESI-negative modes, a neutral loss of water was observed in most cases. As lower sample amounts were required for derivatized plates, and the target zones can be more easily and clearly located, derivatized plates were favored for confirming suspicious findings [42].

## 6.8  THIN-LAYER CHROMATOGRAPHY–DESORPTION ELECTROSPRAY IONIZATION

### 6.8.1  DYES

Desorption electrospray ionization (DESI) was used to obtain mass spectra of dyes, directly from TLC plates. TLC/DESI fundamentals and applications were demonstrated using rhodamines (6G, B, and 123) and federal food, drug, and cosmetic

(FD&C) dyes (erythrosine B, brilliant blue FCF, fast green FCF, and sunset yellow FCF). For the rhodamines, TLC was carried out using RP C8 and RP C2 plates, which were developed using methanol/water (80:20) containing ammonium acetate. For the FD&C dyes, TLC was carried out using RP C18 plates, which were developed using water/acetone (70:30) containing ammonium acetate. The plates were dried and an ES emitter was mounted approximately 4 mm from the curtain plate of the mass spectrometer at a ~50° angle relative to the TLC plate surface. The optimization conditions, such as solvent flow rate, solvent composition, nebulizing gas flow rate, DESI emitter-to-surface distance, and the effect of surface scan rate on signal levels and chromatographic readout resolution, were examined. Positioning of the DESI emitter, TLC plate surface, and the atmospheric sampling orifice of the mass spectrometer were found to be crucial for obtaining maximum analyte signal levels [43].

Rhodamine B, 6G, and 123 were characterized directly from TLC RP C8 plates using a DESI ion source connected to an automated sampling and imaging setup. After resolving, the TLC plate was dried and attached to the sample platform, whereas the DESI emitter was mounted 1–4 mm from the TLC surface at a ~50° angle to the plate. The sampling capillary was 100 µm or less above the TLC surface and ~2 mm back from the position where the DESI plume impacted the surface. The position of the sample platform was controlled manually using a joystick (x/y positioning) and a jog wheel (z positioning). A color webcam was mounted directly over the TLC surface and centered on the DESI emitter and sampling capillary. This camera was used for manual and computer-controlled positioning of the surface in the x/y plane. With computer control, it was possible to perform spot sampling, array sampling, lane scanning, or imaging of the TLC surface. The data acquired during analysis contained mass spectral data, the corresponding surface location data, and the time elapsed since the beginning of the analysis. The webcam image of the surface examined could be loaded with the interrogation path superimposed [44].

## 6.8.2 Drugs

In a paper describing the analysis of FD&C dyes and rhodamine dyes using TLC–DESI technique [43], drugs (caffeine, acetaminophen, and aspirin) were also examined. The drugs were developed on silica gel plates and developed using ethyl acetate/acetic acid (99:1). The DESI experimental setup was identical to that in the dye analysis. In comparison to the dye analysis, it was necessary to spot significantly larger amounts (microgram quantities) of drugs onto the plate in order to obtain high-quality mass spectra. The poorer desorption ionization efficiency of drugs appeared to be related at least in part to the normal-phase stationary phase [43].

## 6.8.3 Alkaloids

Goldenseal and related alkaloids were qualitatively identified and quantitatively determined using TLC/DESI analysis. The TLC separations were performed using aluminum sheets precoated with silica gel 60 $F_{254}$, or using glass-backed silica gel 60 plates. After the application of analytes, the plates were developed in ascending mode in a glass chamber saturated with ethyl acetate/methanol/formic acid/water (50:10:6:3). After development, the plates were dried and placed on a sample platform. Glass-backed TLC plates were secured with plastic lock nuts into a recess in a rectangular plexiglass block attached to the top of the positioning stage. Aluminum-backed plates were secured with double-sided tape to a glass plate mounted into this recess. The DESI emitter was mounted ~3.5 mm from the analyzed surface at an approximately 60° angle to the surface and 4 mm back from the sampling capillary. Standard curves for the fixed-charge alkaloids berberine, palmatine, and hydrastinine were linear over two separate ranges, namely, 2.5–100 and 25–1000 pmol. The detection levels for these three alkaloids, obtained in mass spectral full-scan mode, were ~5 ng for each alkaloid. However, signal levels for hydrastine, which required protonation for detection, were nearly one order of magnitude lower than those of a comparable amount of the fixed-charge alkaloids. Nonetheless, levels of detection were comparable to fluorescence detection and should be adequate for typical sample loadings on conventional TLC and HPTLC plates [45].

## 6.9 THIN-LAYER CHROMATOGRAPHY–ELECTROSPRAY-ASSISTED LASER DESORPTION/IONIZATION

### 6.9.1 DYES

Electrospray-assisted laser desorption/ionization (ELDI) was used under ambient conditions to characterize FD&C dyes separated in the central track on a TLC plate coated with reversed-phase C18 particles. Dyes (erythrosine, erioglaucine, and fast green FCF) were developed using 500-mM ammonia solution/acetone (70:30). After development, the TLC plates were air-dried or dried in an oven for 15 min prior to further ELDI analysis. The TLC plates were then placed on an acrylic sample holder, which was set in front of the sampling skimmer of an ion trap mass analyzer. The sample holder was then moved slowly using a syringe pump. A pulsed nitrogen laser ablated a trail as it traversed the center of the TLC plate. The desorbed sample molecules entered into an ESI plume and were ionized through their interactions with the charged species generated by electrospray. The detection limits were estimated using the solutions containing different concentrations of erythrosine (from $10^{-3}$ to $10^{-7}$ M). The molecular ion of this compound at $m/z$ 835 was detected only when the concentration of erythrosine in the solution was higher than $10^{-6}$ M. The calibration curve, based on the peak area of $m/z$ 835 versus the concentration of the sample spots, showed a linear relationship between $10^{-3}$ and $10^{-6}$ M. However, it has been suggested that only semiquantitative analysis should be performed using this method because the ion intensity of an analyte on a TLC plate varies by the laser power, laser focusing size, thickness and composition of the silica gel, and diffusion coefficient of the analyte on the TLC plate during ELDI analysis [46].

### 6.9.2 DRUGS

Drug extracts containing acetaminophen, chlorpheniramine, and ethenzamide were developed on aluminum-backed TLC plates using ethyl acetate/acetic acid/chloroform

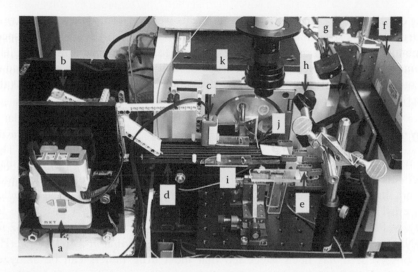

**FIGURE 6.1** Photograph of the combination of LEGO-made TLC plate delivery system and ELDI/MS. This system contains several parts including (a) a control box, (b) TLC plate storage box and dealing system, (c) light sensor, (d) conveyer, (e) collecting box, (f) pulsed laser, (g) reflector, (h) focusing lens, (i) electrospray, (j) inlet of MS, and (k) CCD. (Reprinted with permission from Cheng, S.C. et al. *Anal. Chem.*, 84: 5864–5868. Copyright 2012, American Chemical Society.)

(98:1:1). Afterward, the dried plates were analyzed using an ELDI source combined with an automatic TLC plate delivery system constructed from LEGO building blocks, which is shown in Figure 6.1. The building blocks contained 612 elements and several electronic parts such as motors, ultrasonic sensor, touch sensors, and color sensor. The plate delivery system consisted of a dealing system, a conveyor, and a collecting box. This system was integrated with an ELDI source by setting it in front of the inlet of a mass analyzer. As the TLC plate moved through, the surface of the TLC plate was laser-irradiated. The mass spectra obtained allowed the identification of the composition of over-the-counter drugs. It has been calculated that this plate delivery system allows for screening of more than 400 TLC plates in a 24-h period [47].

## 6.10  THIN-LAYER CHROMATOGRAPHY–EASY AMBIENT SONIC SPRAY IONIZATION

### 6.10.1  Semipolar Compounds

An easy ambient sonic spray ionization (EASI) source uses gentle sonic spray ionization to create charged droplets, which are formed due to the sonic spray causing a statistical imbalance in the distribution of charges. It was used for on-spot detection and analyte characterization on TLC plates. To test its usefulness, an equimolar mixture of three semipolar nitrogenated molecules (allyl phenylamine, phenylamine, and ethylpyridine) was applied to commercial TLC aluminum sheets and resolved using ethyl acetate/hexane (2:8). MS experiments were performed on a Q-Trap triple quadrupole mass spectrometer equipped with a homemade EASI source. All spectra obtained showed a major ion corresponding to the protonated molecule. The advantage of the EASI technique is its superior ability to form intact protonated or deprotonated molecules with little or no dissociation, which grandly simplifies the detection of particular compounds [48].

### 6.10.2 DRUGS

The usefulness of an EASI source was also tested in the fast screening of drug tablets containing propranolol or amlodipine. The commercial drug tablets were ground, dissolved in water, neutralized with ammonium hydroxide, and extracted with ethyl acetate. The ethyl acetate solution was applied onto a TLC plate for analysis. For propranolol, intense signals at $m/z$ 260 for $[M+H]^+$ and $m/z$ 282 for $[M+Na]^+$ were observed, whereas for amlodipine, a signal at $m/z$ 409 for $[M+H]^+$ was observed. It has been suggested that most drug tablets can be analyzed directly by EASI with no chromatographic separation, and that TLC–EASI may be used for multidrug tablets or for forensic fingerprinting analysis of counterfeit tablets [48].

## 6.11   THIN-LAYER CHROMATOGRAPHY–DIRECT ANALYSIS IN REAL TIME IN ANALYSIS OF SMALL ORGANIC COMPOUNDS

High-resolution mass spectra of individual spots on a TLC plate were obtained quickly and easily at atmospheric pressure with zero sample preparation using a DART ionization source. An artificial mixture of four organic compounds (cinnamaldehyde, phenolphthalein, acetaminophen, and caffeine) was resolved on standard, commercially available 200-μm silica gel polyester backing plates with UV254 indicator. For mass spectra analysis, the spots were visualized under a UV lamp and circled with a pencil. The TLC slide was then cut with scissors through the center of the four spots, and the edge of the TLC slide was held so that the gas stream grazed the center of each spot, beginning at the bottom of the slide and ending at the compound that traveled the furthest. On all high-resolution mass spectra, the most intense signals were observed for $[M+H]^+$ ions [49].

## 6.12   THIN-LAYER CHROMATOGRAPHY–LASER-INDUCED ACOUSTIC DESORPTION/ELECTROSPRAY IONIZATION

### 6.12.1   DYES

Laser-induced acoustic desorption (LIAD) is a technique developed for desorbing and ionizing organic and biological materials from solid substrates under vacuum. After irradiation of a pulsed laser beam to the rear of a thin metal foil, the resulting ablation creates large-amplitude acoustic shock waves that propagate through the foil. It has been suggested that molecules predeposited on the other side of the foil would be detached through the actions of the acoustic shock wave, which concurrently would ensure that the molecules do not break apart [50–53]. Methods of LIAD in combination with ESI were used to rapidly characterize chemical compounds separated on TLC plates. A mixture of three dyes (fast green FCF, erythrosine, and eriochromcyanin R) was developed on RP C18 TLC plates using a 65% acetone solution containing 1.5% formic acid. After development and air-drying, the rear side of the TLC plate was covered with a thin film of glycerol, and then the plate was taped tightly to a glass microscope slide. A pulsed Q-switched Nd/YAG laser beam was transmitted through the microscope glass slide and irradiated the rear side of the TLC plate. The desorbed analyte molecules entered the ESI plume, generated by the electrospray capillary, which was aligned parallel to and 2–3 mm above the surface of the TLC plate. The dye standards were detected in negative-ion mode as singly charged or doubly charged ions [54].

### 6.12.2 Psychoactive Drugs

Similarly to dye standards, drug standards (3,4-methylenedioxy-$N$-methylamphetamine, lysergic acid diethylamide, flunitrazepam) were resolved on a normal-phase TLC plate using chloroform/methanol (9:1). After drying, LIAD/ESI analysis was performed using the same procedure as for dye standards. All drugs were detected in positive-ion mode as [M+H]$^+$ ions [54].

## 6.13 THIN-LAYER CHROMATOGRAPHY–PLASMA-ASSISTED MULTIWAVELENGTH LASER DESORPTION IONIZATION

### 6.13.1 Dyes

The thin-layer chromatography–plasma-assisted multiwavelength laser desorption ionization (TLC–PAMLDI) technique successfully integrates TLC, the multiwavelength laser ablation, and the excited state plasma from a DART ion source. It has proved to be effective in the simple separation and selective identification of low-molecular-weight compounds. Specifically, a mixture of dyes (rhodamine B, fluorescein, and Sudan III) was resolved on a glass-backed TLC plate using dichloromethane/ethanol/ammonia (66.1:33.1:0.8). After drying, the plate was immobilized on an automated three-dimensional platform and TLC–PAMLDI parameters such as laser wavelength, plasma temperature, and distances between DART exit, ablation point, and ions transfer tube were optimized. The positive PAMLDI mass spectra were recorded using visible laser light (532 nm), and showed signals corresponding to rhodamine B ($m/z$ 443), fluorescein ($m/z$ 333), and Sudan III ($m/z$ 353) [55].

### 6.13.2 Drugs

TLC–PAMLDI techniques have also been used to produce mass spectra of drug standard samples from glass-backed TLC plates. Quinine, gliclazide, and chloramphenicol were developed using hexane/ethanol/formic acid (64.7:32.4:2.9). After optimization of all measurement conditions, the mass spectra were recorded using

UV laser light (355   nm). Mass spectra of each spot were obtained, which showed signals of quinine (*m/z* 325), gliclazide (*m/z* 324), or chloramphenicol (*m/z* 323) [55].

## 6.14   THIN-LAYER CHROMATOGRAPHY–ATMOSPHERIC-PRESSURE CHEMICAL IONIZATION

### 6.14.1   DRUGS

A mixture of caffeine and acetaminophen was resolved on TLC silica gel 60 aluminum sheets in two development steps. In the first step, the mobile phase consisted of cyclohexane/acetic acid/trichloromethane (86:7:7), whereas in the second step, it consisted of cyclohexane/methanol/acetic acid/ethyl acetate (59:6:6:29). The TLC plate was than ablated with a laser (213 nm) in an ablation cell. The ablated sample material was transferred to an APCI source by nitrogen flow through polyamide tubing. This setup allowed for spatially resolved analysis of a TLC plate. The position and the shape of the fluorescence signal spots were consistent with the ion images for caffeine (*m/z* 195) and acetaminophen (*m/z* 152). Furthermore, an intensity increase from the outside to the inside of the spots was perceived in the ion images of these compounds. These increases in intensity indicate an increase in the amount of analyte in the sample and allow for the estimation of the relative amount of the analyte [56].

### 6.14.2   TERPENES

Extracts from fresh leaves of *Leonurus japonicus* were resolved on a TLC silica gel 60 glass-backed plate using 2D elution. The first development solvent system was chloroform/methanol (5:1), whereas the second was chloroform/ethyl acetate (1:1). Two particular spots were present on the TLC plates only if the plant extracts were dried at lower temperatures. To identify these two compounds, spots of interest were extracted with a CAMAG TLC–MS interface using methanol as an extraction solvent and transferred directly to an APCI source. The more polar of the two compounds showed a peak at *m/z* 333 and the other showed a signal at *m/z* 331 in positive-ion mode APCI-TOF. These two compounds were determined to have formulas of $C_{20}H_{28}O_4$ $[M+H-H_2O]^+$ and $C_{20}H_{26}O_4$ $[M+H-H_2O]^+$, respectively, by high-resolution APCI-TOF. The final structures of these compounds were determined by NMR spectroscopy. Both compounds were labdane diterpenes, which have not been previously reported [57].

Ursolic, oleanolic, and betulinic acids as well as miscellaneous vegetable extracts were developed on RP C18 plates using *n*-hexane/ethyl acetate (5:1). A TLC–MS approach was employed to confirm the presence of the acids in the plant extracts studied. A CAMAG TLC–MS interface was used for the elution of compounds from TLC plates into the ion trap mass spectrometer with an APCI source. Mass spectra were recorded in negative-ion mode. In order to differentiate between the isomeric ursolic, oleanolic, and betulinic acids by means of MS, tandem and triple MS experiments were performed. Betulinic acid could be readily distinguished from ursolic and oleanolic acids. MS/MS/MS spectra of the two latter acids varied mainly in the intensities of the produced ions, but due to the poor reproducibility of these spectra, it was not possible to distinguish these two acids by MS [58].

## 6.15 THIN-LAYER CHROMATOGRAPHY–NO EXTERNAL ION SOURCE IN ANALYSIS OF SMALL ORGANIC MOLECULES

Direct analysis of spots from TLC plates, without the need of an external ion source, was developed using the aluminum plate backing as a spray tip. The practical benefits of this technique were demonstrated by detection of by-products of organic reactions (synthesis of aziridine derivative), by identification of degradation products (degradation of Schiff base *N*-(diphenylmethylene)glycine *tert*-butyl ester under acidic conditions), and by accurate confirmation of spots when UV filters (avobenzone, octisalate, and octocrylene) in sunscreens were analyzed by TLC. In all these analyses, after resolving the TLC plate, the spots of interest were cut out, and one side of each was shaped into a tip with an angle of 60°. The TLC piece was mounted in front of the mass spectrometer at a distance of 4 mm from the tip of the sampling orifice. The spray voltage was directly applied to the aluminum backing of the TLC plate piece using a clamp. After applying the spray voltage, 20-μL spray solvent (methanol with 0.1% formic acid) was dispensed onto the spot using a plastic pipette tip, and then, mass spectra were acquired. A high-resolution time-of-flight MS method was used because the method is of particular interest for rapid identification or confirmation of spots from TLC plates. Mass spectra obtained using the presented method were of high quality. The main advantage of the presented procedure lies in the rapid and unambiguous confirmation of analyte identity [59].

## 6.16 THIN-LAYER CHROMATOGRAPHY–DIELECTRIC BARRIER DISCHARGE IONIZATION IN ANALYSIS OF PYRAZOLE DERIVATIVES

Six pyrazole derivatives were developed on TLC aluminum-backed silica gel 60 plates using dichloromethane/diethyl ether (10:1). The TLC plate was then cut through the center of all spots, resulting in a narrow strip, and then, a heating element with a diameter similar to the size of each spot was attached to the bottom of a particular spot. The strip was then heated from the bottom and held manually so that the plasma released from the DBD ion source would emerge just above the marked spot. The sample switching was very fast because it required only the movement of the heating element. Each spectrum obtained represented the major ion corresponding to the protonated molecule with little or no background ions. The structures of the analytes were confirmed by MS/MS analysis of all compounds. The detection limit was estimated to be 100 ng/spot [60].

## 6.17 CONCLUSIONS

The TLC–MS combination method provides additional mass spectroscopic characterization data of resolved compounds, therefore eliminating the need of using appropriate standards. The great advantage of TLC–MS is the fact that the TLC plate, after development, can be physically transferred considerable distances. Therefore, TLC resolution can be performed in a laboratory even when it does not possess a mass spectrometer, or analysis could even be performed outside the laboratory. Moreover, TLC plates can be stored for a long time, which means that MS characterization can be performed when the need arises.

Over the years, many "indirect sampling" and "direct sampling" TLC–MS techniques have been developed. Because "direct sampling" TLC–MS techniques offer fast and, in some examples, fully automated analysis with almost no sample preparation, their usability is very high. Although many "direct sampling" TLC–MS techniques have been developed, only two of them are readily available: TLC–ESI and TLC–MALDI. TLC–ESI owes its popularity to the CAMAG TLC–MS interface, which is a commercially available device and allows for fast connection to mass spectrometers with ESI (and APCI) ion sources. Recently, a paper describing practical advice for use of this TLC–MS interface has been published [61]. The main drawback of this technique is significant intensity of background mass signals coming from the plate, solvents, or any contamination. These background signals can be so intense that they lead to ion suppression [61]. For TLC–MALDI technique, a commercially available plate adapter has been developed, allowing relatively fast mounting of a TLC plate into a MALDI mass spectrometer. Nevertheless, MALDI analysis of a TLC plate requires application of a matrix on a TLC plate and lowering the pressure in the mass spectrometer for the time of analysis, which overall makes it a time-consuming process. These drawbacks of TLC–ESI and TLC–MALDI are rather serious, and therefore, there is a need to develop new TLC–MS techniques.

Many ambient techniques have been applied to produce mass spectra directly from TLC plates. These techniques are still only generally available in laboratories that use custom-built setups. Most are plasma-based setups that produce ions with no or only slight fragmentation, and are usually dedicated to producing ions directly from solid surfaces. These features point toward the techniques potentially becoming commercially available in the future.

# REFERENCES

1. Fuchs, B., Süß, R., Nimptsch, A., and Schiller, J. 2009. MALDI-TOF–MS directly combined with TLC: A review of the current state. *Chromatographia*, 69: 95–105.
2. Peterson, B.L. and Cummings, B.S. 2006. A review of chromatographic methods for the assessment of phospholipids in biological samples. *Biomed. Chromatogr.*, 20: 227–243.
3. Sherma, J. 2008. Planar chromatography. *Anal. Chem.*, 80: 4253–4267.
4. Wall, P.E. *Thin-Layer Chromatography: A Modern Practical Approach*. The Royal Society of Chemistry, Cambridge, UK, Chapter 1.
5. Somsen, G.W., Morden, W., and Wilson, I.D. 1995. Planar chromatography coupled with spectroscopic techniques. *J. Chromatogr. A*, 703: 613–665.
6. Cheng, S.C., Huang, M.Z, and Shiea, J. 2011. Thin layer chromatography–mass spectrometry. *J. Chromatogr. A*, 1218: 2700–2711.
7. Wilson, I.D. 1999. The state of the art in thin-layer chromatography–mass spectrometry: A critical appraisal. *J. Chromatogr. A*, 856: 429–442.

8. Morlock, G. and Schwack, W. 2010. Coupling of planar chromatography to mass spectrometry. *Trends Anal. Chem.*, 29: 1157–1171.
9. Sherma, J. 2010. Planar chromatography. *Anal. Chem.*, 82: 4895–4910.
10. Poole, C.F. 2003. Thin-layer chromatography: Challenges and opportunities. *J. Chromatogr. A*, 1000: 963–984.
11. Tuzimski, T. 2011. Application of different modes of thin-layer chromatography and mass spectrometry for the separation and detection of large and small biomolecules. *J. Chromatogr. A*, 1218: 8799–8812.
12. Fuchs, B., Süß, R., Teuber, K., Eibisch, M., and Schiller, J. 2011. Lipid analysis by thin-layer chromatography—A review of the current state. *J. Chromatogr. A*, 1218: 2754–2774.
13. Van Beek, T., Tetala, K.R., Koleva, I., Dapkevicius, A., Exarchou, V., Jeurissen, S.F., Claassen, F., and van der Klift, E.C. 2009. Recent developments in the rapid analysis of plants and tracking their bioactive constituents. *Phytochem. Rev.*, 8: 387–399.
14. Oka, H., Ito, Y., Ikai, Y., Kagami, T., and Ken-ichi, H. 1998. Mass spectrometric analysis of tetracycline antibiotics in foods. *J. Chromatogr. A*, 812: 309–319.
15. Fuchs, B. 2012. Analysis of phospolipids and glycolipids by thin-layer chromatography–matrix-assisted laser desorption and ionization mass spectrometry. *J. Chromatogr. A*, 1259: 62–73.
16. Morlock, G. and Chernetsova, E. 2012. Coupling of planar chromatography with direct analysis in real time mass spectrometry. *Cent. Eur. J. Chem.*, 10: 703–710.
17. Pasilis, S.P. and Van Berkel, G.J. 2010. Atmospheric pressure surface sampling/ionization techniques for direct coupling of planar separations with mass spectrometry. *J. Chromatogr. A*, 1217: 3955–3965.
18. Unger, S.E., Vincze, A., Cooks, R.G., Chrisman, R., and Rothman, L.D. 1981. Identification of quaternary alkaloids in mushroom by chromatography/secondary ion mass spectrometry. *Anal. Chem.*, 53: 976–981.
19. Oriňák, A., Oriňáková, R., Arlinghaus, H.F., Vering, G., and Hellweg, S. 2006. Postchromatographic TOF-SIMS identification of diterpenes. *Surf. Interface Anal.*, 38: 599–603.
20. Stoll, M.S., Hounsell, E.F., Lawson, A.M., Chai, W., and Feizi, T. 1990. Microscale sequencing of O-linked oligosaccharides using mild periodate oxidation of alditols, coupling to phospholipid and TLC–MS analysis of the resulting neoglycolipids. *Eur. J. Biochem.*, 189: 499–507.
21. Stanley, M.S. and Busch, K.L. 1987. Positive secondary-ion mass spectra and thin-layer chromatography–mass spectrometry of phenothiazine drugs. *Anal. Chim. Acta*, 194: 199–209.
22. Hanisch, F.G. and Peter-Katalinic, J. 1992. Structural studies on fetal mucins from human amniotic fluid. *Eur. J. Biochem.*, 205: 527–535.
23. Chang, T.T., Lay, J.O., and Francel, R.J. 1984. Direct analysis of thin-layer chromatography spots by fast atom bombardment mass spectrometry. *Anal. Chem.*, 56: 109–111.
24. Gusev, A.I., Proctor, A., Rabinovich, Y.I., and Hercules, D.M. 1995. Thin-layer chromatography combined with matrix-assisted laser desorption/ionization mass spectrometry. *Anal. Chem.*, 67: 1805–1814.
25. Mehl, J.T., Gusev, A.I., and Hercules, D.M. 1997. Coupling protocol for thin layer chromatography/matrix-assisted laser desorption ionization. *Chromatographia*, 46: 358–364.
26. Bischoff, A., Eibisch, M., Fuchs, B., Süss, R., Schürenberg, M., Suckau, D., and Schiller, J. 2011. A simple TLC–MALDI method to monitor oxidation products of phosphatidylcholines and -ethanolamines. *Acta Chromatogr.*, 23: 365–375.
27. Kouzel, I.U., Pirkl, A., Pohlentz, G., Soltwisch, J., Dreisewerd, K., Karch, H., and Müthing, J. 2013. Progress in detection and structural characterization of glycosphingolipids in crude lipid extracts by enzymatic phospholipid disintegration combined

with thin-layer chromatography immunodetection and IR–MALDI mass spectrometry. *Anal. Chem.*, 86: 1215–1222.

28. Kuwayama, K., Tsujikawa, K., Miyaguchi, H., Kanamori, T., Iwata, Y., and Inoue, H. 2012. Rapid, simple, and highly sensitive analysis of drugs in biological samples using thin-layer chromatography coupled with matrix-assisted laser desorption/ionization mass spectrometry. *Anal. Bioanal. Chem.*, 402: 1257–1267.

29. Tseng, M.C., Obena, R., Lu, Y.W., Lin, P.C., Lin, P.Y., Yen, Y.S., Lin, J.T., Huang L.D., Lu, K.L., Lai. L.L., Lin, C.C., and Chen, Y.J. 2010. Dihydrobenzoic acid modified nanoparticle as a MALDI-TOF MS matrix for soft ionization and structure determination of small molecules with diverse structures. *J. Am. Soc. Mass Spectrom.*, 21: 1930–1939.

30. Chen, C.C., Yang, Y.L., Ou, C.L., Chou, C.H., Liaw, C.C., and Lin, P.C. 2013. Direct monitoring of chemical transformations by combining thin layer chromatography with nanoparticle-assisted laser desorption/ionization mass spectrometry. *Analyst*, 138: 1379–1385.

31. Leriche, E.D., Hubert-Roux, M., Grossel, M.C., Lange, C.M., Afonso, C., and Loutelier-Bourhis, C. 2014. Direct TLC/MALDI-MS coupling for modified polyamidoamine dendrimers analyses. *Anal. Chim. Acta*, 808: 144–150.

32. Salo, P.K., Salomies, H., Harju, K., Ketola, R.A., Kotiaho, T., Yli-Kauhaluoma, J., and Kostiainen, R. 2005. Analysis of small molecules by ultra thin-layer chromatography–atmospheric pressure matrix-assisted laser desorption/ionization mass spectrometry. *J. Am. Soc. Mass Spectrom.*, 16: 906–915.

33. Salo, P.K., Vilmunen, S., Salomies, H., Ketola, R.A., and Kostiainen, R. 2007. Two-dimensional ultra-thin-layer chromatography and atmospheric pressure matrix-assisted laser desorption/ionization mass spectrometry in bioanalysis. *Anal. Chem.*, 79: 2101–2108.

34. Van Berkel, G.J., Sanchez, A.D., and Quirke, J.M.E. 2002. Thin-layer chromatography and electrospray mass spectrometry coupled using a surface sampling probe. *Anal. Chem.*, 74: 6216–6223.

35. Kertesz, V., Ford, M. J., and Van Berkel, G.J. 2005. Automation of a surface sampling probe/electrospray mass spectrometry system. *Anal. Chem.*, 77: 7183–7189.

36. Vovk, I., Popović, G., Simonovska, B., Albreht, A., and Agbaba, D. 2011. Ultra-thin-layer chromatography mass spectrometry and thin-layer chromatography mass spectrometry of single peptides of angiotensin-converting enzyme inhibitors. *J. Chromatogr. A*, 1218: 3089–3094.

37. Rothenhöfer, M., Scherübl, R., Bernhardt, G., Heilmann, J., and Buschauer, A. 2012. Qualitative and quantitative analysis of hyaluronan oligosaccharides with high performance thin layer chromatography using reagent-free derivatization on amino-modified silica and electrospray ionization-quadrupole time-of-flight mass spectrometry coupling on normal phase. *J. Chromatogr. A*, 1248: 169–177.

38. Chen, Y. and Schwack, W. 2013. Planar chromatography mediated screening of tetracycline and fluoroquinolone antibiotics in milk by fluorescence and mass selective detection. *J. Chromatogr. A*, 1312: 143–151.

39. Kampalanonwat, P., Supaphol, P., and Morlock, G.E. 2013. Electrospun nanofiber layers with incorporated photoluminescence indicator for chromatography and detection of ultraviolet-active compounds. *J. Chromatogr. A*, 1299: 110–117.

40. Smrke, S. and Vovk, I. 2013. Comprehensive thin-layer chromatography mass spectrometry of flavanols from *Juniperus communis* L. and *Punica granatum* L. *J. Chromatogr. A*, 1289: 119–126.

41. Krüger, S., Urmann, O., and Morlock, G.E. 2013. Development of a planar chromatographic method for quantitation of anthocyanes in pomace, feed, juice and wine. *J. Chromatogr. A*, 1289: 105–118.

42. Chen, Y. and Schwack, W. 2014. Rapid and selective determination of multi-sulfon-amides by high-performance thin layer chromatography coupled to fluorescent densitometry and electrospray ionization mass detection. *J. Chromatogr. A*, 1331: 108–116.
43. Van Berkel, G.J., Ford, M.J., and Deibel, M.A. 2005. Thin-layer chromatography and mass spectrometry coupled using desorption electrospray ionization. *Anal. Chem.*, 77: 1207–1215.
44. Van Berkel, G.J. and Kertesz, V. 2006. Automated sampling and imaging of analytes separated on thin-layer chromatography plates using desorption electrospray ionization mass spectrometry. *Anal. Chem.*, 78: 4938–4944.
45. Van Berkel, G.J., Tomkins, B.A., and Kertesz, V. 2007. Thin-layer chromatography–desorption electrospray ionization mass spectrometry: Investigation of goldenseal alkaloids. *Anal. Chem.*, 79: 2778–2789.
46. Lin, S.Y., Huang, M.Z., Chang, H.C., and Shiea, J. 2007. Using electrospray-assisted laser desorption–ionization mass spectrometry to characterize organic compounds separated on thin-layer chromatography plates. *Anal. Chem.*, 79, 8789–8795.
47. Cheng, S.C., Huang, M.Z., Wu, L.C., Chou, C.C., Cheng, C.N., Jhang, S.S., and Shiea, J. 2012. Building blocks for the development of an interface for high-throughput thin layer chromatography/ambient mass spectrometric analysis: A green methodology. *Anal. Chem.*, 84: 5864–5868.
48. Haddad, R., Milagre, H.M.S., Catharino, R.R., and Eberlin, M.N. 2008. Easy ambient sonic-spray ionization mass spectrometry combined with thin-layer chromatography. *Anal. Chem.*, 80: 2744–2750.
49. Smith, N.J., Domin, M.A., and Scott, L.T. 2008. HRMS directly from TLC slides. A powerful tool for rapid analysis of organic mixtures. *Org. Lett.*, 10: 3493–3496.
50. Lindner, B. and Seydel, U. 1985. Laser desorption mass spectrometry of nonvolatiles under shock wave conditions. *Anal. Chem.*, 57: 895–899.
51. Menezes, V., Takayama, K., Ohki, T., and Gopalan, J. 2005. Laser-ablation-assisted microparticle acceleration for drug delivery. *Appl. Phys. Lett.*, 87: 163504.
52. Golovlev, V.V., Allman, S.L., Garrett, W.R., Taranenko, N.I., and Chen, C.H. 1997. Laser-induced acoustic desorption. *Int. J. Mass Spectrom. Ion Processes*, 169–170: 69–78.
53. Peng, W.P., Yang, Y.C., Kang, M.W., Tzeng, Y.K., Nie, Z., Chang, H.C., Chang, W., and Chen, C.H. 2006. Laser-induced acoustic desorption mass spectrometry of single bioparticles. *Angew. Chem. Int. Ed.*, 45: 1423–1426.
54. Cheng, S.C., Huang, M.Z., and Shiea, J. 2009. Thin-layer chromatography–laser-induced acoustic desorption/electrospray ionization mass spectrometry. *Anal. Chem.*, 81: 9274–9281.
55. Zhang, J., Zhou, Z., Yang, J., Zhang, W., Bai, Y., and Liu, H. 2011. Thin layer chromatography–plasma assisted multiwavelength laser desorption ionization mass spectrometry for facile separation and selective identification of low molecular weight compounds. *Anal. Chem.*, 84: 1496–1503.
56. Herdering, C., Reifschneider, O., Wehe, C.A., Sperling, M., and Karst, U. 2013. Ambient molecular imaging by laser ablation atmospheric pressure chemical ionization mass spectrometry. *Rapid Commun. Mass Spectrom.*, 27: 2595–2600.
57. Fuchino, H., Daikonya, A., Kumagai, T., Goda, Y., Takahashi, Y., and Kawahara, N. 2013. Two new labdane diterpenes from fresh leaves of *Leonurus japonicus* and their degradation during drying. *Chem. Pharm. Bull.*, 61: 497–503.
58. Naumoska, K., Simonovska, B., Albreht, A., and Vovk, I. 2013. TLC and TLC–MS screening of ursolic, oleanolic and betulinic acids in plant extracts. *J. Planar Chromatogr.*, 26: 125–131.
59. Himmelsbach, M., Waser, M., and Klampfl, C. 2014. Thin layer chromatography–spray mass spectrometry: A method for easy identification of synthesis products and UV filters from TLC aluminum foils. *Anal. Bioanal. Chem.*, 406: 3647–3656.

60. Cegłowski, M., Smoluch, M., Babij, M., Gotszalk, T., Silberring, J., and Schroeder, G. 2014. Dielectric barrier discharge ionization in characterization of organic compounds separated on thin-layer chromatography plates. *PLoS One*, 9: e106088.
61. Morlock, G.E. 2014. Background mass signals in TLC/HPTLC–ESI–MS and practical advices for use of the TLC–MS interface. *J. Liq. Chromatogr. Relat. Technol.*, 37: 2892–2914.

# 7 Interfacing TLC with Laser-Based Ambient Mass Spectrometry

Sychyi Cheng and Jentaie Shiea

## CONTENTS

## 7.1 INTRODUCTION

Laser, an acronym for "light amplification by stimulated emission of radiation," is a light source that generates highly amplified and coherent electromagnetic radiation through stimulated emission. Because of the inherent properties of monochromic light—high power density and spatial resolution, a laser beam can be used to sample chemical compounds in very small and defined areas [1,2]. Although laser-based surface sampling mechanisms are not fully understood, analytes on surfaces are known to be directly ablated, desorbed, or vaporized by laser irradiation without tedious sample pretreatment. This greatly shortens analytical times and reduces the use of hazardous reagents. The application of lasers in mass spectrometry (MS) was first reported in 1963, when a pulsed ruby laser was used to desorb analytes from the surfaces of conductors, semiconductors, and insulators followed by MS detection [3]. Since then, various lasers, such as gas lasers, solid-state lasers, and excimer lasers, have been utilized in different MS techniques to characterize organic and inorganic compounds on different surfaces. Characterization of chemical compounds on thin-layer chromatographic (TLC) plates by MS has been an important area of analytical chemistry due to its ability to analyze complex samples [4,5]. Because analytes are mainly adsorbed on TLC gel particles rather than eluting out of the stationary phase as in liquid chromatography (LC) and gas chromatography (GC), a laser beam is therefore used to remove analytes from the TLC gel bed for subsequent MS detection. Laser-based sampling in TLC–MS approaches can be operated in vacuum and ambient conditions; however, it is more convenient to characterize analytes on TLC plates in their native environment (i.e., atmospheric pressure and room temperature) [6,7]. This chapter describes the development of ambient laser-based TLC–MS approaches for direct and indirect sampling, including their setups, mechanisms, and applications.

Laser desorption (LD) of analytes on sample surfaces is one of the most promising technologies for directly sampling organic and inorganic compounds. This sampling technique combined with an ionization source, such as chemical ionization (CI) and photoionization (PI), has been used to successfully characterize chemical compounds on separated TLC plates [8,9]. In one study, LD was used to desorb phenanthrene on silica gel plates followed by transportation with a stream of reagent gas for analyte ionization via CI processes under vacuum conditions [8]. In another study, a Nd/YAG laser (266 nm) combined with a resonant two-photon ionization (R2PI) source was used to characterize polyaromatic hydrocarbons (PAHs), carboxylic acids, amino acids, peptides, catecholamines, and drug molecules on silica TLC plates [9].

Laser desorption ionization (LDI), matrix-assisted laser desorption ionization (MALDI), and surface-assisted laser desorption ionization (SALDI) are desorption ionization (DI) techniques that generate analyte ions by means of direct laser irradiation [10]. They have been used to characterize analyte spots on TLC plates with and without the assistance of organic and inorganic matrices. In LDI, zones of interest are directly irradiated by a pulsed laser beam, which produces analyte ions through ion-molecule reactions (IMRs) with protons and charged species generated in the desorption region [11,12]. For TLC–MALDI, an organic matrix solution, such as saturated sinapinic acid, 2,5-dihydrobenzoic acid, and α-cyano-4-hydroxycinnamic acid, is applied on the TLC plate [13,14]. Energy from the pulsed laser beam is first absorbed by the matrix and then transferred to analytes to generate analyte ions. Instead of using organic matrices as those used in MALDI, micrometer- and nanometer-sized inorganic matrices such as $TiO_2$, Co, carbon, graphite, and magnetic nanoparticles are employed in TLC–SALDI to minimize spectral interferences from matrix ions in lower mass ranges [15,16]. TLC–LDI/MS has been used to characterize berberine, plamatine, PAHs, purines, sugars, and amines [11,12]. MALDI/MS has been used to characterize dyes, peptides, proteins, alkaloids, gangliosides, lipids, and cyanobacterial toxins on TLC plates with detection limits in the nanogram (ng)–picogram (pg)/spot range [13,14,17–22]. Studies that used SALDI/MS to characterize peptides and herbicides on TLC plates reported detection limits for bradykinin and porphyrins of 25 ng and 500 pg, respectively [15,23–25]. Due to the high spatial resolution of the laser beam, LDI and MALDI have been used to acquire chromatographic information and molecular images of samples on TLC plates [11,26].

Although laser-based TLC–MS approaches performed under vacuum conditions including LD–CI, LD–PI, LDI, MALDI, and SALDI can characterize analytes on TLC plates, it is difficult for these techniques to detect volatile compounds. In addition, the size of the ionization sources in vacuum limits the size of the TLC plates. Furthermore, the fall of gel particles during analysis may damage the turbo pumps of the MS instrument. Finally, the introduction of TLC plates from ambient to vacuum conditions is time-consuming and labor-intensive, which is disadvantageous for high-throughput analysis. Obviously, characterizing TLC plates using ambient mass spectrometry is a solution to these problems, as analytes are both separated and detected in their native environment.

## 7.2 LASER-BASED THIN-LAYER CHROMATOGRAPHY–MASS SPECTROMETRY APPROACHES PERFORMED UNDER AMBIENT CONDITIONS

Directly sampling chemical compounds on TLC plates via laser irradiation in a vacuum has been demonstrated by LD–CI, LD–R2PI, LDI, MALDI, and SALDI. Because a laser beam is capable of sampling surface analytes in ambient conditions, atmospheric pressure ionization (API) sources, such as electrospray ionization (ESI) and atmospheric pressure chemical ionization (APCI), are employed to ionize laser-desorbed neutrals. Electrospray laser desorption ionization (ELDI) [27], plasma-assisted multiwavelength laser desorption ionization (PAMLDI) [28], laser desorption atmospheric pressure chemical ionization (LD–APCI) [29], laser desorption-dual electrospray and atmospheric pressure chemical ionization (LD–ESI + APCI) [30], laser-induced acoustic desorption electrospray ionization (LIAD–ESI) [31], and laser-induced acoustic desorption dielectric barrier discharge ionization (LIAD–DBDI) [32] are techniques that combine a laser beam and an API source (Table 7.1). They have been demonstrated to directly characterize analyte spots on TLC plates, providing several benefits: (1) it is easier to interface TLC with MS under ambient conditions than in a vacuum; (2) the size of the TLC plate is not limited by the vacuum chamber; (3) sample switching is fast, allowing for high-throughput analysis; and (4) volatile, semivolatile, and nonvolatile compounds can be characterized. In the following, each of the laser-based ambient mass spectrometric (AMS) techniques for direct analysis of analytes on TLC plates will be introduced.

### 7.2.1 ELECTROSPRAY LASER DESORPTION IONIZATION

Electrospray laser desorption ionization (ELDI) is a technique developed for characterizing solid, liquid, and gas samples without or with minimal sample pretreatment [33]. An ELDI source consists of a sample plate, a laser beam, and an electrospray unit. Unlike MALDI, no application of organic matrix on the sample is needed before laser desorption. In ELDI, a pulsed UV or IR laser beam is used to vaporize and desorb analytes on solid surfaces; the desorbed analytes are subsequently ionized in an ESI plume positioned several millimeters above the laser spot. The ionization mechanisms of ELDI are similar to those of fused droplet-electrospray ionization (FD–ESI) [34], where charged solvent (e.g., methanol and water) species such as $H^+$,

## TABLE 7.1
### Abbreviations for Different Laser-Based TLC–AMS Approaches

| Technique | Acronym | API Source | Spatial Resolution | TLC Image | Reference |
|---|---|---|---|---|---|
| Electrospray laser desorption ionization | ELDI | ESI | $100 \times 150$ µm[b] | Yes | 27 |
| Plasma-assisted multi-wavelength laser desorption ionization | PAMLDI | DART | 150 µm[a] | No | 28 |
| Laser desorption atmospheric pressure chemical ionization | LD-APCI | Corona discharge | 50 µm[a] | No | 29 |
| Laser desorption–dual electrospray and atmospheric pressure chemical ionization source | LD–ESI+APCI | ESI + plasma-APCI | 200 µm[a] | No | 30 |
| Laser-induced acoustic desorption electrospray ionization | LIAD-ESI | ESI | 1.3 mm[a] | No | 31 |
| Laser-induced acoustic desorption dielectric barrier discharge ionization | LIAD-DBDI | DBDI | 1.3 mm[a] | No | 32 |

[a] Diameter of desorption area.
[b] Desorption area.

$H_3O^+$, $(H_2O)_nH_3O^+$, $CH_3OH_2^+$, cluster solvent ions, and charged droplets generated in an ESI plume are reacted with neutral analytes to produce singly- and multiply-charged analyte ions. ELDI/MS has been used to directly characterize organic and biological compounds including peptides, proteins, drugs, synthetic polymers, dyes, and lipids on various surfaces such as stainless steel, paper, currency, tissue sections, and even CDs [33,35–39]. Molecular images of plant slices have been obtained by integrating ELDI with an XYZ moving stage [38]. Furthermore, viscous, hydrophilic, and hydrophobic sample solutions can also be analyzed by ELDI/MS after adding fine carbon powders into the liquid, a technique also known as liquid-ELDI/MS [40,41].

Interfacing TLC with ELDI/MS was first reported in 2007 to characterize organic compounds on separated $C_{18}$- and silica-TLC plates [27]. Figure 7.1 shows the schematic illustration of TLC–ELDI/MS. The TLC plate is placed on a sample holder and moved using a syringe pump operated at a speed of ~4 mm/min. A pulsed nitrogen laser operated at a wavelength of 337 nm, a pulse frequency of 10 Hz, a pulse duration of 5 ns, and an energy of ~150 μJ is used to irradiate the TLC gel bed at an incident angle of 30°. An aqueous solution of 50% methanol with 0.1% acetic acid was used as the ESI solution for positive ion detection, while a solution of 50% methanol is used for negative ion detection. Because the organic matrix used in MALDI and SALDI is not employed in ELDI, problems including lateral diffusion of sample spots along the TLC plate and interference of matrix ions at low mass ranges are not observed in TLC–ELDI/MS. Samples including mixtures of dyes, amines, and extracts of drug tablets have been successfully separated and characterized by TLC–ELDI/MS. The detection limit for organic compounds such as FD&C Red dye is in the ng range, for which a linear response from several ng to μg ($R^2 = 0.9886$) is found. Molecular images of phosphatidylcholine and sphingomyelin on a silica TLC plate can be obtained with the use of an XYZ stage for precise movement [7].

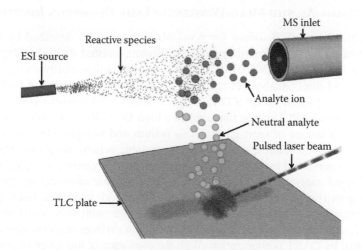

**FIGURE 7.1** Schematic illustration of the TLC ELDI–MS setup.

### 7.2.2 High-Throughput Thin-Layer Chromatography–Electrospray Laser Desorption Ionization/Mass Spectrometry Analysis

Although ELDI/MS is able to characterize chemical compounds on separated TLC plates, sample switching for TLC–ELDI/MS is still time-consuming and labor-intensive because the TLC plate mounted on the sample stage must be manually replaced. This problem is also encountered in other TLC–AMS approaches. To fulfill high-throughput TLC–ELDI/MS analysis, an automatic system has been developed that is capable of dealing, delivering, and collecting TLC plates through an ELDI source [42]. This TLC–MS system consists of a TLC plate storage box, plate-dealer, conveyer belt, light sensor, and TLC plate collection box. The prototype of the TLC plate delivery system was first designed, constructed, and modified using LEGO building blocks. With its advantages of being readily available, cheap, reusable, and easy to assemble and disassemble, the use of LEGO blocks to construct a new system is undoubtedly a green methodology. After demonstrating its usability, materials such as metal, Teflon, and durable electronic components were used to improve the performance and stability of the system. A TLC–ELDI/MS analysis starts by dispensing the first TLC plate from the storage box onto a conveyer belt, which is subsequently moved toward the ELDI ionization region. As the first plate passes the light sensor, the ELDI laser beam is triggered to desorb analytes on the gel bed followed by MS analysis; meanwhile, the second plate is dispensed from the storage box for the next analysis. After ELDI/MS detection, analyzed plates are sent to the plate collection box. Samples including a mixture of dyes and extracts of drug tablets separated on aluminum TLC plates were successfully analyzed to demonstrate the capability of this high-throughput TLC–ELDI/MS system. The reproducibility (RSD, $n = 4$) of the system for chlorpheniramine was calculated to be 12.8%. Since the analysis of a TLC plate 4 cm long was completed within 2.5 min, more than 400 TLC plates could be screened in a day.

### 7.2.3 Plasma-Assisted Multi-Wavelength Laser Desorption Ionization

Other than using an ESI source for postionization, analytes desorbed by LD can also be ionized by APCI-based approaches. Plasma-assisted multiwavelength laser desorption ionization (PAMLDI) is a technique combining multiwavelength laser desorption and direct analysis in real time (DART) [28]. The setup of PAMLDI is similar to that of ELDI except a DART source is utilized for postionization. DART is a plasma-based APCI source that applies a high DC voltage to a needle electrode to discharge a stream of inert gas such as helium and nitrogen [43]. Analyte ionization occurs when reactive species (e.g., metastable helium molecules, $H_3O^+$, and $(H_2O)_nH_3O^+$) generated by DART come into contact with gaseous analytes, forming singly charged analyte ions through a series of gas-phase chemical reactions such as Penning ionization, proton transfer reaction, charge-exchange reactions, and ion-molecule reactions. In PAMLDI, a Nd/YAG laser system with three wavelengths (i.e., 1064, 532, and 355 nm) was used to irradiate sample surfaces at an incident angle of 45° followed by DART postionization. With the assistance of fine graphite powder for LD, chemical compounds such as stearic acid, cholic acid, cortisone, and octadecylamine on paper surfaces were successfully characterized by PAMLDI/MS [44].

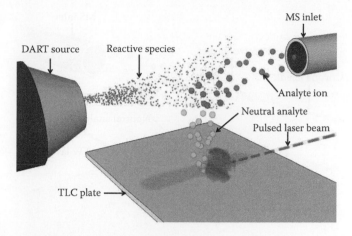

**FIGURE 7.2**    Schematic illustration of the TLC PAMLDI/MS setup.

For molecular imaging analysis, an average pixel size of 60 μm × 60 μm was achieved by this approach [45].

The combination of TLC and PAMLDI/MS was first introduced in 2012 to characterize mixtures [28]. A schematic illustration of TLC–PAMLDI/MS is shown in Figure 7.2. A homemade TLC plate holder and a three-dimensional automatic control platform were used to manipulate the positions of the TLC plates. A pulsed Nd/YAG laser beam with an intensity of several millijoule (mJ) was used to scan the TLC plates. The needle electrode of the DART source was set at 6 kV to discharge helium gas flowed at 2.3 L/min. Analyte ions were characterized by an ion trap mass analyzer. It has been reported that the internal energies of metastable helium were increased when the helium gas temperature was higher than 450°C, resulting in better MS responses. In addition, the strongest signals for rhodamine B, sudan III, and methyl violet were obtained when a 532-nm laser beam was used for desorption. Various samples including dye mixtures, drug standards, and tea extracts separated on normal-phase silica TLC plates were tested and characterized by TLC–PAMLDI/MS with an average detection limit of 5 ng/mm².

### 7.2.4  LASER DESORPTION–ATMOSPHERIC PRESSURE CHEMICAL IONIZATION

Laser desorption atmospheric pressure chemical ionization (LD–APCI) combines a laser system and an APCI source to desorb and ionize small chemical compounds on TLC plates (Figure 7.3) [29]. Vaporization and desorption of analytes from the TLC gel bed was achieved by surface heating with a continuous wave (CW) diode laser operated at 808 nm. It was reported that a laser power density of $10^6$ W/cm² enables desorption of analytes from white TLC plates. Furthermore, the application of a graphite suspension (10 mg/mL in isopropanol) on the TLC gel decreased the CW laser power required for analyte desorption to $10^4$ W/cm². Thermally desorbed analytes were postionized by reacting with charged species generated by corona discharge of the air. The TLC LD–APCI/MS approach was first used to characterize

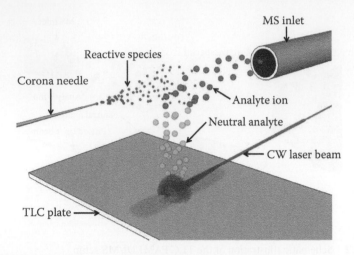

**FIGURE 7.3**   Schematic illustration of the TLC LD–APCI/MS setup.

reserpine on a glass-based TLC plate without actual separation [46]. A glass tube with a length of 10 cm and an XY stage was later used to modify the existing LD–APCI/MS system to perform full plate detection [29]. Analytes desorbed by the CW laser were transferred from the desorption area to the ionization region via a glass tube, where the temperature of the glass tube was maintained at 350°C by a heated wire to reduce sample loss during analyte transfer. TLC LD–APCI/MS has been used to characterize a mixture of lecithin and sphingomyelin (SPM) on separated silica TLC plates with a linear coefficient ($R^2$) of 0.9991 over a range of 0–1.0 μg.

### 7.2.5   Laser Desorption–Dual Electrospray and Atmospheric Pressure Chemical Ionization Source

The aforementioned TLC–AMS approaches (including ELDI, PAMLDI, and LD–APCI) are techniques coupling a laser beam to an ESI or an APCI source. ELDI is useful for characterizing thermally labile, nonvolatile, and polar compounds over an extensive mass range, whereas PAMLDI and LD–APCI are useful for characterizing nonpolar or less polar compounds with lower molecular weights. Although different TLC–AMS approaches with different ionization sources are useful for providing complementary information on analytes on TLC plates, it inevitably increases the analytical time because the sample has to be analyzed repeatedly using different approaches. To expand the polarity and mass range of detected analytes in a single analysis, an ionization source with both ESI and APCI functions was developed and combined with laser desorption to characterize the analytes on TLC plates. The novel source, termed "dual electrospray and atmospheric pressure chemical ionization" (dual ESI + APCI), was constructed by combining an ESI emitter and a plasma-APCI source [47]. A fused silica capillary was inserted into a stainless steel column enclosed in a glass tube. A high DC voltage was applied to an acidic methanol solution flowing through the silica capillary, while a high AC voltage was applied to a ring electrode attached to the glass tube to discharge an inert gas flowing between the glass tube and the stainless steel column. This concentric arrangement of the ESI plume and the APCI plasma in the source ensured that the reactive species generated from both ESI and plasma-APCI simultaneously exited the source to react with analytes through ESI and APCI processes including Penning ionization and ion–molecule reactions (Equations 7.1 through 7.3).

$$He^* + M \rightarrow M^{\bullet+} + N_2 + e^- \tag{7.1}$$

$$M + H_3O^+ \rightarrow MH^+ + H_2O \tag{7.2}$$

$$M + \text{charged droplet} \rightarrow MH_n^n + \tag{7.3}$$

Because the high voltages required for ESI and plasma-APCI are independently applied and controlled, the dual ion source can be operated in ESI-only, APCI-only, or ESI + APCI modes to characterize polar, nonpolar, or both polar and nonpolar compounds, respectively. Laser systems, including a CW laser and a pulsed laser, have been combined with the dual-ion source to characterize chemical compounds on surfaces, where the desorbed analytes are introduced into the ESI and/or APCI plumes for postionization. In addition, analytes on sample surfaces can also be directly desorbed and ionized by directing the ESI + APCI plume toward the sampling area, an approach also known as desorption ESI + APCI [47]. Chemical compounds including PAHs, peptides, drugs, diesel oils, and essential oils on stainless-steel and paper surfaces have been characterized by the dual ionization source.

Figure 7.4 displays the schematic illustration of the TLC–LD/ESI + APCI/MS setup. LD followed by postionization via dual ESI + APCI has been utilized to characterize chemical compounds including methylene blue, ferrocene, and ferrocenealdehyde on silica TLC plates (Figure 7.5a) [30]. For ESI-only mode, methylene blue $((M–Cl)^+, m/z\ 284)$ and ferrocenealdehyde $((M+H)^+, m/z\ 215)$ ions were characterized, while ferrocene ions were not (Figure 7.5b). For APCI-only mode, ferrocene $(M^{\bullet+},$

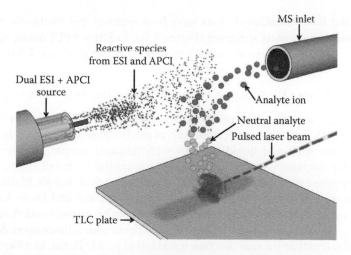

**FIGURE 7.4** Schematic illustration of the TLC–LD/ESI + APCI/MS setup.

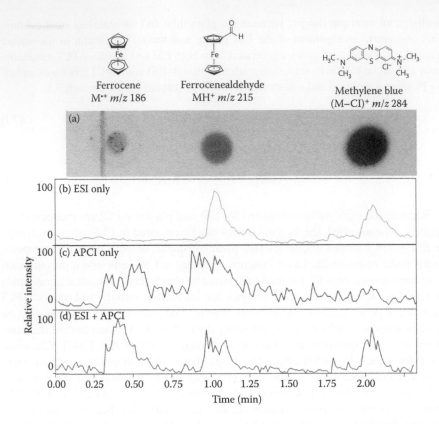

**FIGURE 7.5** (a) Photograph of methylene blue, ferrocene, and ferrocenealdehyde spots on a silica TLC plate. (b–d) Extracted ion chromatograms of methylene blue, ferrocene, and ferrocenealdehyde ($m/z$ 186 + 215 + 284); operation of the dual ESI + APCI source in (b) ESI-only, (c) APCI-only, and (d) ESI + APCI modes, respectively.

$m/z$ 186) and ferrocenealdehyde ions were both detected, but methylene blue ions were not seen on the mass spectrum (Figure 7.5c). In ESI + APCI mode, methylene blue, ferrocene, and ferrocenealdehyde ions were all detected (Figure 7.5d).

### 7.2.6 LASER-INDUCED ACOUSTIC DESORPTION–ELECTROSPRAY IONIZATION

Laser-induced acoustic desorption–electrospray ionization mass spectrometry (LIAD–ESI/MS) is a technique combining an electrospray and a pulsed laser beam to characterize solid and liquid samples with minimal sample preparation [48]. Although the instrumental setup of LIAD–ESI is similar to that of ELDI, the laser intensity required for LIAD (i.e., $10^8$ W/cm$^2$) is higher than that for ELDI, and the desorption mechanism of LIAD is also different from that of LD. In LIAD, the sample is not desorbed by direct laser irradiation, but by acoustic and shock waves induced by the laser irradiation. A pulsed laser beam with a flux energy of several mJ is used to irradiate the rear of a thin metal foil (e.g., Al, Ti, Cu, and Ta; 5–25 μm thickness) to generate acoustic and shock waves [48–50]. These laser-induced

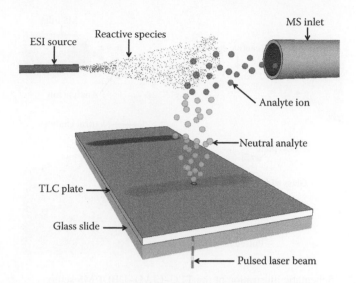

**FIGURE 7.6**   Schematic illustration of the TLC–LIAD–ESI/MS setup.

acoustic and shock waves propagate through the metal substrate to desorb analytes deposited on the other side. LIAD has been demonstrated to desorb analytes without producing analyte fragments (which are always generated during direct laser irradiation). The desorbed analytes are postionized in an ESI plume positioned several millimeters above the sample surface, forming singly and multiply charged analyte ions. LIAD–ESI/MS has been used to analyze biological fluids and solids for chemical compounds including proteins, peptides, dyes, lipids, and amino acids [48].

Integration of TLC and LIAD was reported in 2009 for characterization of analytes on separated $C_{18}$ and silica TLC plates (Figure 7.6) [31]. Because a TLC plate is much thicker than the metal foil reported in previous studies, a larger laser density (i.e., $2.1 \times 10^9$ W/cm$^2$) is needed for analyte desorption in TLC–LIAD/ESI/MS. In addition, a viscous solution such as glycerol and polyethylene glycol is applied between a glass slide and the aluminum side of the TLC plate to efficiently transfer acoustic and shock waves. An aqueous ESI solution of 50% methanol with 0.1% acetic acid was used for position ion detection, whereas 100% methanol was used for negative ion detection. It was found that the diameter of the ablated area (i.e., 1.3 mm for normal-phase silica TLC plates and 3 mm for reverse-phase $C_{18}$ TLC plates) on the TLC gel bed was bigger than the laser spot (i.e., 0.35 mm) at the rear of the aluminum plate. Thus, the TLC–LIAD/ESI approach provides a lower spatial resolution than TLC–ELDI/MS. TLC–LIAD–ESI/MS has been used to characterize mixtures of drugs, dyes, and essential oils with detection limits in the ng levels.

### 7.2.7   LASER-INDUCED ACOUSTIC DESORPTION–DIELECTRIC BARRIER DISCHARGE IONIZATION

Similar to that of LIAD–ESI, the combination of LIAD and APCI has been developed and used to characterize analytes on TLC plates [32]. A schematic illustration

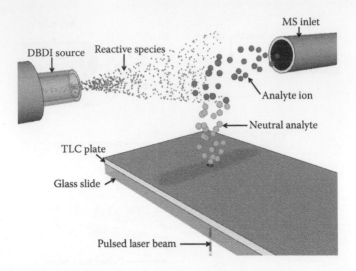

**FIGURE 7.7**    Schematic illustration of the TLC–LIAD–DBDI/MS setup.

of TLC–LIAD–APCI/MS is shown in Figure 7.7. In this approach, a dielectric barrier discharge ionization (DBDI) source was utilized to generate plasma by applying a high AC voltage (i.e., 9.7 $kV_{pp}$, 19 kHz) to a stream of nitrogen gas heated at 200°C. A glass slide and glycerol solution was used to improve the desorption efficiency of analytes on TLC plates. A pulsed IR laser beam operated at 1064 nm and 2 Hz was used to irradiate the underneath of an aluminum TLC plate to desorb analyte spots deposited on the other side. The desorbed analytes were postionized via reactions with charged species generated by DBDI and then detected by MS. Since DBDI is useful for ionizing less-polar and nonpolar compounds, TLC–LIAD–DBDI/MS has been used to characterize a mixture of aromatic compounds including carbazole, triphenylphosphine, and fluoranthene, showing radical and protonated analyte ions in the mass spectra (Figure 7.8). Complex samples such as essential and crude oils were also separated and detected without sample pretreatment.

## 7.3  CONCLUSION

Laser-based AMS approaches that combine laser irradiation and API sources (including ESI and APCI) are capable of direct characterization of chemical and biochemical compounds without tedious sample preparation, are time- and labor-saving, and allow high-throughput analysis. These approaches have been utilized to analyze complex samples separated on TLC plates. Sampling of analytes via laser irradiation of a focused area provides a means for scanning TLC plates to obtain chromatographic information and molecular images of chemical compounds, which is useful for precisely realizing the distribution of analytes on separated TLC plates. Because only a small portion of the analytes is desorbed from the gel bed for MS detection, the sensitivities of laser-based TLC–AMS approaches are obviously poorer than conventional methods where the analyte spots are scraped, extracted,

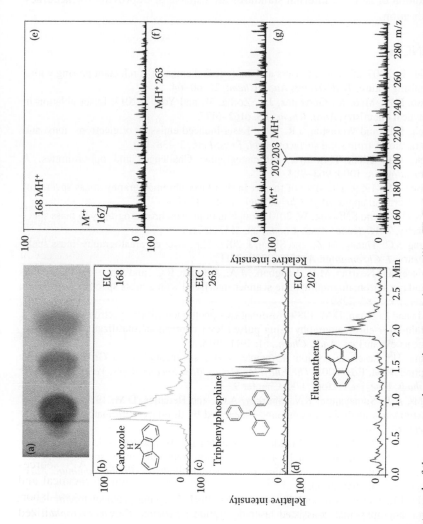

**FIGURE 7.8** (a) Photograph of three separated aromatic compounds on a silica TLC plate. Extracted ion chromatograms of (b) carbazole (MH+, m/z 168), (c) triphenylphosphine (MH+, m/z 263), and (d) fluoranthene (M+·, m/z 202), and LIAD–DBDI mass spectra of (e) carbazole, (f) triphenylphosphine, and (g) fluoranthene.

concentrated, and filtered for MS detection. It must be cautioned that some of the detached TLC gel particles may enter the MS; this may damage the vacuum system of MS. An ion funnel system that enables the manipulation and focusing of ions at ambient pressure will be useful for preventing the gel particles from entering into the MS orifice and reducing the loss of analyte ions, improving the detection limit of laser-based TLC–AMS approaches. Furthermore, quantification strategies such as the addition of isotopic internal standards are capable of improving the accuracy of quantification.

## REFERENCES

1. Smith, B. 2007. 25 years of lasers and analytical chemistry: A reluctant pairing with a promising future, *TrAC-Trends Anal. Chem.*, 26: 60–64.
2. Russo, R.E., Mao, X., Gonzalez, J.J., Zorba, V., and Yoo, J. 2013. Laser ablation in analytical chemistry, *Anal. Chem.*, 85: 6162–6177.
3. Honig, R.E. and Woolston, J.R. 1963. Laser-induced emission of electrons, ions, and neutral atoms from solid surfaces, *Appl. Phys. Lett.*, 2: 138–139.
4. Poole, C.F. 2003. Thin-layer chromatography: Challenges and opportunities, *J. Chromatogr. A*, 1000: 963–984.
5. Wilson, I.D. 1999. The state of the art in thin-layer chromatography–mass spectrometry: A critical appraisal, *J. Chromatogr. A*, 856: 429–442.
6. Morlock, G. and Schwack, W. 2010. Coupling of planar chromatography to mass spectrometry, *TrAC-Trends Anal. Chem.*, 29: 1157–1171.
7. Cheng, S.C., Huang, M.Z., and Shiea, J. 2011. Thin layer chromatography–mass spectrometry, *J. Chromatogr. A*, 1218: 2700–2711.
8. Ramaley, L., Nearing, M.E., Vaughan. M.A., Ackman, R.G., and Jamieson, W.D. 1983. Thin-layer chromatographic plate scanner interfaced with a mass spectrometer, *Anal. Chem.*, 55: 2285–2289.
9. Li, L. and Lubman, D.M. 1989. Resonant two-photon ionization spectroscopic analysis of thin-layer chromatography using pulsed laser desorption/volatilization into supersonic jet expansions, *Anal. Chem.*, 61: 1911–1915.
10. Rohrs, H., Laser desorption: Principles and instrumentation, in Gross, M.L. and Caprioli, R.M. Eds. 2007. *The Encyclopedia of Mass Spectrometry, Vol. 6, Ionization Methods*, Elsevier, Oxford, UK, Chapter 9.
11. Kubis, A.J., Somayajula, K.V., Sharkey, A.G., and Hercules, D.M. 1989. Laser mass spectrometric analysis of compounds separated by thin-layer chromatography, *Anal. Chem.*, 61: 2516–2523.
12. Shariatgorji, M., Spacil, Z., Maddalo, G., Cardenas, L.B., and Ilag, L.L. 2009. Matrix-free thin-layer chromatography–laser desorption ionization mass spectrometry for facile separation and identification of medicinal alkaloids, *Rapid Commun. Mass Spectrom.*, 23: 3655–3660.
13. Mehl, J.T., Gusev, A.I., and Hercules, D.M. 1997. Coupling protocol for thin layer chromatography–matrix-assisted laser desorption ionization, *Chromatographia*, 46: 358–364.
14. Gusev, A.I., Proctor, A., Rabinovich, Y.I., and Hercules, D.M. 1995. Thin-layer chromatography combined with matrix-assisted laser desorption/ionization mass spectrometry, *Anal. Chem.*, 67: 1805–1814.
15. Chen, Y.C., Shiea, J., and Sunner, J. 1998. Thin-layer chromatography–mass spectrometry using activated carbon, surface-assisted laser desorption/ionization, *J. Chromatogr. A*, 826: 77–86.

16. Crecelius, A., Clench, M.R., Richards, D.S., and Parr, V. 2002. Thin-layer chromatography–matrix-assisted laser desorption ionization-time-of-flight mass spectrometry using particle suspension matrices, *J. Chromatogr. A,* 958: 249–260.
17. Santos, L.S., Haddad, R., Hoehr, N.F., Pilli, R.A., and Eberlin, M.N. 2004. Fast screening of low molecular weight compounds by thin-layer chromatography and "on-spot" MALDI-TOF mass spectrometry, *Anal. Chem.,* 76: 2144–2147.
18. Dreisewerd, K., Müthing, J., Rohlfing, A., Meisen, I., Vukelić, Z., Peter-Katalinić, J., Hillenkamp, F., and Berkenkamp, S. 2005. Analysis of gangliosides directly from thin-layer chromatography plates by infrared matrix-assisted laser desorption/ionization orthogonal time-of-flight mass spectrometry with a glycerol matrix, *Anal. Chem.,* 77: 4098–4107.
19. Meisen, I., Distler, U., Müthing, J., Berkenkamp, S., Dreisewerd, K., Mathys, W., Karch, H., and Mormann M. 2009. Direct coupling of high-performance thin-layer chromatography with UV spectroscopy and IR-MALDI orthogonal TOF MS for the analysis of cyanobacterial toxins, *Anal. Chem.,* 81: 3858–3866.
20. Fuchs, B., Süß, R., Nimptsch, A., and Schiller, J. 2009. MALDI–TOF–SIMS combined with TLC: A review of the current state, *Chromatographia,* 69: S95–S105.
21. Meisen, I., Mormann, M., and Müthing, J. 2011. Thin-layer chromatography, overlay technique and mass spectrometry: A versatile triad advancing glycosphingolipidomics, *Biochim. Biophys. Acta,* 1811: 875–896.
22. Fuchs, B. 2012. Analysis of phospolipids and glycolipids by thin-layer chromatography–matrix-assisted laser desorption and ionization mass spectrometry, *J. Chromatogr. A,* 1259: 62–73.
23. Chen, Y.C. and Wu, J.Y. 2001. Analysis of small organics on planar silica surfaces using surface-assisted laser desorption/ionization mass spectrometry, *Rapid Commun. Mass Spectrom.,* 15: 1899–1903.
24. Wu, J.Y. and Chen, Y.C. 2002. A novel approach of combining thin-layer chromatography with surface-assisted laser desorption/ionization (SALDI) time-of-flight mass spectrometry, *J. Mass Spectrom.,* 37: 85–90.
25. Chen, C.C., Yang, Y.L., Ou, C.L., Chou, C.H., Liaw, C.C., and Lin, P.C. 2013. Direct monitoring of chemical transformations by combining thin layer chromatography with nanoparticle-assisted laser desorption/ionization mass spectrometry, *Analyst,* 138: 1379–1385.
26. Gusev, A.I., Vasseur, O.J., Proctor, A., Sharkey, A.G., and Hercules, D.M. 1995. Imaging of thin-layer chromatograms using matrix-assisted laser desorption/ionization mass spectrometry, *Anal. Chem.,* 67: 4565–4570.
27. Lin, S.Y., Huang, M.Z., Chang, H.C., and Shiea, J. 2007. Using electrospray-assisted laser desorption/ionization mass spectrometry to characterize organic compounds separated on thin-layer chromatography plates, *Anal. Chem.,* 79: 8789–8795.
28. Zhang, J., Zhou, Z., Yang, J., Zhangm, W., Bai, Y., and Liu, H. 2012. Thin layer chromatography–plasma assisted multiwavelength laser desorption ionization mass spectrometry for facile separation and selective identification of low molecular weight compounds, *Anal. Chem.,* 84: 1496–1503.
29. Peng, S., Edler, M., Ahlmann, N., Hoffmann, T., and Franzke, J. 2005. A new interface to couple thin-layer chromatography with laser desorption–atmospheric pressure chemical ionization mass spectrometry for plate scanning, *Rapid Commun. Mass Spectrom.,* 19: 2789–2793.
30. Shiea, J., Cheng, S.C., Jhang, S.S., and Hung, R.H. 2014. Detection of polar and non-polar compounds on TLC plate using laser desorption–electrospray + atmospheric pressure chemical ionization/mass spectrometry (LD/ESI + APCI/MS), *HPTLC 2014,* Lyon, France, July 2–4, Abstract O-8.
31. Cheng, S.C., Huang, M.Z., and Shiea, J. 2009. Thin-layer chromatography–laser-induced acoustic desorption/electrospray ionization mass spectrometry, *Anal. Chem.,* 81: 9274–9281.

32. Cheng, S.C. and Shiea, J. 2014. Thin layer chromatography–laser-induced acoustic desorption/atmospheric pressure chemical ionization mass spectrometry, *HPTLC 2014*, Lyon, France, July 2–4, Abstract P-28.

33. Shiea, J., Huang, M.Z., Hsu, H.J., Lee, C.Y., Yuan, C.H., Beech, I., and Sunner J. 2005. Electrospray-assisted laser desorption/ionization mass spectrometry for direct ambient analysis of solids, *Rapid Commun. Mass Spectrom.*, 19: 3701–3704.

34. Shiea, J., Chang, D.Y., Lin, C.H., and Jiang, S.J. 2001. Generating multiply charged protein ions by ultrasonic nebulization/multiple channel-electrospray ionization mass spectrometry, *Anal. Chem.*, 73: 4983–4987.

35. Huang, M.Z., Hsu, H.J., Wu, C.I. Lin, S.Y., Ma, Y.L., Cheng, T.L., and Shiea, J. 2007. Characterization of the chemical components on the surface of different solids with electrospray-assisted laser desorption ionization mass spectrometry, *Rapid Commun. Mass Spectrom.*, 21: 1767–1775.

36. Peng, I.X., Shiea, J., Ogorzalek Loo., R.R., and Loo, J.A. 2007. Electrospray-assisted laser desorption/ionization and tandem mass spectrometry of peptides and proteins, *Rapid Commun. Mass Spectrom.*, 21: 2541–2546.

37. Cheng, S.C., Lin, Y.S., Huang, M.Z., and Shiea, J. 2010. Applications of electrospray laser desorption ionization mass spectrometry for document examination, *Rapid Commun. Mass Spectrom.*, 24: 203–208.

38. Huang, M.Z., Cheng, S.C., Jhang, S.S., Chou, C.C., Cheng, C.N., Shiea, J., Popov, IA., and Nikolaev, EN. 2012. Ambient molecular imaging of dry fungus surface by electrospray laser desorption ionization mass spectrometry, *Int. J. Mass Spectrom.*, 325–327: 172–182.

39. Kao, Y.Y., Cheng, C.N., Cheng, S.C., Ho, H.O., and Shiea, J. 2013. Distinguishing authentic and counterfeit banknotes by surface chemical composition determined using electrospray laser desorption ionization mass spectrometry, *J. Mass Spectrom.*, 48: 1129–1135.

40. Cheng, C.Y., Yuan, C.H., Cheng, S.C., Huang, M.Z., Chang, H.C., Cheng, T.L., Yeh, CS., and Shiea, J. 2008. Electrospray-assisted laser desorption/ionization mass spectrometry for continuously monitoring the states of ongoing chemical reactions in organic or aqueous solution under ambient conditions, *Anal. Chem.*, 80: 7699–7705.

41. Shiea, J., Yuan, C.H., Huang, M.Z., Cheng, S.C., Ma, Y.L., Tseng, W.L., Chang H.C., and Hung, W.C. 2008. Detection of native protein ions in aqueous solution under ambient conditions by electrospray laser desorption/ionization mass spectrometry, *Anal. Chem.*, 80: 4845–4852.

42. Cheng, S.C., Huang, M.Z., Wu, L.C., Chou, C.C., Cheng, C.N., Jhang, S.S., and Shiea, J. 2012. Building blocks for the development of an interface for high-throughput thin layer chromatography–ambient mass spectrometric analysis: A green methodology, *Anal. Chem.*, 84: 5864–5868.

43. Cody, R.B., Laramée, J.A., and Durst, H.D. 2005. Versatile new ion source for the analysis of materials in open air under ambient conditions, *Anal. Chem.*, 77: 2297–2302.

44. Zhang, J., Li, Z., Zhang, C., Feng, B., Zhou, Z., Bai, Y., and Liu, H. 2012. Graphite-coated paper as substrate for high sensitivity analysis in ambient surface-assisted laser desorption/ionization mass spectrometry, *Anal. Chem.*, 84: 3296–3301.

45. Feng, B., Zhang, J., Chang, C., Li, L., Li, M., Xiong, X., Guo, C., Tang, F., Bai, Y., and Liu, H. 2014. Ambient mass spectrometry imaging: Plasma assisted laser desorption ionization mass spectrometry imaging and its applications, *Anal. Chem.*, 86: 4164–4169.

46. Peng, S., Ahlmann, N., Kunze, K., Nigge, W., Edler, M., Hoffmann, T., and Franzke, J. 2004. Thin-layer chromatography combined with diode laser desorption/atmospheric pressure chemical ionization mass spectrometry, *Rapid Commun. Mass Spectrom.*, 18: 1803–1808.

47. Cheng, S.C., Jhang, S.S., Huang, M.Z., and Shiea, J. 2015. Simultaneous detection of polar and nonpolar compounds by ambient mass spectrometry with a dual electrospray and atmospheric pressure chemical ionization source, *Anal. Chem.*, 87: 1743–1748.
48. Cheng, S.C., Cheng, T.L., Chang, H.C., and Shiea, J. 2009. Using laser-induced acoustic desorption/electrospray ionization mass spectrometry to characterize small organic and large biological compounds in the solid state and in solution under ambient conditions, *Anal. Chem.*, 81: 868–874.
49. Zinovev, A.V., Veryovkin, I.V., Moore, J.F., and Pellin, M.J. 2007. Laser-driven acoustic desorption of organic molecules from back-irradiated solid foils, *Anal. Chem.*, 79: 8232–8241.
50. Nyadong, L., McKenna, A.M., Hendrickson, C.L., Rodgers, R.P., and Marshall, A.G. 2011. Atmospheric pressure laser-induced acoustic desorption chemical ionization Fourier transform ion cyclotron resonance mass spectrometry for the analysis of complex mixtures, *Anal. Chem.*, 83: 1616–1623.

# 8 TLC–MS Analysis Using Solvent Elution of Compounds from Chromatographic Media

*Alen Albreht and Irena Vovk*

## CONTENTS

## 8.1 INTRODUCTION

Thin-layer chromatography (TLC) is a truly versatile analytical tool that is used in many industrial areas but, more importantly, also in scientific fields such as medicinal and pharmaceutical analysis, food quality and safety, organic synthesis, phytochemistry, forensics, environmental chemistry, and many other branches of life sciences. It is a complementary technique to other well-established separation techniques such as high-performance liquid chromatography (HPLC), gas chromatography (GC), capillary electrophoresis (CE), and others. The basic concept of TLC is to separate compounds on a planar chromatographic adsorbent as the developing solvent moves up the plate by capillary action, carrying the analytes alongside. The identity of compounds can afterward be tentatively determined according to their $R_F$ values (migration distances), bioluminescence, intrinsic colors or colors that arise from nonspecific chemical derivatizations, and according to their ultraviolet–visible (UV–Vis) or fluorescence spectra. However, by combination of TLC with additional techniques such as mass spectrometry (MS), one can identify individual analytes with increased certainty. At first, mostly experimental analysts made use of TLC–MS, which aided in the structural elucidation of (unknown) compounds and was not considered reliable for quantitative analysis. However, the innovations and the development of analytical instrumentation soon changed that.

Interfacing TLC with MS can be achieved in four different ways: (1) the compounds of interest are extracted or eluted, respectively, from the chromatographic adsorbent, redissolved in a secondary solvent and introduced into the MS as a discrete sample; (2) the analytes are introduced into the MS still interconnected with the chromatographic matrix; (3) the entire intact chromatogram is placed inside an ion source of the MS and, consequently, the surface of the plate can be fully mapped; and (4) the analytes are eluted from the chromatographic plate and introduced into the MS in a simultaneous fashion. However, the purpose of this chapter is not to give an exhaustive review on every aspect of TLC–MS, but rather to present the development and basic concepts of elution-based online TLC–MS. Advantages and challenges of this approach and a comparison with the conventional offline TLC–MS will be covered. For a more general survey on TLC–MS, the reader is directed elsewhere [1–6].

## 8.2   A BRIEF HISTORICAL OVERVIEW

An indirect elution-based TLC–MS analysis has been known for decades. In the beginning, this approach was employed as an alternative technique for the analysis of nonvolatile and labile analytes that could not be thermally desorbed from the chromatographic media and subsequently analyzed by electron ionization (EI) or chemical ionization mass spectrometry (CI–MS), respectively. Toward the end of 1960s, offline TLC–MS approach was already well established and it usually included scraping the adsorbent from the TLC support and extraction of nonvolatile compounds into a secondary solvent, which was eventually introduced into the inlet of an MS analyzer. On the other hand, progress and innovation in the field of online coupling was slow and mostly based on advances of HPLC–MS instrumentation, which received considerably more attention at that time compared to TLC–MS. In contrast to the well-established HPLC–MS and GC–MS, TLC–MS requires an interface that has to ensure a stable liquid sample introduction into the MS from a static planar, open chromatogram. The appearance of atmospheric pressure ionization MS marked an important turning point at which several direct elution-based interfaces started to emerge.

The first device for direct quantitative elution of compounds from TLC plates was introduced as early as 1975 [7]. The so-called "Eluchrom" used a circular sampling probe to extract the spots from a developed TLC plate. The adsorbent was scraped off in a ring around the area of interest to allow a tight seal for the elution cylinder. As the solvent flowed through the layer, it extracted the compounds, which were collected in a glass vessel. Although the device was not coupled with an MS, this study can be considered an early pioneering work in the evolution of online elution-based TLC–MS. Based on this groundwork, in 2004 Luftmann devised an online TLC–MS interface in the form of an elution head extraction device [8]. It delivered high MS sensitivity as the elution of sample from the chromatographic plate was brought to completion. Various improvements that ensued in the following years enabled a broader applicability of this interface. This was the first commercially available online TLC–MS interface, which was patented in 2002 and traded under the name "ChromeXtrakt" by ChromAn. In 2009, an upgraded device simply called "TLC–MS Interface" was introduced by CAMAG and replaced the former. Today, this tool is the most widely utilized elution-based TLC–MS interface in the world. However, it does have some deficiencies. It offers rather low-spatial resolution and, consequently, it also lacks imaging capability.

In 1998, Anderson and Busch presented an offline TLC–MS probe composed of an array of microcapillaries [9]. This device lacked the general sensitivity of Luftmann's device because it only sampled the uppermost layer of the TLC plate. Nevertheless, it also planted the idea of MS imaging of sample spots from the developed TLC plates by an elution-based approach. Van Berkel further developed this concept in 2002 [10]. A liquid microjunction surface sampling probe enabled stepwise as well as continuous sampling mode of operation, which theoretically could be used for imaging analyses of whole TLC plates. The spatial resolution was a function of scan speed and the nature of the eluting solvent. This device underwent many improvements in the following years; however, it has been never commercialized.

A few additional, somewhat exotic, online TLC–MS approaches were also brought forward in the early beginning of this millennium and these included mostly couplings between continuous or overrun TLC with MS [11–13]. The design of these interfaces imitates conventional HPLC–MS in which all compounds are consecutively eluted from the chromatographic media and fed into the MS inlet. Only a number of individual research groups put their interest into the development of these concepts, which can prove cumbersome or laborious.

The operation and characteristics of all of the mentioned elution-based interfaces will be addressed in more detail in the next section of this chapter.

## 8.3 ONLINE SOLVENT ELUTION TLC–MS

Indirect or offline elution-based TLC–MS approach has been well established for quite some time. This laborious and time-consuming procedure usually involves removal of the analyte-containing adsorbent from the developed chromatographic plate, extraction of compound into a secondary solvent, filtration and/or centrifugation, and finally introduction of the sample solution into the MS system. The complete process might have a detrimental effect on compounds that prove unstable when exposed to light, heat, acids or bases, oxidants, etc. On the other hand, in direct or online elution-based TLC–MS analysis, the sample is extracted from the plates and subjected to MS analysis in a simultaneous fashion. This significantly speeds up and simplifies the overall analysis. Online TLC–MS under ambient conditions, such as solvent elution, also overcomes many obstacles that burden most vacuum-based approaches: (1) chromatographic plates of various sizes can be employed without any custom modifications to the ion source; (2) atmospheric pressure enables fast chromatogram switching, which results in high-throughput analysis; and (3) all volatile and nonvolatile analytes can be analyzed. Therefore, continuous-type ion sources, which operate under atmospheric pressure (e.g., electrospray [ESI], atmospheric pressure chemical ionization [APCI], and atmospheric pressure photoionization [APPI]), are ideal for online solvent elution TLC–MS. This is not surprising as, in some way, this technique mimics the well-established HPLC–MS.

The main function of an online TLC–MS interface is to free the sample molecules that are adsorbed on the chromatographic adsorbent and transport them from the plates to the MS source in a liquid or gaseous phase. What separates outstanding interfaces from ordinary ones is their ease and speed of operation, high sensitivity and specificity, broad compatibility with various types of TLC plates and stationary phases, good spatial resolution, affordability, and automation. Different online elution-based TLC–MS concepts have been devised. In many cases, they evolved from successful offline approaches. In this respect, the work from Anderson and Busch surely presents an important stepping-stone [9]. This offline interface consists of an array of extraction microcapillaries, although a larger probe with a single channel was originally prepared (Figure 8.1). The suitable extraction solvent is supplied to the TLC spot (band) through these small capillary tubes, which form the extraction probe. The probe does not come in contact with the developed TLC plate, only the solvent diffuses into the uppermost layer of the plate, which enables the dissolution and extraction of compounds into the solvent. The analyte-containing eluate is then drawn by capillary action up into the adsorbent material, which surrounds the inlet capillary tubes. The sample is then acquired by a subsequent reextraction from the adsorbent material. This configuration enables 2D imaging of samples on the developed plates and the resolution is limited by the number of microcapillaries. An improvement of the single channel probe includes: (1) an additional procedure of isolation of the sample spot by a ring of wax to prevent the solvent from spreading

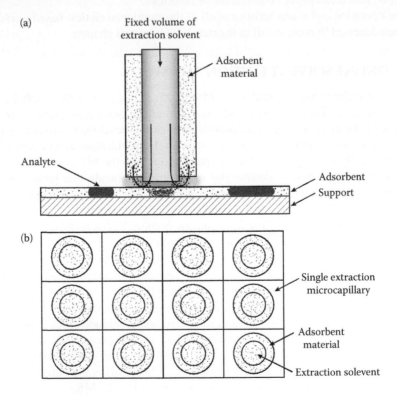

**FIGURE 8.1** Schematic representation of a single capillary probe (a) and a cross section of a microcapillary array (b).

across the plate and (2) a concomitant increase in extraction efficiency due to incorporation of a worm solvent.

One of the first online elution-based TLC–MS interfaces is represented by a microjunction surface sampling probe, which extracts compounds from reversed phase (RP) C8 and C18 TLC plates (Figure 8.2) [10]. The chromatograms can be scanned in a stepwise or continuous sampling mode. The probe has two coaxial capillary channels and is positioned perpendicularly to the TLC surface at a distance of approximately 50 µm above the plate. The probe's outer channel serves as an inlet for the extraction solvent and the extracted analytes are transferred to the MS system through the inner channel by self-aspiration. This is achieved because of a local vacuum created by pneumatic nebulization along with the electrostatic field created by applying a high-ESI voltage. The space between the probe and the plate represents a small but stable liquid microjunction where the extraction into the solvent takes place. It is crucial for the solvent to be contained within the probe confines so that no flooding of the stationary phase occurs. Therefore, a compromise in solvent system that balances analyte solubility and phase wettability is required. The lack of an appropriate extraction solvent can pose a serious drawback of this approach. A solvent with a high-contact angle with the stationary phase usually insufficiently extracts the analytes from the TLC matrix, which can markedly affect the MS sensitivity. On the other hand, solvents with good solubility characteristics cause considerable leakage, which renders the TLC–MS analysis impossible. Nonetheless, by having an appropriate approach, this technique can serve as a convenient tool in qualitative and quantitative TLC–MS analysis [14,15]. The procedure was subsequently optimized to extend the analytical utility also to wettable surfaces without any flooding of TLC

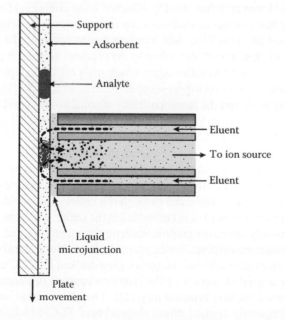

**FIGURE 8.2**    Schematic representation of a liquid-microjunction surface sampling probe.

or HPTLC plates, respectively [16]. This involved coating of hydrophilic silica and cellulose plates in a hydrophobic layer, which enabled online TLC–MS. The same is achieved by blotting the analytes from a developed hydrophilic plate to a topmost surface of a hydrophobic adsorbent, from which the compounds can be sampled in the usual fashion [17]. An important step toward automation of this technique is represented by an implementation of the monitoring and automated adjustment of the sampling probe-to-surface distance [18].

A related technique, which is based on the same liquid microjunction principle, is called liquid extraction surface analysis (LESA) and is best used in combination with chip-based nano-ESI [19,20]. Again, for polar extraction solvents (relatively high-water percentage), a hydrophobic stationary phase is crucial for the formation of the liquid junction. The mode of operation is fairly simple and automated. A small amount of extraction solvent is at first aspirated into a conductive pipette tip by its immersion into the solvent reservoir. The tip is then moved to the TLC plate and the extraction solvent is dispensed onto the sample spot in the form of a drop. Quickly after, the analyte containing solvent is aspirated back into the pipette, which is then moved to the ESI ionization chip. The nano-ESI is initiated by applying the appropriate high voltage to the pipette tip and gas pressure on the liquid. Although it seems straightforward at first glance, this technique provides some challenges. A highly aqueous elution solvent provides poor analyte solubility, and hence, solvent composition is always chosen in a way that positions it on the brink of phase wettability. This has a profound negative effect on method sensitivity. Additionally, the extraction solvent should ideally enable effective ionization of compounds. Given the compromised approach, this is rather difficult to achieve, and therefore, LESA is clearly still in its infancy and it has a long way to go before it can be used routinely in the laboratory. However, it has already attracted some attention [21].

Another probe that samples analytes directly from the developed chromatographic plates was designed [8]. This TLC–MS interface can be considered a simplified and improved analog of "Eluchrom" described in the previous section. It uses an elution head encircled with a sharp metallic edge, which seals off the sampled area by cutting into the sorbent until it firmly presses against the solid support (Figure 8.3). This solves the flooding issue and the incompatibility of some common solvent extraction systems with different stationary phases. Nevertheless, leakages still occurred at first in rare cases when RP C8 or C18 stationary phases were used [22]. However, this inconvenience was dealt with in time by further improvements. The interface utilizes the following principle of operation. The elution solvent pumped by an LC pump is delivered to the elution head through an inlet capillary. The analytes are extracted from the isolated area and transferred through the outlet capillary directly into the MS ion source. An inline filter frit is embedded at the outlet, which prevents any particulate matter (mostly chromatographic sorbent) from entering and damaging the MS system. Although the original device was only amenable to aluminum foils, subsequent modifications also allowed the use of glass-backed HPTLC and TLC plates [22]. Yet another upgraded version of the interface enabled full automation, which resulted in improved method repeatability [23]. The elution-head interface is currently the most frequently applied direct elution-based TLC–MS interface [24–38]. This technique, however, does not enable continuous scanning of chromatograms

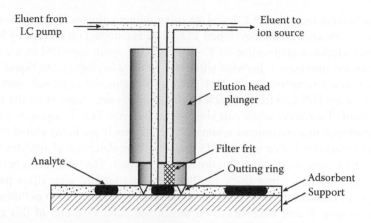

**FIGURE 8.3** Schematic representation of an elution-head based interface. It comprises a sharp edge, which effectively seals the sampled area.

because the elution head has to be manually lowered onto the layer and raised again after each extraction cycle. Moreover, the chromatographic resolution is dependent on the geometry of the cutting tool—the narrower the probe, the better the resolution. Compared to some vacuum-based TLC–MS interfaces, elution head-based solvent extraction device does not preserve the original chromatogram, but again, high-extraction yields allow for high sensitivity with low limits of detection. It can be used for qualitative [39–47] as well as for quantitative analysis [48–52]. Accurate, repeatable, and precise quantitative results were elegantly obtained for the determination of caffeine in pharmaceutical and energy drink samples using stable isotope dilution analysis [53]. Since elution of compounds proceeds independent of the MS ion source, this technique is therefore nondestructive and can alternatively be applied for compound isolation, which can eventually be further subjected to diverse chromatographic, chemical, and spectroscopic analyses [24,54]. This probe was also successfully applied in the analysis of urinary analytes, which were analyzed by TLC–MS using an innovative online gradient solvent elution of the samples from an undeveloped plate [55]. The method provides satisfactory resolution of analytes and reduction of ion suppression stemming from interfering compounds. In another study, this interface was utilized for direct quantitative analysis of dried blood spots (DBS) and gave good bioanalytical results [56]. The method demonstrated superior sensitivity compared to that of manual extraction, which allowed for direct analysis of drugs in DBS samples at physiologically relevant concentrations. Even lower limits of quantitation in DBS analysis can be achieved by combining direct elution of the blood spot with online SPE–LC–MS/MS [57].

Right around the time when the cutting metallic-edge probe was introduced, Prošek et al. demonstrated a similar functioning online TLC–MS extraction device of their own [58]. This interface also uses a cutting extraction head, which isolates the sample area from the surroundings and therefore prevents diffusion of solvent and analyte throughout the TLC adsorbent. Somewhat laborious but computer-controlled elution of compounds is accomplished with two syringes that pump solvent into and withdraw solvent from the TLC layer. Working with an aliquot loop injection, only 10% of the substance on the developed TLC plate is detected on average by MS.

Another elution-based online TLC–MS coupling again uses ESI as a constituent part of the interface, otherwise witnessed in the aforementioned liquid-microjunction surface sampling probe [11]. This unconventional approach mimics the operation of an HPLC–MS, in which the compounds are eluted from the column and detected. Therefore, when carrying out an overrun TLC analysis, the plate is being developed in a continuous manner and compounds are being eluted from the end of a miniaturized plate into the MS system, where detection of analytes occurs. Two distinct setups are possible (Figure 8.4). In the first, TLC analysis is performed in a 2-mm wide and 1-mm thick capillary channel packed with silica particles. Although the channel of these dimensions can hardly be referred to as "thin-layer" chromatography, it still deserves to be mentioned here. One end of this channel is connected to the developing solvent reservoir, and two bound optical fibers are sticking out on the other end to a distance of 5 mm. They measure 125 μm in diameter and are buried in the layer. At this side of the chromatogram, a makeup solution

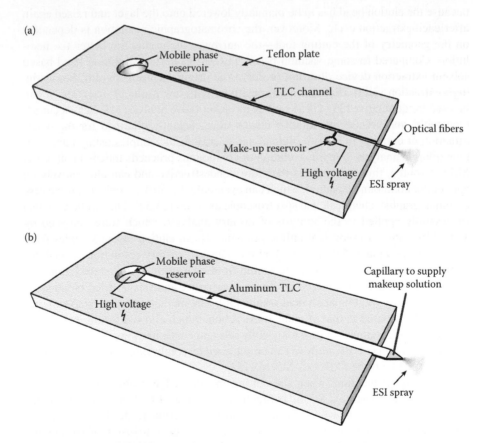

**FIGURE 8.4** Schematic representation of two overrun TLC systems based on (a) capillary TLC channel with optical fibers and (b) sharpened aluminum TLC strip.

is also continuously supplied to assist the transfer and ionization of analytes for MS analysis. A platinum wire is inserted into the makeup reservoir and a high voltage is applied to induce ESI of the solution flowing through the fibers. These are positioned 10–15 mm away from the MS inlet. The second overrun TLC–MS configuration includes aluminum-backed TLC strips. The sorbent is scraped off at the far eluting end of the strip, which is additionally sharpened and positioned in front of the MS inlet. The blunt end of the strip is inserted into the developing solvent reservoir and a makeup solution is continuously supplied to the sharp end via a capillary. A high potential is applied to the developing solvent by inserting a platinum electrode into the reservoir and, consequently, the electrospray is generated at the sharp end of the TLC strip. In a bigger TLC system, the aluminum plate is dried after the development and each individual spot is cut out, sharpened, and placed in front of the MS inlet. After application of the spray voltage via a metal clamp, a small amount of spray solvent is dispensed onto the spot and an MS spectrum is acquired [59]. The analysis in the first two described setups takes place in an open chamber, which can significantly affect the separation efficiency due to the loss of developing solvent through evaporation. However, only up to 1 µL of sample and 200 µL of developing solvent are needed per analysis, which considerably reduces operational costs. Additionally, these interfaces are some of a few, which do not require an external ion source.

Forced-flow layer liquid chromatographic techniques such as overpressured layer chromatography (OPLC) and rotation planar chromatography (RPC) can also be coupled to MS via an elution-based interface. Again, both techniques utilize overrun or continuous development, respectively. In OPLC, the stationary phase is sealed between a solid support, to which it is bound, and an inert membrane sheet that is applied onto the plate under external pressure. The mobile phase is pumped through the layer at a constant speed and compounds eluting at the OPLC system outlet are introduced directly into the MS ion source [12,60]. In RPC, the sample is applied in the center of a circular chromatographic plate, which is then spun at approximately 1000 rpm. The developing solvent is also being continuously applied to the center of the plate and instead of just capillary action, this technique uses centrifugal force to move the eluent outward. The analytes separate from each other in the form of concentric rings, which are finally eluted from the plate in a consecutive fashion and introduced into the MS inlet [13]. Only a small part of the effluent actually reaches the MS; the rest is directed to a fraction collector, which collects the analytes for further analyses. In all continuous TLC–MS approaches, the $R_F$ values cannot be defined and are replaced with $t_R$, a parameter that is well established in HPLC and GC. Since compounds are eluted quantitatively from the plates, these techniques offer high-MS sensitivity, given that no contaminants from the chromatographic matrix suppress the analyte signal.

Elution-based TLC–MS approaches, with the exception of microjunction surface sample probe, enable transfer of the entire sample from TLC plate into the MS inlet, regardless of the sample depth distribution within the TLC layer. Therefore, the sample flux with these total consumption interfaces comes close to that obtained in column chromatography, which considerably increases the sensitivity. Unlike with some surface sampling TLC–MS interfaces (ambient as well as vacuum), this increased sensitivity also enables tandem MS analysis, which is crucial if the sample is plagued by a strong matrix or if structurally analogous compounds have similar $R_F$ values [38,48]. However, elution-based TLC–MS devices lack the high-spatial resolution and imaging capability that is readily attainable with some vacuum-based interfaces, such as MALDI, for instance. A universal interface that would elegantly combine both high sensitivity and high spatial resolution unfortunately has not been made available yet.

### 8.3.1 OFFLINE VERSUS ONLINE TLC–MS

An offline "scrape-and-extract" TLC–MS approach has been used for a long time in organic synthesis, phytochemical analysis, food analysis, pharmaceutical and medical analysis, life sciences, and related areas. This approach nowadays is often prejudicially regarded as a rudimental and outdated TLC–MS technique, but some beneficial aspects can often still make it the preferred choice. In offline mode, there are practically no limitations to the solvents and additives being used for most stages of the analysis as long as the unwanted chemicals are removed somewhere along the way to introduction of the sample into MS. This includes MS noncompatible solvents and buffers such as phosphate buffer and triethylammonium acetate, for instance. This allows for optimal extraction and stability of analytes before, during, and after TLC analysis. Therefore, if care is exercised, labile compounds can be transferred from the TLC plate to the MS with negligible analyte loss, and the sample can additionally be concentrated in a small amount of secondary solvent, which again increases method sensitivity. However, offline TLC–MS is frequently a laborious and time-consuming undertaking that is unfortunately ideal for the introduction of errors into the analysis, which are otherwise minimized in an online approach. Moreover, prolonged exposure times of analytes to acids and bases, light, heat, or oxidants can lead to oxidation, degradation, and isomerization products and similar artifacts [45,61]. Online elution-based TLC–MS enables rapid transfer of compounds from the developed plate to the MS, which reduces the risk of analyte deterioration.

However, there is a disadvantage that is typical for both elution-based TLC–MS approaches—low-spatial resolution. This deteriorates the inherent resolution of the chromatogram and makes utilization of HPTLC and UPLC plates unreasonable. Resolution in indirect analysis is determined by the operator's meticulous scraping of adsorbent from the solid support. Especially in the case of UTLC plates, it can be quite challenging to physically separate individual analyte containing bands and still attain high enough sensitivity. In direct TLC–MS analysis, the resolution is a function of probe/elution-head dimensions and scan speed in the case of microjunction surface sampling probe. The elution-based interface devised by Anderson and Busch could theoretically generate high-imaging resolution, which would be governed only by the number of microcapillaries that constitute the probe. When high resolution is essential, one can always reach for a desorption-based interface or extend the developing TLC distance. In the latter case, the interband space increases, which enables selective analyte sampling.

In the end, each approach—either offline or online elution-based TLC–MS—has its advantages and disadvantages. The technique that will be most suitable to our needs will largely depend on the type of sample at hand and on the information that we endeavor to obtain.

## 8.3.2 Pitfalls and Challenges of Online Approach

Although online solvent elution TLC–MS is an indispensable tool for an analytical chemist, it is nonetheless hampered by a few obstacles. Some were briefly mentioned in the previous section, but here we take a deeper look into the current challenges of this technique.

When doing TLC–MS, one should always keep in mind that the TLC plate submitted to MS analysis does not contain only the sample molecules but also adsorbent, which is in excess, binder, and often the fluorescent indicator. In cases where functionalized silica is utilized, traces of organic compounds might also be present. Additionally, residual solvents and salts from the developing solvent system are usually left behind after the development of the plate as well. On top of that, the eluent used for the extraction of the analyte from the adsorbent can additionally introduce a plethora of different organic and inorganic contaminants. All of the above-mentioned interferences are invariably present at any location on the TLC plate and can have a detrimental influence on an MS spectrum, causing the analyte signal to plummet in the high spectral background. Therefore, the complexity of this mixture should be minimized in order to achieve satisfactory analytical results. Solvents used for the development and for the subsequent elution of compounds from the TLC plate should be of the highest purity or at least nonvolatile impurities that accompany these chemicals should be kept to a minimum. The same applies to raw materials, which are used if TLC plates are made in-house. Even when commercial TLC or HPTLC plates are utilized, the MS background of plates from different batches is mostly irregular (Figure 8.5) [38]. Discrepancies between various plate manufacturers are even more pronounced. The impurities can cause serious ion suppression in the MS ion source and this can be rather strongly dependent on the chemistry of the adsorbent. For example, it was shown that silica gel plates could give much higher background noise than cellulose stationary phase [62]. Even recently introduced MS grade silica gel TLC plates, which are designed specifically for minimal MS noise, do not always rise to their expectations. Therefore, to remove as many contaminants as possible, it is advisable to prewash the plates with a suitable solvent system prior to TLC analysis [12]. However, in offline TLC–MS, such inconveniences can be circumvented altogether by applying additional purification steps, which diminish the influence of contaminants and interfering compounds, respectively.

Caution must be exercised when prewashing, developing, and elution solvent systems are being selected as they may contain impurities and ion suppressants, but many additional parameters also have to be considered. First, every chemical that reaches the ion source must be MS compatible. Inorganic salts and nonvolatile components left behind from the developing solvent should be removed prior to MS analysis. Moreover, the elution solvent should be comprised of only volatile solvents and buffers; otherwise damage to the MS system can easily occur. Additional parameters that affect the choice of chemicals are their chemical and physical properties. In the case of microjunction surface sampling probe, the selection of an appropriate solvent

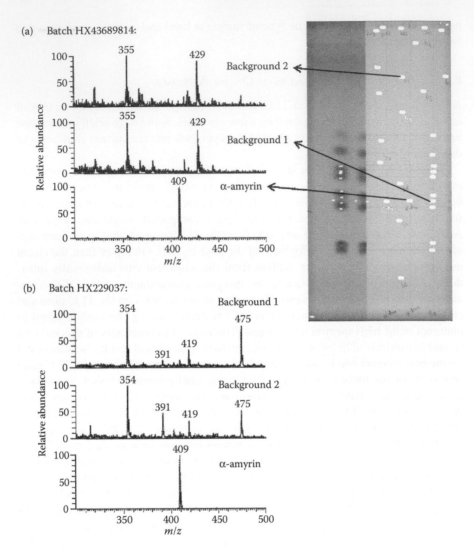

**FIGURE 8.5** Background mass spectra acquired at different $R_F$ values from two different batches of HPTLC $C_{18}$ RP plates ((a) batch HX43689814; (b) batch HX229037) predeveloped with acetone and developed in ethyl acetate-acetonitrile (3:2, v/v) and mass spectrum of α-amyrin eluted from the corresponding plate. (From Naumoska, K. and Vovk, I. 2015. *J. Chromatogr. A*, 1381: 229–238. With permission.)

is a compromise between good analyte solubility and stationary phase wettability. Excellent extraction properties of the solvent often lead to TLC leakages, but on the other hand, solvents forming a high-contact angle with the stationary phase usually insufficiently extract the compounds, which results in inadequate MS sensitivity. To compensate for the low sample flux, a nonscanning mass analyzer should be used to maximize ion transmission; otherwise, the sensitivity of the TLC–MS method is additionally degraded.

Even though the uncontrolled flooding of the plates is associated primarily with the microjunction surface sampling probe, this problem can also occur with the most widespread TLC–MS interface—a plunger-based elution-head probe. This happens in two distinct cases. The inline filter frit at the probe outlet will get blocked every so often. Consequently, the pressure inside the sealed area exponentially rises to the point at which the elution head can no longer contain the eluent, so it starts to leak at the probe-plate juncture, spreading through the chromatographic layer. For this reason, the frit has to be properly regenerated by periodic backflushing. In the second case, the wetting of the TLC phase is a result of an inadequate seal of the sampled area. The TLC–MS interface is optimized for TLC and HPTLC plates, so when ultrathin-layer chromatographic (UTLC) plates are used, a tight seal cannot be generated between the thin 10-μm monolithic layer and the elution head. However, there is a simple and elegant solution to this problem. An ordinary filter paper, prewashed with the elution solvent and dried, can be placed on top of the sample to be extracted (Figure 8.6). The plunger is then lowered and the elution head tightly presses the filter paper against the UTLC plate and properly isolates the sampling area [37]. The elution solvent can also flood TLC and HPTLC plates if there is a distortion in the stationary phase in the close vicinity of the sampled area. This is usually observed when bands with similar $R_F$ values are consecutively sampled. When the elution head cuts into the stationary phase, it slightly thrusts the external adsorbent outward, which causes minor wrinkling of the layer. Cracks may appear and if the next sample is extracted in a way in which the elution head partially overlaps with the impaired phase, the solvent will flood the plate. It is actually advised that two neighboring bands should be sampled at least a couple of millimeters apart. This requirement renders total acquisition or imaging of a single TLC track by elution-head probe impossible. One way of getting around this issue is by implementing a successive

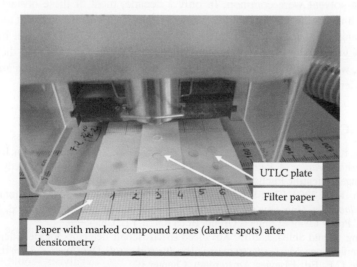

**FIGURE 8.6** UTLC–MS by modified use of CAMAG TLC–MS interface. (From Vovk, I. et al. 2011. *J. Chromatogr. A*, 1218: 3089–3094. With permission.)

zigzag sampling from two adjacent tracks, which represent equivalent samples [62]. However, switching to an alternative TLC–MS interface might prove a better option.

TLC–MS has long been used for qualitative but not for quantitative analysis. In the last couple of years, much has changed, although some pitfalls remain. Manual positioning of extraction probes can substantially contribute to the overall analytical error. Relative standard deviation of multiple replicate extractions can be as high as 18%, which is indicative of poor repeatability [22]. In addition, devices that sample only the topmost layer of the chromatogram were in the past also considered unsuitable for evaluation of compound concentration because the analyte is unevenly distributed along the thickness of the layer. Today, quantitation by online elution-based TLC–MS is carried out largely based on an isotopically labeled internal standard, which compensates for the positioning error and markedly improves the accuracy of the analytical measurement.

Compared to densitometry and desorption-based approaches (atom and ion bombardment, laser light beam, spray beam, excited gas beam) where only a few micrometers of the plate surface is being sampled, elution-based TLC–MS is a destructive technique as it extracts all or most of the sample, respectively. This sets aside one of the main advantages of TLC, which is the possibility to reevaluate chromatograms at a later time (i.e., after weeks or months).

In conclusion, elution-based online TLC–MS is just over a decade-old technique. What started out as an indirect "scrape-and-extract" approach soon matured into a semiautomated online technique that, to be quite honest, had some limitations in the beginning. Various approaches suffered from specific drawbacks and these included: (1) glass-backed plates were not amenable to TLC–MS analysis; (2) only one type of adsorbent could be used; (3) sample flux into the MS was small and sensitivity was consequently compromised, therefore, higher sample concentrations were necessary; (4) quantitation was not feasible; and (5) floodings of chromatographic plates with the elution solvent were common. In only a decade, most of these obstacles were overcome and elution-based online TLC–MS is now becoming a frequent and indispensable analytical tool. Some challenges of this technique still remain, but these will surely give birth to further advances, innovations, and automation in the field of TLC–MS, which will only enforce the use of this invaluable technique in analytical and life sciences.

## REFERENCES

1. Bush, K.L. 2001. Planar chromatography with mass spectrometric detection, In: *Planar Chromatography: A Retrospective View for the Third Millennium*, Nyiredy, S., Ed., Springer Scientific Publisher, Budapest, Chapter 14.
2. Bush, K.L. 2003. Thin-layer chromatography coupled with mass spectrometry, In: *Handbook of Thin Layer Chromatography*, 3rd ed., Sherma, J. and Fried, B., Eds., CRC Press/Taylor & Francis Group, Boca Raton, FL, Chapter 9.
3. Cheng, S. and Shiea, J. 2015. Advanced spectroscopic detectors for identification and quantification: Mass spectrometry, In: *Instrumental Thin-layer Chromatography*, Poole, C.F., Ed., Elsevier, Amsterdam, Chapter 10.
4. Cheng, S.C., Huang, M.Z., and Shiea, J. 2011. Thin layer chromatography–mass spectrometry, *J. Chromatogr. A*, 1218: 2700–2711.

5. Morlock, G. and Schwack, W. 2010. Coupling of planar chromatography to mass spectrometry, *Trends Anal. Chem.*, 29: 1157–1171.

6. Wilson, I.D. 1999. The state of the art in thin-layer chromatography–mass spectrometry: A critical appraisal, *J. Chromatogr. A*, 856: 429–442.

7. Falk, H. and Krummen, K. 1975. A new method for the quantitative evaluation of thin-layer chromatograms, *J. Chromatogr.*, 103: 279–288.

8. Luftmann, H. 2004. A simple device for the extraction of TLC spots: Direct coupling with an electrospray mass spectrometer, *Anal. Bioanal. Chem.*, 378: 964–968.

9. Anderson, R.M. and Busch, K.L. 1998. Thin-layer chromatography coupled with mass spectrometry: Interfaces to electrospray ionization, *J. Planar Chromatogr.*, 11: 336–341.

10. Van Berkel, G.J., Sanchez, A.D., and Quirke, J.M.E. 2002. Thin-layer chromatography and electrospray mass spectrometry coupled using a surface sampling probe, *Anal. Chem.*, 74: 6216–6223.

11. Hsu, F.L., Chen, C.H., Yuan, C.H., and Shiea, J. 2003. Interfaces to connect thin-layer chromatography with electrospray ionization mass spectrometry, *Anal. Chem.*, 75: 2493–2498.

12. Chai, W., Leteux, C., Lawson, A.M., and Stoll, M.S. 2003. On-line overpressure thin-layer chromatographic separation and electrospray mass spectrometric detection of glycolipids, *Anal. Chem.*, 75: 118–125.

13. Van Berkel, G.J., Llave, J.J., De Apadoca, M.F., and Ford, M.J. 2004. Rotation planar chromatography coupled on-line with atmospheric pressure chemical ionization mass spectrometry, *Anal. Chem.*, 76: 479–482.

14. Ford, M.J. and Van Berkel, G.J. 2004. An improved thin-layer chromatography–mass spectrometry coupling using a surface sampling probe electrospray ion trap system, *Rapid Commun. Mass Spectrom.*, 18: 1303–1309.

15. Ford, M.J., Deibel, M.A., Tomkins, B.A., and Van Berkel, G.J. 2005. Quantitative thin-layer chromatography–mass spectrometry analysis of caffeine using a surface sampling probe electrospray ionization tandem mass spectrometry system, *Anal. Chem.*, 77: 4385–4389.

16. Walworth, M.J., Stankovich, J.J., Van Berkel, G.J., Schulz, M., Minarik, S., Nichols, J., and Reich, E. 2011. Hydrophobic treatment enabling analysis of wettable surfaces using a liquid microjunction surface sampling probe/electrospray ionization–mass spectrometry system, *Anal. Chem.*, 83: 591–597.

17. Walworth, M.J., Stankovich, J.J., Van Berkel, G.J., Schulz, M., and Minarik, S. 2012. High-performance thin-layer chromatography plate blotting for liquid microjunction surface sampling probe mass spectrometric analysis of analytes separated on a wettable phase plate, *Rapid Commun. Mass Spectrom.*, 26: 37–42.

18. Kertesz, V., Ford, M.J., and Van Berkel, G.J. 2005. Automation of a surface sampling probe/electrospray mass spectrometry system, *Anal. Chem.*, 77: 7183–7189.

19. Kertesz, V. and Van Berkel, G.J. 2010. Fully automated liquid extraction-based surface sampling and ionization using a chip-based robotic nanoelectrospray platform, *J. Mass Spectrom.*, 45: 252–260.

20. Himmelsbach, M., Varesio, E., and Hopfgartner, G. 2014. Liquid extraction surface analysis (LESA) of hydrophobic TLC plates coupled to chip-based nanoelectrospray high-resolution mass spectrometry, *Chimia*, 68: 150–154.

21. Park, H., Zhou, Y., and Costello, C.E. 2014. Direct analysis of sialylated or sulfated glycosphingolipids and other polar and neutral lipids using TLC–MS interfaces, *J. Lipid Res.*, 55: 773–781.

22. Alpmann, A. and Morlock, G. 2006. Improved online coupling of planar chromatography with electrospray mass spectrometry: Extraction of zones from glass plates, *Anal. Bioanal. Chem.*, 386: 1543–1551.

23. Luftmann, H., Aranda, M., and Morlock, G.E. 2007. Automated interface for hyphenation of planar chromatography with mass spectrometry, *Rapid Commun. Mass Spectrom.*, 21: 3772–3776.

24. Adhami, H.R., Scherer, U., Kaehlig, H., Hettich, T., Schlotterbeck, G., Reich, E., and Krenn, L. 2013. Combination of bioautography with HPTLC–MS/NMR: A fast identification of acetylcholinesterase inhibitors from galbanum, *Phytochem. Anal.*, 24: 395–400.

25. Altmaier, S. and Schulz, M. 2015. Fast analysis of "dirty" samples with monolithic silica LC and silica gel TLC stationary phases, *LC–GC Europe*, 1: 34–39.

26. Aranda, M. and Morlock, G. 2006. Simultaneous determination of riboflavin, pyridoxine, nicotinamide, caffeine and taurine in energy drinks by planar chromatography-multiple detection with confirmation by electrospray ionization mass spectrometry, *J. Chromatogr. A*, 1131: 253–260.

27. Bertrams, J., Müller, M.B., Kunz, N., Kammerer, D.R., and Stintzing, F.C. 2013. Phenolic compounds as marker compounds for botanical origin determination of German propolis samples based on TLC and TLC–MS, *J. Appl. Bot. Food Qual.*, 86: 143–153.

28. Chen, Y. and Schwack, W. 2013. Planar chromatography mediated screening of tetracycline and fluoroquinolone antibiotics in milk by fluorescence and mass selective detection, *J. Chromatogr. A*, 1312: 143–151.

29. Glavnik, V., Simonovska, B., Albreht, A., and Vovk, I. 2012. TLC and HPLC screening of *p*-coumaric acid, *trans*-resveratrol, and pterostilbene in bacterial cultures, food supplements and wine, *J. Planar Chromatogr.*, 25: 251–258.

30. Klingelhöfer, I. and Morlock, G.E. 2014. Sharp-bounded zones link to the effect in planar chromatography–bioassay–mass spectrometry, *J. Chromatogr. A*, 1360: 288–295.

31. Klöppel, A., Grasse, W., Brümmer, F., and Morlock, G.E. 2008. HPTLC coupled with bioluminescence and mass spectrometry for bioactivity-based analysis of secondary metabolites in marine sponges, *J. Planar Chromatogr.*, 21: 431–436.

32. Mathon, C., Ankli, A., Reich, E., Bieri, S., and Christen, P. 2014. Screening and determination of sibutramine in adulterated herbal slimming supplements by HPTLC–UV densitometry, *Food Addit. Contam. A*, 31: 15–20.

33. Meriane, D., Genta-Jouve, G., Kaabeche, M., Michel, S., and Boutefnouchet, S. 2014. Rapid identification of antioxidant compounds of *Genista saharae* Coss. & Dur. by combination of DPPH scavenging assay and HPTLC–MS, *Molecules*, 19: 4369–4379.

34. Sajewicz, M., Wojtal, Ł., Natić, M., Staszek, D., Waksmundzka-Hajnos, M., and Kowalska, T. 2011. TLC–MS versus TLC–LC–MS fingerprints of herbal extracts. Part I. Essential oils, *J. Liq. Chromatogr. Relat. Technol.*, 34: 848–863.

35. Sajewicz, M., Staszek, D., Natić, M., Wojtal, Ł., Waksmundzka-Hajnos, M., and Kowalska, T. 2011. TLC–MS versus TLC–LC–MS fingerprints of herbal extracts. Part II. Phenolic acids and flavonoids, *J. Liq. Chromatogr. Relat. Technol.*, 34: 864–887.

36. Sajewicz, M., Staszek, D., Natić, M., Waksmundzka-Hajnos, M., and Kowalska, T. 2011. TLC–MS versus TLC–LC–MS fingerprints of herbal extracts. Part III. Application of the reversed-phase liquid chromatography systems with $C_{18}$ stationary phase, *J. Chromatogr. Sci.*, 49: 560–566.

37. Vovk, I., Popović, G., Simonovska, B., Albreht, A., and Agbaba, D. 2011. Ultra-thin-layer chromatography mass spectrometry and thin-layer chromatography mass spectrometry of single peptides of angiotensin-converting enzyme inhibitors, *J. Chromatogr. A*, 1218: 3089–3094.

38. Naumoska, K. and Vovk, I. 2015. Analysis of triterpenoids and phytosterols in vegetables by thin-layer chromatography coupled to tandem mass spectrometry, *J. Chromatogr. A*, 1381: 229–238.

39. Chen, Y. and Schwack, W. 2014. High-performance thin-layer chromatography screening of multi class antibiotics in animal food by bioluminescent bioautography and electrospray ionization mass spectrometry, *J. Chromatogr. A*, 1356: 249–257.

40. Chen, Y. and Schwack, W. 2014. Rapid and selective determination of multi-sulfonamides by high-performance thin layer chromatography coupled to fluorescent densitometry and electrospray ionization mass detection, *J. Chromatogr. A*, 1331: 108–116.
41. Cretu, G.C. and Morlock, G.E. 2014. Analysis of anthocyanins in powdered berry extracts by planar chromatography linked with bioassay and mass spectrometry, *Food Chem.*, 146: 104–112.
42. Krüger, S., Urmann, O., and Morlock, G.E. 2013. Development of a planar chromatographic method for quantitation of anthocyanes in pomace, feed, juice and wine, *J. Chromatogr. A*, 1289: 105–118.
43. Morlock, G.E., Meyer, S., Zimmermann, B.F., and Roussel, J.M. 2014. High-performance thin-layer chromatography analysis of steviol glycosides in *Stevia* formulations and sugar-free food products, and benchmarking with (ultra) high-performance liquid chromatography, *J. Chromatogr. A*, 1350: 102–111.
44. Naumoska, K., Simonovska, B., Albreht, A., and Vovk, I. 2013. TLC and TLC–MS screening of ursolic, oleanolic and betulinic acids in plant extracts, *J. Planar Chromatogr.*, 26: 125–131.
45. Rodić, Z., Simonovska, B., Albreht, A., and Vovk I. 2012. Determination of lutein by high-performance thin-layer chromatography using densitometry and screening of major dietary carotenoids in food supplements, *J. Chromatogr. A*, 1231: 59–65.
46. Rothenhöfer, M., Scherübl, R., Bernhardt, G., Heilmann, J., and Buschauer, A. 2012. Qualitative and quantitative analysis of hyaluronan oligosaccharides with high performance thin layer chromatography using reagent-free derivatization on amino-modified silica and electrospray ionization-quadrupole time-of-flight mass spectrometry coupling on normal phase, *J. Chromatogr. A*, 1248: 169–177.
47. Yili, A., Yimamu, H., Ghulameden, S., Qing, Z.H., Aisa, H.A., and Morlock, G.E. 2014. Determination of antidiabetic polysaccharides of *Ocimum basilicum* seeds indigenous to Xinjiang of China by high-performance thin-layer chromatography-UV–Vis-mass spectrometry, *J. Planar Chromatogr.*, 27: 11–18.
48. Jautz, U. and Morlock, G. 2006. Efficacy of planar chromatography coupled to (tandem) mass spectrometry for employment in trace analysis, *J. Chromatogr. A*, 1128: 244–250.
49. Jautz, U. and Morlock, G. 2007. Validation of a new planar chromatographic method for quantification of the heterocyclic aromatic amines most frequently found in meat, *Anal. Bioanal. Chem.*, 387: 1083–1093.
50. Morlock, G. and Schwack, W. 2006. Determination of isopropylthioxanthone (ITX) in milk, yoghurt and fat by HPTLC–FLD, HPTLC–ESI/MS and HPTLC–DART/MS, *Anal. Bioanal. Chem.*, 385: 586–595.
51. Chernetsova, E.S., Revelsky, I.A., and Morlock, G.E. 2011. Fast quantitation of 5-hydroxymethylfurfural in honey using planar chromatography, *Anal. Bioanal. Chem.*, 401: 325–332.
52. Ramesh, B., Hari babu, K., Sarma, V.U.M., and Devi, P.S. 2011. Development and validation of a HPTLC–ESI/MS method for the simultaneous determination of ramipril, hydrochlorothiazide and telmisartan in tablet dosage form, *J. Pharm. Res.*, 4: 4541–4545.
53. Aranda, M. and Morlock, G. 2007. New method for caffeine quantification by planar chromatography coupled with electrospray ionization mass spectrometry using stable isotope dilution analysis, *Rapid Commun. Mass Spectrom.*, 21: 1297–1303.
54. Oellig, C. and Schwack, W. 2012. Planar solid phase extraction clean-up for pesticide residue analysis in tea by liquid chromatography-mass spectrometry, *J. Chromatogr. A*, 1260: 42–53.
55. Devenport, N.A., Reynolds, J.C., Weston, D.J., Wilson, I.D., and Creaser, C.S. 2012. Direct extraction of urinary analytes from undeveloped reversed-phase thin layer

chromatography plates using a solvent gradient combined with on-line electrospray ionisation ion mobility–mass spectrometry, *Analyst*, 137: 3510–3513.

56. Abu-Rabie, P. and Spooner, N. 2009. Direct quantitative bioanalysis of drugs in dried blood spot samples using a thin-layer chromatography mass spectrometer interface, *Anal. Chem.*, 81: 10275–10284.

57. Heinig, K., Wirz, T., and Gajate-Perez, A. 2010. Sensitive determination of a drug candidate in dried blood spots using a TLC–MS interface integrated into a column-switching LC–MS/MS system, *Bioanalysis*, 2: 1873–1882.

58. Prosek, M., Milivojevic, L., Krizman, M., and Fir, M. 2004. On-line TLC–MS, *J. Planar Chromatogr.*, 17: 420–423.

59. Himmelsbach, M., Waser, M., and Klampfl, C.W. 2014. Thin layer chromatography–spray mass spectrometry: A method for easy identification of synthesis products and UV filters from TLC aluminium foils, *Anal. Bioanal. Chem.*, 406: 3647–3656.

60. Mincsovics, E., Ott, P.G., Alberti, A., Böszörményi, A., Héthelyi, E.B., Szöke, E., Kéry, A., Lemberkovics, E., and Móricz, A.M. 2013. In-situ clean-up and OPLC fractionation of chamomile flower extract to search active components by bioautography, *J. Planar Chromatogr.*, 26: 172–179.

61. Meléndez-Martínez, A.J., Vicario, I.M., and Heredia, F.J. 2007. Geometrical isomers of violaxanthin in orange juice, *Food Chem.*, 104: 169–175.

62. Smrke, S. and Vovk, I. 2013. Comprehensive thin-layer chromatography mass spectrometry of flavanols from *Juniperus communis* L. and *Punica granatum* L., *J. Chromatogr. A*, 1289: 119–126.

# 9 Recording of Mass Spectra from Miniaturized Layers (UTLC–MS)

*Tim T. Häbe and Gertrud E. Morlock*

## CONTENTS

## 9.1 SCOPE OF ULTRATHIN-LAYER CHROMATOGRAPHY–MASS SPECTROMETRY LAYERS: INTRODUCTION TO MINIATURIZED PLANAR CHROMATOGRAPHY

A new dimension in planar chromatography started in 2001 with the introduction of miniaturized ultrathin-layer chromatography (UTLC) layers. In contrast to TLC/HPTLC layers, the different layers developed so far do not use irregular particulate adsorbents, and thus provide the benefit that no classical binder is needed to fix the layer material on the carrier substrate which may contribute to background signals in the mass spectra. Faster separations, lower limits of detection, a reduced amount of analyte (several nanoliters), and low-mobile phase consumption were reached in various applications throughout the further development of different layer materials and production techniques (Table 9.1). Compared to HPTLC, the separation number is reduced for most layers because of the shorter migration distance and smaller specific surface area for adsorption. However, recent developments mitigated this disadvantage and showed an improved performance along with a multiple plate usage at an increased mechanical stability [1,2].

### 9.1.1 Monolithic UTLC Layers

First layers of a 10-μm thin monolithic silica gel structure with 1- to 2-μm macropores and 3- to 4-nm mesopores were manufactured by hydrolytic polycondensation of liquid alkoxysiloxane films coated on glass substrates. Separations were performed for steroids, pesticides, dyestuffs, amino acids, pharmaceutically active ingredients, phenols, and plasticizers [3,4]. Besides this commercially available monolithic UTLC product, which resulted from these studies and was used for several hyphenations to MS [5–10], the sol–gel synthesis process was further improved to provide a high homogeneity, reproducibility, and mechanical stability of the layer material. Optimized synthesis is still used to build up monolithic stationary phases with new characteristics, and synthetic dyes and food dyes were separated on a 100-μm thin layer [11,12].

For the separation of peptides and proteins followed by MALDI-TOF–MS detection, porous polymer monoliths were prepared by UV-initiated photografting of the respective monomer solutions. Plates were produced as 50- to 200-μm thin poly(butyl methacrylate-*co*-ethylene dimethacrylate) layers and as 50-μm thin poly(glycidyl methacrylate-*co*-ethylene dimethacrylate) layers with a gradient of hydrophobicity for 2D separations [13,14]. Thermally initiated polymerization was used for the production of 50-μm thin poly(4-methylstyrene-*co*-chloromethylstyrene-*co*-divinylbenzene) layers. The specific surface area of this styrene-containing polymer was further increased by hypercrosslinking via Friedel–Crafts alkylation, resulting in a higher separation performance [15].

### 9.1.2 Electrospun UTLC Layers

Electrospinning of (composite) polymer solutions, applied under high voltage onto the flexible carrier foil, is another process creating a nanofiber meshwork mat with fiber diameters mostly between 150 and 400 nm. A respectable range of mostly 15- to 25-μm ultrathin layer mats of different polymers and carbon nanofibers has been created through the deposition of the (composite) polymer solutions via the electrically charged jet, directed on the grounded rotating carrier foil. Electospun ultrathin-layer phases made of polyacrylonitrile (PAN) were prepared for the separation of laser dyes, steroidal compounds, and β-blockers [16,17]. With the same concept, ultrathin-layer phases made of electrospun glassy carbon nanofibers and of polyvinyl alcohol

**TABLE 9.1**
**Overview of Miniaturized UTLC Layers (Typical Values for Dimensions and Materials Are Given) Compared to HPTLC Layers**

| First Report | UTLC | | | | | | | HPTLC |
| --- | --- | --- | --- | --- | --- | --- | --- | --- |
| | 2001 [5] | 2001 [47] | 2007 [49] | 2008 [28] | 2009 [56] | 2011 [60] | 2011 [63] | 1975 [3] |
| Layer type | Monolithic layer | Monolayer on channel bottom | Ordered (non)porous pillar arrays | Nanostructured layer | Electrospun mat | Carbon-nanotube-templated microfabrication (CNT-M) | Submicrometer particulate layer with cross linked polymer brushes | Particulate layer |
| Technique of fabrication | Polymerization on glass plate (sol–gel process) and opt. photografting | DRIE of Si-wafer surface and coating | Mid/deep-UV lithography, DRIE of Si-wafer sur- and coating | GLAD of inorganic oxides on glass plates | Electrospinning of (composite) polymer solutions on aluminium foil | Coating CNTs with silica by (pseudo) atomic layer deposition plus second coating | Slurry overlay on Si-wafer and brush coating by polymerization | Slurry overlay on various carriers (glass plate, aluminium or polymer foil) and coatings |
| Layer icon | | | | | | | | |
| Layer structure | Monolithic texture with 1–2 µm macropores | Monolayered porous silicon bottom of a nanochannel (0.7 µm wide, 0.3 µm deep) | Monolayer coating or monolithic silica shell of cylindrical pillars (Ø 4 µm, 10 µm high, spaced 0.3–1.7 µm) in a 70 µm nanochannel | Column array of verticals, posts, helices, zig-zags or blades (spaced 2–50 nm) with (an)isotropic structure | Spun mat of nanofibers (Ø 200–400 nm, cm to m long) forming cylindric channels | Silica coated (20–60 nm) herring-bone hedge array (3–4 µm wide, spaced 4–7 µm) forming channels (50–100 µm long) | Nonporous particles coated with a polymer brush layer | Particles of Ø 5–7 µm |
| Layer thicknesses (µm) | 10–50 | Monolayer 0.05–0.3 | Monolayer or 0.5 µm porous shell | 1.3–7 | 15–25 | 50 | 15 | 50–200 |

*(Continued)*

**TABLE 9.1 (Continued)**
**Overview of Miniaturized UTLC Layers (Typical Values for Dimensions and Materials Are Given) Compared to HPTLC Layers**

| First Report | UTLC | | | | | | | HPTLC |
| --- | --- | --- | --- | --- | --- | --- | --- | --- |
| | 2001 [5] | 2001 [47] | 2007 [49] | 2008 [28] | 2009 [56] | 2011 [60] | 2011 [63] | 1975 [3] |
| Adsorbent types | Silica gel, poly (4-methyl-tyrene-co-chloromethyl-styrene-co-divinylbenzene) | C8, C18 | C8; C18 [50] | Silica, zirconia alumina, titania, C18 | Glassy carbon, polyvinyl alcohol, polyacrylonitrile | Silica, amino | Polyacrylamide; poly(GMA-co-DECDMA-NH$_2$) [64] | Silica, amino, cyano, diol, C2, C8, C18, cellulose, etc. |
| Layer geometry (mm) | 60 × 36 or 30 × 33 | 0.7 × 20 | 0.14 × 40; 10 × 30 [50] | 25 × 25 or 100 × 20 | 30 × 60, individually sliceable | 12 × 60 | 25 × 25 | 200 × 100, individually sliceable |
| Adsorbent pore diameter | 3–4 nm, BET (mesopores) | 10–20 nm | n.a. | <2 nm | 9 nm, BET | | Nonporous (hard core) | 6 nm, BET |
| Pore volume | 0.3 mL/g (specific) | ε = 0.85 (internal porosity) | ε ≥ 0.4 (external porosity) | – | 0.05 cm$^3$/g (cumulative, BJH) | | – | 0.75 mL/g (specific) |
| Surface area (m$^2$/g, BET) | 350 | 150 | 23% carbon coverage [50] | 150 | 22 | | 150/240 nm high-brush layer [64] | 500 |
| Flow | Capillary | Shear-driven | Pressure-driven; capillary [50] | Capillary | Capillary | Capillary | Capillary | Capillary |
| Typical migration distance [mm] | 10–30 | 2–8 | 1.5–30 | 3–10 | 30 | 2–40 | 19; 30 [64] | 50–70 |
| Development times/speed | 1–6 min | <1.5 s | 0.03–3.8 mm/s | 1–10 min | 5–10 min | 1 min | 10 min; 100 s [64] | 15–40 min |

*Source:*   Reprinted from Morlock, G.E., *J. Chromatogr. A*, 1382, 87–96, 2015. Copyright 2015, with permission from Elsevier.

were used for the separation of laser dyes and amino acids [18,19]. The flexibility of this layer production technique was furthermore increased by the preparation of carbon nanotube (CNT) and carbon nano-rod-filled PAN composite nanofibers to utilize their strong π–π interactions with aromatic analytes for the separation of polycyclic aromatic hydrocarbons [20].

Chromatography on polymer-based layers and their hyphenation to elution-based MS is only possible with nonsolvents of the polymer. Further ultrathin layer processing yielded calcined nanofibers produced by electrospinning of a solution of silica nanoparticles dispersed in polyvinylpyrrolidone followed by heating for calcination and selective removal of the polymer [21]. The application range was further expanded by producing PAN layers equipped with an incorporated photoluminescence indicator and used for the separation of preservatives. This was also the first application of this kind of UTLC layer hyphenated with ESI–MS [1].

### 9.1.3  GLAD-Fabricated UTLC Layers

The computer-controlled glancing-angle deposition (GLAD) technique for the deposition of porous nanostructured thin-layers of $SiO_2$ in 2008 blazed the trail to produce nanostructured chromatographic structures with engineered shapes like helices, spirals, vertical posts, blades, and chevrons in the nanometer scale by growing nanocolumns to a layer thickness of 1–7 μm. These layers with in-plane anisotropic nanostructures showed a decoupling effect where the analyte migration direction (dye solution) was decoupled from the direction of the solvent front movement [22–24]. Morphological and material modifications on this kind of layer were performed, like the implementation of a concentration zone, the introduction of polarity-adjustable reversed phase layers, the creation of metal oxide layers ($Al_2O_3$, $ZrO_2$, $TiO_2$, and ZnO) and surface modifications [24–27]. These ultrathin layers were used for the separation of carotenoids, synthetic food dyes, and sugars. The separated dyes Brilliant Black BN and tartrazine and applied glucose were detected by ESI–MS directly from such UTLC layers using the TLC–MS Interface [27,28].

### 9.1.4  Carbon Nanotube-Templated Microfabrication of UTLC Layers

The CNT-templated microfabrication of porous silicon–carbon UTLC layers is another technique to produce 3D-shaped chromatographic structures. These layers can be designed as herringbone CNT pattern by the lithographic patterning of the CNT growth catalyst. The nanoscale dimensions are achieved by the diameter and spacing of the CNTs grown on this catalyst. The first types of this UTLC layer were produced by the infiltration of silicon to the nanotube framework designed as 4-μm wide hedges, spaced by 7-μm channels for a directed solvent flow. Subsequent thermal oxidation for the removal of CNTs and conversion of the silicon yielded in a robust silica structure of around 30-μm height, used for the separation of lipophilic dyes [29]. The fabrication process was subsequently improved to avoid volume distortion of the microfeatures during the oxidation step and to prepare amino UTLC

phases by treatment with 3-aminopropyltriethoxysilane for the separation of fluorescent dyes [30]. The detailed surface characterization and the effect of the growth
catalyst thickness were investigated further to increase the separation performance
of different dye solutions and analgesics [31–33].

The separation performance was determined to be 170,000 and 200,000
theoretical plates $m^{-1}$ for a separation of two fluorescent dyes on a 50-µm thin
amino-silane-coated plate, and to be 40,000–140,000 theoretical plates $m^{-1}$ for
a separation of lipophilic dyes on a 50-µm thin uncoated silica plate [34]. The
latter separation was optimized on a 50-µm thin silicon nitride-based layer with
3-µm wide hedges, spaced by 5-µm channels, yielding 86% reduced migration
time compared to HPTLC. For the first time, UTLC–DART–MS studies were performed with this kind of layer. Also, water soluble food dyes were separated on this
layer showing a reduced mobile phase consumption of only 400 µL and a separating efficiency of up to 233,000 theoretical plates $m^{-1}$. During DART–MS studies
and the mobile phase optimization period, a single plate was used for 25 separations interrupted by rinsing/washing steps without loss of separation performance.
Two fluorescent dyes were also separated for the first UTLC–DESI–MSI study
with this kind of layer [2].

### 9.1.5  OTHER MINIATURIZED UTLC LAYERS

The brush-gel polymer film is a submicrometer particulate layer with cross-linked
polymer brushes. Nonporous particles with diameter of 350 nm, 700 nm, or 900 nm,
modified with polyacrylamide, were applied on a silicon wafer as slurry to obtain
a 15-µm thin layer. Coating with polyacrylamide brushes increased the capillary
force for increased mobile-phase velocity and the overall separation performance.
Three fluorescence-labeled proteins were separated with a sinapinic acid containing
mobile phase for subsequent detection via MALDI [35]. A second modification of
this brush-gel polymer was manufactured by cross-linking poly(glycidyl methacry-
late) and di(ethylene glycole)dimethacrylate to graft the thin layer covalently on the
glass substrate and to manipulate the separation characteristic. The separation of a
fluorescent dye mixture was performed on this layer and the ability for a multiple
reuse was shown [36].

Shear-driven chromatography (SDC) with porous silicon monolayers at the bottom of microchannels, being 0.7 µm wide and 0.3 µm deep, is another UTLC technique, which theory was first described in 1999 [37]. In this application, the mobile
phase is not propulsed by pressure or capillary action but by shear-driven forces
due to a moving wall element over the microchannels. First flow channels were
simply prepared by laser-jet printing on a transparency sheet. The toner particle
lines formed the 8-µm high wall elements and were moved underneath the stationary phase consisting of commercial RP-HPLC beads embedded in a polyacrylic
polymer matrix. This method was used to separate a mixture of Rhodamine B and
PN Black 151 at a mean fluid velocity of 0.1 mm $s^{-1}$ [38]. State-of-the-art microchannels are prepared by deep reactive ion etching (RIE) of a 0.3 µm deep and
0.7 µm wide channel followed by a silanization reaction. Sample loading through
integrated inlets were performed by an automated injection system and separations

were shown for coumarins [39,40]. The latest approaches are silica channels with a sub-100 nm depth, yielding 50,000–100,000 theoretical plates for Rhodamine 110 and Rhodamine 575 [41].

Porous and nonporous shell pillar-array columns are another layer type produced by UV-lithography, deep RIE, and followed by optional reverse phase surface coating. Silicon pillars with a diameter of 4.4 μm and a height of 11.5 μm were fabricated and oxidized to provide a maximum of silanol groups. Reverse phase coating was achieved by covalently coating with a monolayer of hydrophobic C8-chains. The layer is mounted between two sealing plates to enable a pressure-driven mobile-phase flow to separate three coumarin dyes within 3 s [42]. The pillar diameters were further decreased to a total outer diameter of 3.4 μm including a hydrophobic porous silica coating with C8-chains for the advanced separation of coumarin dyes [43]. The pillar and channel geometry were further reduced and the surface coating optimized, especially for C18 coating, leading to lower plate heights using a fluorescent tracer band and a capillary-based mobile phase flow [44,45].

However, the latter two separation techniques are still restricted to fluorescent substances as the loading capacity is too low for other optical detection modes. As all these layers are still in their infancy, separation performance and detection modes have to be studied. Among these, the hyphenation to MS would be an adequate detection technique.

## 9.2   OVERVIEW OF APPROACHES AND MASS SPECTRA OF UTLC–MS

Due to the open planar surface of UTLC layers, especially ambient desorption- or elution-based techniques were used to transfer analytes from the layer to the ionization region (Table 9.2). In addition, MALDI applications under vacuum were reported and the introduction of the whole ultrathin layer plate was possible without any special mounting devices, due to the small plate dimension. As UTLC–MS is a very new hyphenation, only a few applications of MS detection were reported after separation of different substances on UTLC layers. In addition, desorption- or elution-based approaches for detecting analytes without a separation directly from the UTLC layer are mentioned to show the capabilities of this hyphenation technique. However, as there is no chromatography (separation), it may not be termed UTLC–MS.

### 9.2.1   UTLC–TIME-OF-FLIGHT-SECONDARY ION MASS SPECTROMETRY

Monolithic silica UTLC plates were used in 2005 for the detection of gibberellic acid applied on this layer. The thin-layer background signals contained mainly $m/z$ 27.99063 and $m/z$ 45.00111 corresponding to the silica material. For gibberellic acid, $m/z$ values were 91, 105, 165, and 181 [5]. On the same layer, abietic acid and gibberellic acid were separated and eluted to a SIMS-compatible silver channel followed by TOF-SIMS detection with limits of detection of 1 and 4 ng, respectively. For gibberellic acid, $m/z$ values were 77, 91, 128, 136, 152,

**TABLE 9.2**

**Overview of UTLC–MS Applications for Different Plate Materials and Recorded Mass Signals of Compounds**

| Method and UTLC Layer | Compounds | m/z and Assignment | Reference |
|---|---|---|---|
| TOF-SIMS | Gibberellic acid | 91, 105, 165, 181 | Oriňák et al. [5] |
| Monolithic silica (Merck) | Abietic acid | 43, 91, 105, 121, 131, 136, 259 | Talian et al. [8] |
|  | Gibberellic acid | 77, 91, 128, 136, 152,165,181 | Talian et al. [8] |
| MALDI–IMS | Abietic acid | 302 [M]+ |  |
| Monolithic silica (Merck) | Gibberellic acid | 369 [M+Na]+ |  |
|  | Metoprolol | 268 [M+H]+, 290 [M+Na]+ | Salo et al. [6] |
|  | Midazolam | 326 [M+H]+ |  |
|  | Triazole 1 | 230 [M+H]+, 252 [M+Na]+ |  |
|  | Triazole 2 | 236 [M+H]+, 258 [M+Na]+ |  |
|  | Triazole 3 | 146 [M+H]+ |  |
|  | Triazole 4 | 186 [M+H]+, 208 [M+Na]+ |  |
|  | Verapamil | 455 [M+H]+ |  |
|  | N-desalkyl-flurazepam | 289 [M+H]+, 311 [M+Na]+ | Salo et al. [7] |
|  | Diazepam | 285 [M+H]+, 307 [M+Na]+ |  |
|  | Lorazepam | 321 [M+H]+, 343 [M+Na]+ |  |
|  | Midazolam | 326 [M+H]+ |  |
|  | Nitrazepam | 282 [M+H]+ |  |
|  | Oxazepam | 287 [M+H]+, 309 [M+Na]+ |  |
|  | Triazolam | 343 [M+H]+, 365 [M+Na]+ |  |
| Monolith of poly(butyl methacrylate-co-ethylene dimethacrylate) | Methylene blue | 284.044 [M]+ | Bakry et al. [13] |
|  | Angiotensin II | 1049.115, 1309.727 |  |
|  | [Sar1,Ile8]-Angiotensin II | 970.597, 1159.904 |  |
|  | Neurotensin | 1321.984, 1933.509 |  |

(Continued)

**TABLE 9.2 (*Continued*)**

**Overview of UTLC–MS Applications for Different Plate Materials and Recorded Mass Signals of Compounds**

| Method and UTLC Layer | Compounds | *m/z* and Assignment | Reference |
|---|---|---|---|
| | Cytochrome c | 12396.015 | |
| | Insulin (labeled) | 6301.446 | |
| | Lysozyme | 14396.651 | |
| | Myoglobin | 16995.835 | |
| | Myoglobin (labeled) | 17568.993 | |
| Monolith of poly(glycidyl methacrylate-*co*-ethylene dimethacrylate) | Leucine encephalin | 555.6 | Urbanova and Svec [14] |
| | Oxytocin | 1007.2 | |
| Monolith of poly(4-methylstyrene-*co*-chloro-methylstyrene-*co*-divinylbenzene) | [Met⁵]Encephalin | 593.0 | Lv et al. [15] |
| | Melittin | 2882.4 | |
| | Oxytocin | 1297.2 | |
| | Lysozyme | 14831.4 | |
| | Myoglobin | 18090.5 | |
| | Ribonuclease A | 14227.3 | |
| Polyacrylamide modified nonporous silica particles | Cytochrome c | 12239.0 | Zhang et al. [35] |
| | Lysozyme | 14304.0 | |
| | Myoglobin | 16973.0 | |
| ESI-MS | Cilazapril | 418 [M+H]⁺ | Vovk et al. [9] |
| Monolithic silica (Merck) | Cilazaprilat | 390 [M+H]⁺ | |
| | Lisinopril | 406 [M+H]⁺ | |
| | Ramipril | 417 [M+H]⁺ | |
| | Ramiprilat | 389 [M+H]⁺ | |
| | Quinapril | 439 [M+H]⁺ | |
| | Quinaprilat | 411 [M+H]⁺ | |

(*Continued*)

**TABLE 9.2 (*Continued*)**

**Overview of UTLC–MS Applications for Different Plate Materials and Recorded Mass Signals of Compounds**

| Method and UTLC Layer | Compounds | m/z and Assignment | Reference |
|---|---|---|---|
| Electrospun nanofiber | Benzoic acid | 121.1 [M–H]– | Kampalanonwat et al. [1] |
| | Butyl-4-hydircxybenzoate | 193.0 [M–H]– | |
| | Ethyl-4-hydroxybenzoate | 164.9 [M–H]– | |
| | 4-Hydroxybenzoic acid | 136.9 [M–H]– | |
| | Methyl-4-hydroxybenzoate | 151.0 [M–H]– | |
| | Propyl-4-hydroxybenzoate | 179.1 [M–H]– | |
| | Sorbic acid | 223.0 [2M–H]– | |
| Titania and zirconia GLAD | Brilliant Black BN | 194 [M–4Na]4– | Wannenmacher et al. [27] |
| | Taitrazine | 244 [M–2Na]2–, 511 [M–Na]– | |
| Silica GLAD | Glucose | 179 [M–H]–, 181 [M+H]– | Kirchert et al. [28] |
| DESI-MS | Acetylcholine | 146 [M]+ | Kauppila et al. [10] |
| Monolithic silica (Merck) | Diazepam | 285 [M+H]+ | |
| | Dobutamin | 302 [M+]+ | |
| | Midazolam | 326 [M+H]+ | |
| | Testosterone | 289 [M+H]+ | |
| | Verapamil | 455 [M+H]+ | |
| Silicon nitride coated CNT-templated | Basic Blue 7 | 478.3 [M]+ | Kanyal et al. [2] |
| | Rhodamine B | 443.2 [M]+ | |
| DART-MS | Dimethyl Yellow | 226 [M+H]+ | Kanyal et al. [2] |
| Silicon nitride coated CNT-templated | Oracet Red G | 238 [M+H]+ | |
| | Solvent Blue 22 | 305 [M+H]+ | |
| | Solvent Blue 35 | 351 [M+H]+ | |
| | Sudan Red G | 279 [M+H]+ | |

165, and 181 and for abietic acid $m/z$ values were 43, 91, 105, 121, 131, 136, and 259 [8]. As TOF-SIMS is a hard ionization technique, no molecular ions were detected.

## 9.2.2 UTLC–MATRIX-ASSISTED LASER DESORPTION IONIZATION–MASS SPECTROMETRY

First ultrathin-layer chromatography–matrix-assisted laser desorption ionization/mass spectrometry (UTLC–MALDI–MS) studies were performed on the monolithic silica UTLC plate under ambient and vacuum conditions. Separation of midazolam ($m/z$ 326 [M+H]$^+$), verapamil ($m/z$ 455 [M+H]$^+$), metoprolol ($m/z$ 268 [M+H]$^+$), and four 1,2,3-triazoles ($m/z$ 230, 236, 146, and 186; all [M+H]$^+$) were detected by applying an $\alpha$-cyano-4-hydroxycinnamic acid matrix onto the developed plate. The monolithic silica UTLC plates provided 10–100 times better sensitivity compared to HPTLC plates. Benzodiazepines were also detected in the picomole range after 2D UTLC by AP–MALDI–MS, and proved the suitability of this method for difficult bioanalysis (Figure 9.1). The ambient ionization method yielded higher signal intensities and the domination of the deprotonated molecule due to its softer ionization compared to vacuum MALDI (Figure 9.2) [6,7]. Investigations on MALDI matrices were performed for 2,5-dihydroxybenzoic acid (DHB) showing $m/z$ 137 for [M–OH]$^+$ and $m/z$ 155 for [M+H]$^+$ and for ferulic acid (FA) showing $m/z$ 177 for [M–OH]$^+$ and $m/z$ 195 for [M+H]$^+$. Abietic acid ($m/z$ 302 M$^+$) and gibberellic acid were separated to study these matrices, but only the FA matrix enabled clear mass signals on the monolithic silica plate. Gibberellic acid was not clearly identified due to its high fragmentation and the absence of the molecular ion. Nevertheless, as MALDI is a softer ionization technique compared to SIMS, the molecular ions of these substances were mainly found in the mass spectra [8].

Monolithic porous polymer layers made of poly(butyl methacrylate-*co*-ethylene dimethacrylate) were prepared on glass slides and directly on stainless-steel MALDI target plates. The first plate design was used to separate methylene blue ($m/z$ 284.044 M$^+$) and methyl red followed by MALDI without using any additional matrix (Figure 9.3). Two fluorescamine-labeled mixtures, one composed of peptides and another of proteins, were also separated, followed by detection via MALDI-TOF–MS with $\alpha$-cyano-4-hydroxycinnamic acid and sinapinic acid as matrix, respectively. MS-spectra of fluorescamine labeled [Sar$^1$,Ile$^8$]-angiotensin II ($m/z$ 970.597 and 1159.994), angiotensin II ($m/z$ 1049.115 and 1309.727), neurotensin ($m/z$ 1321.984 and 1933.509) showed $m/z$ values for the labeled and unlabeled molecule (Figure 9.4). Labeled insulin ($m/z$ 6301.446) and myoglobin ($m/z$ 17,568.993) were also detected, as well as unlabeled cytochrome c ($m/z$ 12,396.015), lysozyme ($m/z$ 14,396.651), and myoglobin ($m/z$ 16,995.835). The latter protein experiment was also performed with the monolithic layer attached directly on the stainless steel MALDI target plate for the instant transfer of the chromatographed zone into MALDI-TOF–MS [13].

Layers made of poly(glycidyl methacrylate-*co*-ethylene dimethacrylate) with a gradient of hydrophobicity for 2D separations were used to separate the

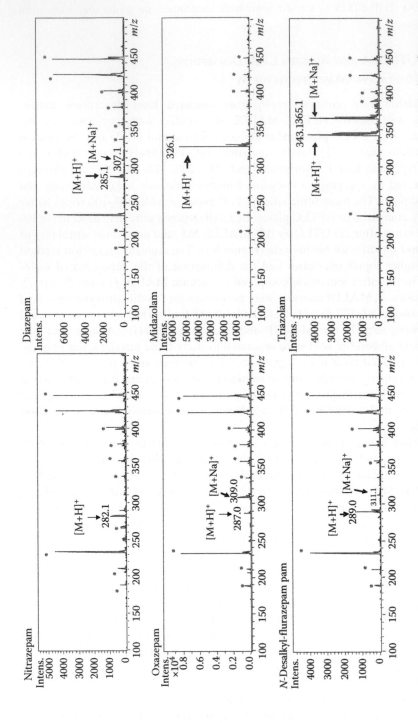

**FIGURE 9.1** MALDI–MS of six benzodiazepines (spiked in urine) separated on monolithic UTLC plates (main matrix ions for α-cyano-4-hydroxycinnamic acid marked with an asterisk). (Reprinted with permission from Salo, P.K. et al., *Anal. Chem.*, 79: 2101–2108. Copyright 2007, American Chemical Society.)

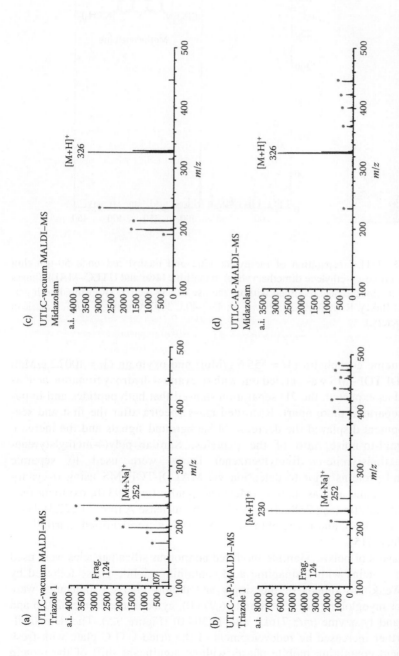

**FIGURE 9.2** Comparison of mass spectra obtained by vacuum MALDI–MS (a and c) and AP-MALDI–MS (b and d) recorded on monolithic silica UTLC plates (10 nmol α-cyano-4-hydroxycinnamic acid sprayed over triazole (a and b) and midazolam (c and d), 1 nmol each). (From Salo, P.K. et al., *J. Am. Soc. Mass Spectrom.*, 16: 906–915, 2005. Copyright 2005. With kind permission from Springer Science+Business Media.)

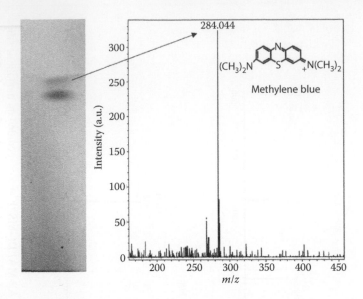

**FIGURE 9.3** UTLC separation of methylene blue and methyl red on a 50-μm thin poly(butyl acrylate-*co*-ethylene dimethacrylate) monolithic layer and UTLC–MALDI mass spectrum of methylene blue recorded without the use of any matrix. (Reprinted with permission from Bakry, R. et al. *Anal. Chem.,* 79: 486–493, 2007. Copyright 2007, American Chemical Society.)

peptides leucine encephalin (*M* = 555.6 g/Mol) and oxytocin (*M* = 1007.2 g/Mol) [14]. MALDI-TOF–MS was carried out with α-cyano-4-hydroxycinnamic acid as matrix, and as expected, the 2D separation showed that both peptides and impurities are separated more apart. Recorded mass spectra after the first and second development displayed the decrease of background signals and the increase of the signal-to-noise ratio of the peptides. Similar poly(4-methylstyrene-*co*-chloromethylstyrene-*co*-divinylbenzene) layers were used to separate peptides and proteins prior to detection via MALDI-TOF–MS using α-cyano-4-hydroxycinnamic acid as matrix. [Met[5]]encephalin (*m/z* 593.0), oxytocin (*m/z* 1297.2), and melittin (*m/z* 2882.4) as well as ribonuclease A (*m/z* 14,227.3), lysozyme (*m/z* 14,831.4), and myoglobin (*m/z* 18,090.5) were identified, partially as matrix adducts [15].

UTLC layers of polyacrylamide-modified nonporous silica particles were used to separate proteins with a sinapinic acid containing mobile phase followed by MALDI. Weak MS signals of the singly and doubly charged molecules were obtained for myoglobin (*m/z* 8514.8 and 16,973.0), cytochrome c (*m/z* 6291.6 and 12,239.0), and lysozyme (*m/z* 7161.1 and 14,304.0) (Figure 9.5). The detectability was further increased by redevelopment of the dried UTLC plate with fresh sinapinic acid containing mobile phase, without significant shift of the protein bands [35].

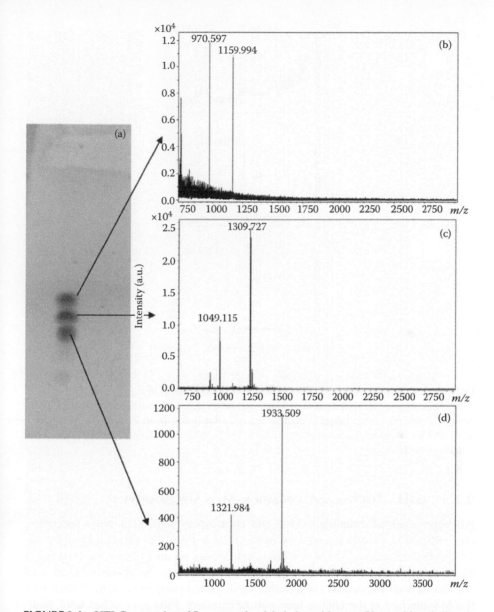

**FIGURE 9.4** UTLC separation of fluorescamine-labeled peptides on a 50-μm thin poly(butyl acrylate-*co*-ethylene dimethacrylate) monolithic layer (a) as well as UTLC–MALDI mass spectrum of [Sar$^1$,Ile$^8$]-angiotensin (b), angiotensin (c), and neurotensin (d) recorded with α-cyano-4-hydroxycinnamic acid as matrix. (Reprinted with permission from Bakry, R. et al. *Anal. Chem.*, 79: 486–493, 2007. Copyright 2007 American Chemical Society.)

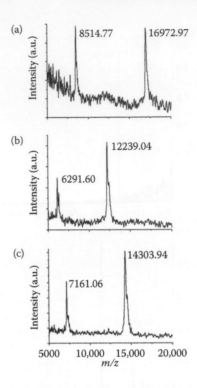

**FIGURE 9.5** UTLC–MALDI–MS spectra of the three proteins myoglobin (a), cytochrome c (b), and lysozyme (c) separated on polyacrylamide modified nonporous silica particles and desorbed/ionized using sinapinic acid as matrix. (Reprinted from Zhang, Z., Ratnayaka, S.N., and Wirth, M.J., *J. Chromatogr. A*, 1218, 7196–7202, 2011. Copyright 2011, with permission from Elsevier.)

### 9.2.3 UTLC–Electrospray Ionization–Mass Spectrometry

All approaches of coupling UTLC and electrospray ionization–mass spectrometry (ESI–MS) were performed by online elution from the ultrathin-layer by the TLC–MS Interface (CAMAG). This interface was mounted between a common high-performance liquid chromatography (HPLC) pump for solvent delivery into the elution head pressed on the ultrathin layer. Eluted compounds were flushed into the MS attached at the elution head outline capillary. First approaches were made for the detection of peptides of angiotensin-converting enzyme inhibitors directly from monolithic silica UTLC plates after elution with methanol at 0.3 mL min$^{-1}$. Lisinopril ($m/z$ 406 [M+H]$^+$), cilazapril ($m/z$ 418 [M+H]$^+$), cilazaprilat ($m/z$ 390 [M+H]$^+$), ramipril ($m/z$ 417 [M+H]$^+$), ramiprilat ($m/z$ 389 [M+H]$^+$), quinapril ($m/z$ 439 [M+H]$^+$), and quinaprilat ($m/z$ 411 [M+H]$^+$) were detected as protonated molecules and sodium/disodium-adducts (Figure 9.6) [9].

Electrospun nanofiber layers were also used as elution substrate for ESI–MS via the TLC–MS Interface. The preservatives sorbic acid ($m/z$ 223 [2M–H]$^-$),

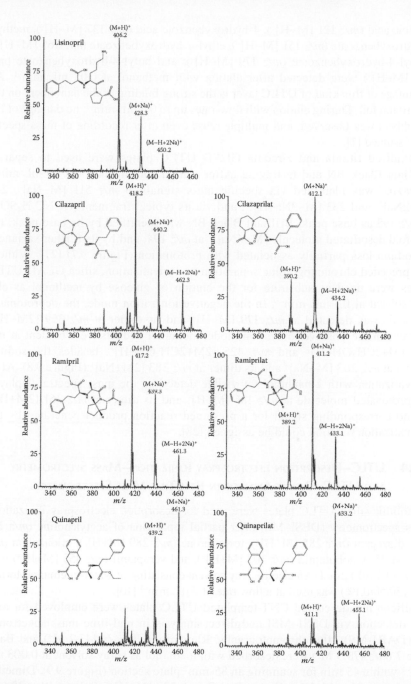

**FIGURE 9.6** UTLC–ESI–MS spectra of prils and prilates recorded on monolithic silica UTLC plates. (Reprinted from Vovk, I. et al., *J. Chromatogr. A*, 1218, 3089–3094, 2011. Copyright 2011, with permission from Elsevier.)

benzoic acid (m/z 121 [M–H]$^-$), 4-hydroxybenzoic acid (m/z 137 [M–H]$^-$), methyl-4-hydroxybenzoate (m/z 151 [M–H]$^-$), ethyl-4-hydroxybenzoate (m/z 165 [M–H]$^-$), propyl-4-hydroxybenzoate (m/z 179 [M–H]$^-$), and butyl-4-hydroxybenzoate (m/z 193 [M–H]$^-$) were detected after elution with methanol at 0.05 mL min$^{-1}$. An advantage of this kind of UTLC layer is the strong binding of the nanofibers on the aluminum foil. During elution with flow-rates up to 0.4 mL min$^{-1}$, no damage of the nanofibers was observed, and multiple reuse even after recording of mass spectra was assumed [1].

Oxidized titania and zirconia GLAD UTLC plates were used to separate Brilliant Black BN and tartrazine. After elution with methanol at 0.1 mL min$^{-1}$, tartrazine was identified via specific mass signals at m/z 511 [M–Na]$^-$, 244 [M–2Na]$^{2-}$ and 233 [M–3Na+H]$^{2-}$, and via its typical fragment [OCNC$_6$H$_4$SO$_3$]$^-$ at m/z 198 as base peak. Brilliant Black BN was identified by its base peak, the fourfold desodiated molecule [M–4Na]$^{4-}$ at m/z 194, and by its further variances of sodium loss partially associated with protonation (Figure 9.7) [27]. Without any preceded chromatographic separation or derivatization, silica GLAD UTLC plates were used as substrate for the elution of glucose by methanol as elution solvent at 0.1 mL min$^{-1}$. In the negative ionization mode, the deprotonated molecule was detected at m/z 179 [M–H]$^-$ and its dimer at m/z 359 [2M–H]$^-$, whereas in the positive ionization mode, methanol adducts were evident at m/z 245 [M+2CH$_3$OH+H]$^+$ and m/z 425 [2M+2CH$_3$OH+H]$^+$, besides the sodium adduct at m/z 203 [M+Na]$^+$ and its dimer at m/z 383 [2M+Na]$^+$ (Figure 9.8). After derivatization with 2-naphthol for visible detection, the mass spectra displayed the protonated molecule at m/z 181 [M+H]$^+$ and its dimer at m/z 361 [2M+H]$^+$, but no corresponding signal for a presumed reaction product generated by the derivatization reaction could be assigned [28].

### 9.2.4   UTLC–Desorption Electrospray Ionization–Mass Spectrometry and UTLC–Direct Analysis in Real-Time Mass Spectrometry

Monolithic silica UTLC plates were used for desorption electrospray ionization–mass spectrometry (DESI–MS) after partial separation of acetylcholine (m/z 146 M$^+$), diazepam (m/z 285 [M+H]$^+$), testosterone (m/z 289 [M+H]$^+$), midazolam (m/z 326 [M+H]$^+$), dobutamin (m/z 302 [M+H]$^+$), and verapamil (m/z 455 [M+H]$^+$) with LODs of 1–100 pmol. An electrospray solvent consisting of water–methanol–formic acid (50/50/0.1%) was used at a flow rate of 7 μL min$^{-1}$ [10].

Silicon nitride coated CNT-templated UTLC plates were employed for analyte detection via DESI–MSI and direct analysis in real-time mass spectrometry (DART-MS) after chromatography. Rhodamine B (m/z 443.2 M$^+$) and Basic Blue 7 (m/z 478.3 M$^+$) were desorbed with methanol as spray solvent at 0.003 mL min$^{-1}$ within 45 min for scanning an 85-mm$^2$ plate section (Figure 9.9). Dimethyl Yellow (m/z 226 [M+H]$^+$), Oracet Red G (m/z 238 [M+H]$^+$), Solvent Blue 35 (m/z 351 [M+H]$^+$), Sudan Red G (m/z 279 [M+H]$^+$), and Solvent Blue 22 (m/z 305 [M+H]$^+$) were detected within 3.5 min with a substantially optimized interface for HPTLC–DART–MS applying a helium flow of 3 L min$^{-1}$ at 500°C (Figure 9.10) [2].

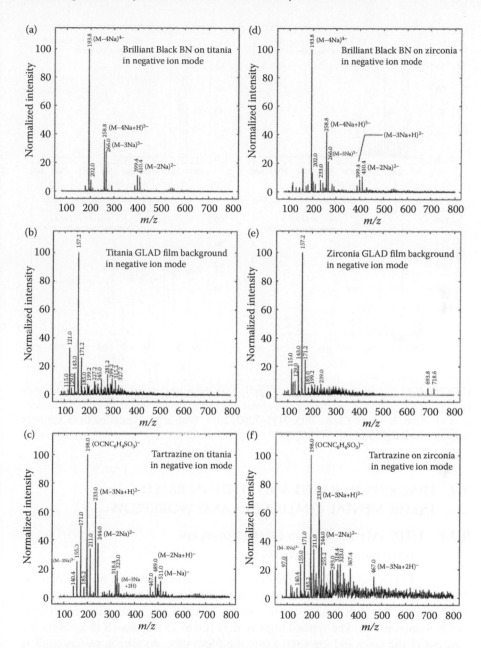

**FIGURE 9.7** UTLC–ESI–MS spectra recorded after separation on nanostructured titania (a–c) and zirconia (d–f) GLAD layers: Brilliant Black BN (a and d), GLAD layer background (b and e), and tartrazine (c and f). (Reprinted from Wannenmacher, J. et al., *J. Chromatogr. A,* 1318, 234–243, 2013. Copyright 2013, with permission from Elsevier.)

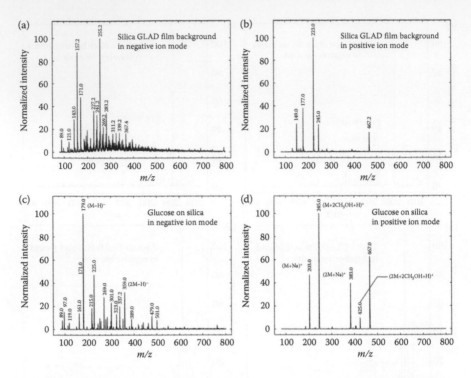

**FIGURE 9.8**  Mass spectra of glucose applied on the nanostructured silica GLAD layer and layer background in negative (a and c) and positive ion mode (b and d). (From Kirchert, S. et al., *Anal. Bioanal. Chem.*, 405, 7195–7203, 2013. With kind permission from Springer Science+Business Media.)

## 9.3  DESORPTION-BASED AND ELUTION-BASED INSTRUMENTAL CHALLENGES AND WORKFLOW

### 9.3.1  UTLC–MATRIX-ASSISTED LASER DESORPTION IONIZATION–MASS SPECTROMETRY

For HPTLC/TLC–MALDI–MS, the development on an aluminum foil is a precondition, which is clamped into the MALDI adapter target. Due to the conductivity of aluminum, the high voltage applied to the MALDI target plate is transferrable to the aluminum foil. The applied high voltage (up to 25 kV) assists in accelerating ions out of the layer and ion source into the flight tube. As silicon wafers used as a carrier for UTLC layers [35] show a good conductivity, the voltage transfer was given. In addition, the direct polymerization and usage of the ultrathin layer on the MALDI target plate [13] enabled a good voltage transfer. Voltage transfer to glass plates is limited due to the low conductivity of the quartz glass, mounted on the target plate by conductive and nonconductive tape [6–8,14]. Nevertheless, the ion transmission rates into the analyzer vacuum stage after desorption/ionization was

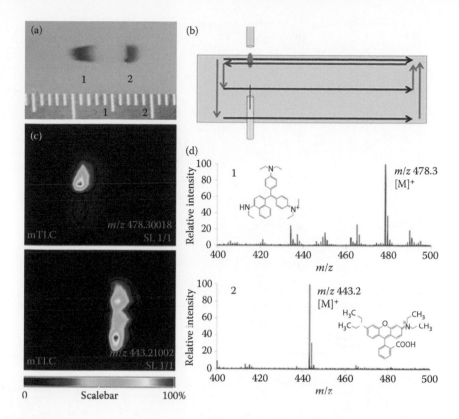

**FIGURE 9.9** Section of the scan area of a separation of Basic Blue 7 (BB7, 1) and Rhodamine B (RhB, 2), each 0.6 µg, on a CNT-templated UTLC plate (a), illustration of the spray impact target route during plate carrier movement for the multiple line-scanning (b), and UTLC–DESI–MSI false color image (c) generated for the molecular ion intensities of BB7 at *m/z* 478.3 and RhB at *m/z* 443.2 (d). (Reprinted from Kanyal, S.S. et al., *J. Chromatogr. A*, 1404, 115–123, 2015. Copyright 2015, with permission from Elsevier.)

high enough for MALDI–MS detection from these plates using vacuum MALDI and AP–MALDI.

A general challenge is the analyte-to-matrix molar ratio as many matrices caused interfering mass peaks at low *m/z* values. High matrix amount decreases selectivity, while a low matrix amount reduces the mass signal intensity and thus detectability. A suitable matrix concentration for UTLC is stated to be 2.66 nmol mm$^{-2}$ of α-cyano-4-hydroxycinnamic acid, which is about 10 times less than compared to HPTLC (22.3 nmol mm$^{-2}$) [6].

The homogenous application of the MALDI matrix is another important issue, solved by different application techniques for UTLC plates thus far. The simple deposition of a few microliters by syringe next to the analyte spot or the spray application over the entire plate was described [13,15]. Another spray-on technique with the Linomat 4 (CAMAG) was performed to apply the matrix solution

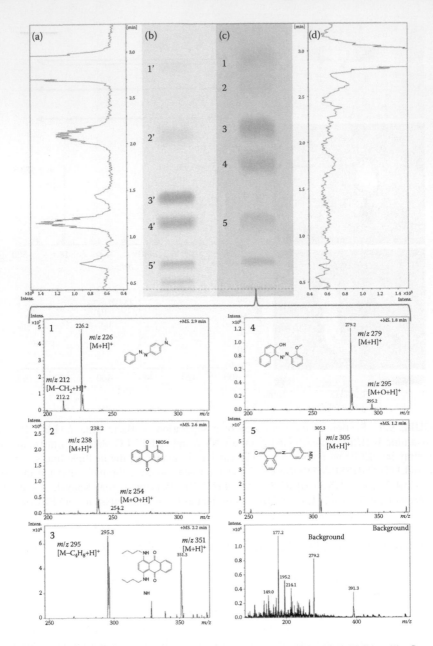

**FIGURE 9.10** DART–MS scanning of the lipophilic dyes Dimethyl Yellow (1), Oracet Red G (2), Solvent Blue 35 (3), Sudan Red G (4), and Solvent Blue 22 (5) showing the TIC chromatogram (a) on an HPTLC plate (b) with higher signal intensities compared to the respective TIC chromatogram (d) on a CNT-templated UTLC plate (c). (Reprinted from Kanyal, S.S. et al., *J. Chromatogr. A*, 1404, 115–123, 2015. Copyright 2015, with permission from Elsevier.)

homogenously only on the sampling zone [6,7]. A further option for matrix deposition was its addition to the sample solution or mobile phase [14]. The first option did not guarantee a sufficient matrix concentration at the analyte spot, due to matrix adsorption on the layer material. In the case of matrix added to the mobile phase, the development with sinapinic acid containing methanol had to be repeated for a sufficient amount of matrix on the plate [35]. The crystallization process and the dimension of matrix crystals are crucial in UTLC. As shown for α-cyano-4-hydroxycinnamic acid, matrix crystals are much smaller in relation to the large, irregularly shaped silica gel particles of TLC plates (Figure 9.11a). But this scale ratio changed for the application of UTLC layers, for which sinapinic acid matrix crystals were much larger than the polyacrylamide modified nonporous silica UTLC particles (Figure 9.11b) [35,46].

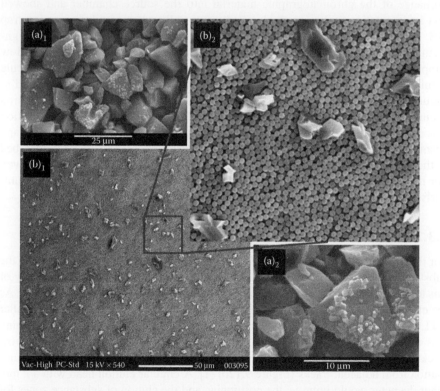

**FIGURE 9.11** Scanning electron microscope (SEM) images at increasing levels of magnification of α-cyano-4-hydroxycinnamic acid crystals on silica TLC particles (a) and of sinapinic acid crystals on polyacrylamide modified nonporous silica UTLC particles (b). (Reprinted from Zhang, Z., Ratnayaka, S.N., and Wirth, M.J., *J. Chromatogr. A*, 1218, 7196–7202, 2011, copyright 2011, with permission from Elsevier; Hayen, H., and Volmer, D.A., *Rapid Commun. Mass Spectrom.*, 19, 711–720, 2005, copyright Wiley-VCH Verlag GmbH & Co. KGaA, reproduced with permission.)

Mounting the UTLC plate into the MALDI interface is a critical procedure and different methods were described. The simplest mounting technique was the precise fixation of the UTLC foil after optional cutting onto modified MALDI target plates by double-sided conductive tape or the fixation of the plate in a milled-out region of the target plate by carbon tape [6,7,14,35]. Plate preparation directly on the MALDI target plate was also described for monolithic porous polymer layers where the polymerization mixture was placed on the stainless steel MALDI target plate prior to photo-initiated polymerization [13].

A disadvantage of vacuum MALDI is the introduction of the whole chromatographic material into the vacuum chamber and thus a long preparation time for plate exchange and pumping-down. In addition, the ionization process of vacuum MALDI is much harder than AP-MALDI, which often resulted in high fragmentation and the absence of molecular ions. In contrast, AP-MALDI enabled a quick exchange of the chromatographic material into the source chamber and showed less fragmentation and more stable results especially when coupled to an ion trap MS, whereas MALDI-TOF MS provided a higher resolution for structural assignment. Formation of clusters or dimers of the analyte and matrix occured at low temperatures, whereas at high-temperatures fragmentation of the analyte molecule dominated. In AP-MALDI, the collisional cooling is more dominant compared to vacuum MALDI, and, therefore, dimers were stabilized and less fragmentation occured. The very thin UTLC layers were advantageous for the MALDI desorption process by the laser pulse. Analytes were located closer to the layer surface and desorption was more efficient with the pulsed laser compared to analytes adsorbed in the deeper parts of the adsorbent layer of the comparatively thick HPTLC layer. For the monolithic silica layer, a 10–100 times better sensitivity was stated in comparison with conventional HPTLC plates [6,7].

### 9.3.2   UTLC–Electrospray Ionization–Mass Spectrometry

For the coupling of UTLC with ESI-MS, the TLC-MS Interface was used to elute the substance bands into the ion source. Besides general advantages in the workflow of this technique, different challenges occur for elutions on UTLC layers as a surface. As the elution head was designed for larger and thicker HPTLC layers, the much smaller UTLC bands have to be targeted exactly and the selectivity with regard to positioning was defined by the smallest 2 mm × 4 mm elution head (Figure 9.12a). For narrow track distances, it was also possible to rotate the head by 90° to avoid cross-contamination from adjacent tracks (Figure 9.12b) [1]. A circular elution head with a 2 mm inner diameter would improve the positioning and the elution of substance zones for coupling to ESI-MS. Such an elution head was already described [47], but is not commercially available yet. For a good positioning, target zones on the monolithic silica layers were marked with a soft pencil directly on the layer, whereas for the almost lucent GLAD layers, zones were marked on the backside of the plate [9,27].

Elution from UTLC layers was handicapped by insufficient sealing of the elution head on the layer, resulting in elution solvent spreading on the layer. As the TLC-MS Interface was designed for much thicker TLC and HPTLC layers, a pressure-tight sealing was achieved by grouted silica gel, when the stainless-steel cutting edge of

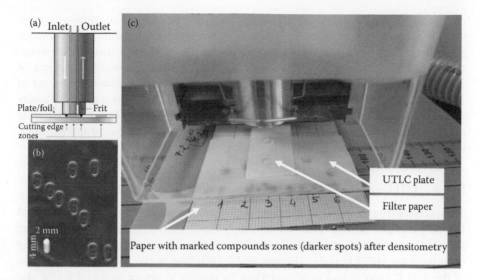

**FIGURE 9.12** Illustration of the elution head-based TLC–MS Interface (a) and layer imprints on the backside of a PAN nanofiber layer after elution (b). Modified use of the interface with filter paper between the elution head and the monolithic silica UTLC plate to avoid leakage of the elution solvent (c). (Reprinted from Kampalanonwat, P., Supaphol, P., and Morlock, G.E., *J. Chromatogr. A*, 1299, 110–117, 2011; Vovk, I. et al., *J. Chromatogr. A*, 1218, 3089–3094, 2013. Copyright 2011 and 2013, with permission from Elsevier.)

the elution head was pressed through the layer onto the plate support material. This problem was prevented for monolithic silica layers by placing a cleaned piece of filter paper on the layer, sealing the cutting edge of the elution head on the layer without hampering the elution quality (Figure 9.12c) [9]. The same problem occurred for GLAD layers, but was avoided by increasing the gas pressure used for the elution head movement and sealing force (no need for a filter paper layer).

A related challenge was the spreading of a small droplet of the residual elution solvent, which was located within the cutting edge and migrated onto the adsorbent when the elution head was lifted after the elution. The small volume of liquid spread to nearby substance zones and partially distorted the chromatographic result [27]. In contrast to HPTLC layers, thinner UTLC layers cannot cope with this after-drop due to the reduced layer thickness and reduced surface activity, resulting in a higher elution power and thus increased zone shift.

### 9.3.3 UTLC–Desorption Electrospray Ionization–Mass Spectrometry

DESI-MS experiments were reported for monolithic silica layers and CNT-templated UTLC plates. An improved sensitivity and detectability was expected compared to HPTLC layers similar to MALDI-MS results. A thinner adsorption layer *per se* mitigated the location of analytes in the deep sorbent layer. Thus, the impact of the DESI solvent spray reached more analyte molecules. The solvent flow rate was crucial for a sufficient desorption rate at a low solvent spreading over the layer. A too high flow rate might smear the substance bands resulting in a low spatial resolution or even the flow (removal) of analytes out of the detection area. For monolithic silica plates, an optimum flow rate was found to be 5–10 μL min⁻¹ using a mixture of water, methanol, and formic acid (50/50/0.1%, *V/V/V*) at a sprayer-to-surface distance of 3–4 mm [10]. For CNT-templated UTLC plates, the methanol flow rate was set to 3 μL min⁻¹ [2]. In contrast to HPTLC plates made of particulate silica gel, both layers were mechanically stable and not abraded by the solvent spray. Therefore, multiple usages of the layer materials are possible at a low contamination of the MS-inlet system with loose silica particles.

### 9.3.4  UTLC–DIRECT ANALYSIS IN REAL-TIME MASS SPECTROMETRY

This solvent-free desorption and ionization method was used on CNT-templated UTLC plates and showed no abrasion of the mechanically stable layer. The scanning procedure was performed on a DART interface for quantitative surface scanning optimized for HPTLC plates (Figure 9.13a) [48]. Due to the lower plate thickness of the UTLC layer, it had to be underlain by spacers to obtain an equal height and the same scan lane alignment compared to HPTLC plates and thus optimum signal intensities (Figure 9.13b). Scanning was performed at the same ion source conditions as for HPTLC plates, but in the direct comparison, signal intensities from the UTLC layer were lower than from HPTLC layers (Figure 9.10a and b). In contrast to other desorption-based techniques like MALDI and DESI, desorption and ionization was weaker on the thinner CNT-templated UTLC plate. Analytes adsorbed deep in the silica hedge pores cannot be reached by the DART gas stream scanning over the upper surface layer. This effect might be more distinct compared to HPTLC layers. However, the lower sensitivity might also result from the conductive coated waver used as support for the UTLC plate and, therefore, due to its thermal and electrical conductivity, leading to an energetic discharge of the metastable helium [2].

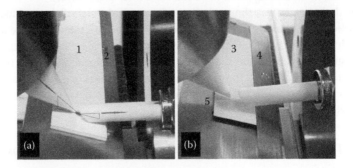

**FIGURE 9.13**  DART–MS recording with the substantially modified DART interface showing the HPTLC setup (a) with the plate (1) aligned at arresters (2) compared to the UTLC setup (b) with mounted CNT-templated UTLC plate (3) aligned at a spacer for scan lane adjustment (4) and underlain by a spacer for height adjustment (5). (From Habe, T.T., and Morlock, G.E., *Rapid Commun. Mass Spectrom.*, 29, 474–484, 2015. Copyright Wiley-VCH Verlag GmbH & Co. KGaA. Reproduced with permission.)

## 9.4  OUTLOOK

The hyphenation of UTLC to MS requires more effort in precise handling than HPTLC, but is generally not limited by its current dimensions. UTLC layers are a dynamic and rapidly developing field of research with numerous basic approaches and with a great potential for further developments in layer materials and chromatographic applications [49,50]. As it is still in its infancy, the drawback in automatic devices for the chromatographic process, similar to HPTLC devices, will be overcome by contemporary technical trends, summarized in the Office Chromatography concept [51]. A major basic challenge in UTLC is the precise deposition of sharp application zones on partially sensitive layers to yield an optimum chromatographic result and precise sampling zones for MS. The sample application in UTLC evolved from the spray-on techniques used in HPTLC to the smoother bubble-jet application by partially or largely modified inkjet printers for precise low nanoliter application zones [27,28,52]. Due to the low analyte amounts, MS is an especially suitable detection mode, whereas other detection modes reach their limit of detection or are restricted to fluorescent analytes, suitable derivatizations or effect-directed analysis. The pros and cons of the different UTLC-MS methods are comparable to TLC/HPTLC-MS methods and have to be considered beside the described instrumental challenges when UTLC-MS is applied. The workflows and classifications described have to be adapted for each analytical task and stationary phase. However, the main advantages of UTLC-MS remain rapidness, reduced solvent consumption, low layer abrasion, reduced background signals, and an increased sensitivity for most layers.

## REFERENCES

1. Kampalanonwat, P., Supaphol, P., and Morlock, G.E. 2013. Electrospun nanofiber layers with incorporated photoluminescence indicator for chromatography and detection of ultraviolet-active compounds, *J. Chromatogr. A*, 1299: 110–117.
2. Kanyal, S.S., Häbe, T.T., Cushman, C.V., Dhunna, M., Roychowdhury, T., Farnsworth, P.B., Morlock, G.E., and Linford, M.R. 2015. Microfabrication, separations, and detection by mass spectrometry on ultrathin-layer chromatography plates prepared via the low-pressure chemical vapor deposition of silicon nitride onto carbon nanotube templates, *J. Chromatogr. A*, 1404: 115–123.
3. Hauck, H. E., Bund, O., Fischer, W., and Schulz, M. 2001. Ultra-thin layer chromatography (UTLC)—A new dimension in thin-layer chromatography, *J. Planar Chromatogr.*, 14: 234–236.
4. Hauck, H.E. and Schulz, M. 2002. Ultrathin-layer chromatography, *J. Chromatogr. Sci.*, 40: 1–3.
5. Oriňák, A., Vering, G., Arlinghaus, H.F., Andersson, J.T., Halas, L., and Oriňáková, R. 2005. New approaches to coupling TLC with TOF-SIMS, *J. Planar Chromatogr.*, 18: 44–50.
6. Salo, P.K., Salomies, H., Harju, K., Ketola, R.A., Kotiaho, T., Yli-Kauhaluoma, J., and Kostiainen, R. 2005. Analysis of small molecules by ultra thin-layer chromatography–atmospheric pressure matrix-assisted laser desorption/ionization mass spectrometry, *J. Am. Soc. Mass Spectrom.*, 16: 906–915.
7. Salo, P.K., Vilmunen, S., Salomies, H., Ketola, R.A., and Kostiainen, R. 2007. Two-dimensional ultra-thin-layer chromatography and atmospheric pressure matrix-assisted laser desorption/ionization mass spectrometry in bioanalysis, *Anal. Chem.*, 79: 2101–2108.

8. Talian, I., Orinák, A., Preisler, J., Heile, A., Onofrejová, L., Kaniansky, D., and Arlinghaus, H.F. 2007. Comparative TOF-SIMS and MALDI TOF-MS analysis on different chromatographic planar substrates, *J. Sep. Sci.*, 30: 2570–2582.

9. Vovk, I., Popović, G., Simonovska, B., Albreht, A., and Agbaba, D. 2011. Ultra-thin-layer chromatography mass spectrometry and thin-layer chromatography mass spectrometry of single peptides of angiotensin-converting enzyme inhibitors, *J. Chromatogr. A*, 1218: 3089–3094.

10. Kauppila, T.J., Talaty, N., Salo, P.K., Kotiaho, T., Kostiainen, R., and Cooks, R.G. 2006. New surfaces for desorption electrospray ionization mass spectrometry: Porous silicon and ultra-thin layer chromatography plates, *Rapid Commun. Mass Spectrom.*, 20: 2143–2150.

11. Frolova, A.M., Chukhlieb, M.A., Drobot, A.V., Kryshtal, A.P., Loginova, L.P., and Boichenko, A.P. 2009. Producing of monolithic layers of silica for thin-layer chromatography by sol-gel synthesis, *TOSURSJ*, 1: 40–45.

12. Frolova, A.M., Konovalova, O.Y., Loginova, L.P., Bulgakova, A.V., and Boichenko, A.P. 2011. Thin-layer chromatographic plates with monolithic layer of silica: Production, physical-chemical characteristics, separation capabilities, *J. Sep. Sci.*, 34: 2352–2361.

13. Bakry, R., Bonn, G. K., Mair, D., and Svec, F. 2007. Monolithic porous polymer layer for the separation of peptides and proteins using thin-layer chromatography coupled with MALDI-TOF-MS, *Anal. Chem.*, 79: 486–493.

14. Urbanova, I. and Svec, F. 2011. Monolithic polymer layer with gradient of hydrophobicity for separation of peptides using two-dimensional thin layer chromatography and MALDI-TOF-MS detection, *J. Sep. Sci.*, 34: 2345–2351.

15. Lv, Y., Lin, Z., Tan, T., and Svec, F. 2013. Preparation of porous styrenics-based monolithic layers for thin layer chromatography coupled with matrix-assisted laser-desorption/ionization time-of-flight mass spectrometric detection, *J. Chromatogr. A*, 1316: 154–159.

16. Clark, J.E. and Olesik, S.V. 2009. Technique for ultrathin layer chromatography using an electrospun, nanofibrous stationary phase, *Anal. Chem.*, 81: 4121–4129.

17. Beilke, M.C., Zewe, J.W., Clark, J.E., and Olesik, S.V. 2013. Aligned electrospun nanofibers for ultra-thin layer chromatography, *Anal. Chim. Acta*, 761: 201–208.

18. Clark, J.E. and Olesik, S.V. 2010. Electrospun glassy carbon ultra-thin layer chromatography devices, *J. Chromatogr. A*, 1217: 4655–4662.

19. Lu, T. and Olesik, S.V. 2013. Electrospun polyvinyl alcohol ultra-thin layer chromatography of amino acids, *J. Chromatogr. B*, 912: 98–104.

20. Fang, X. and Olesik, S.V. 2014. Carbon nanotube and carbon nanorod-filled polyacrylonitrile electrospun stationary phase for ultrathin layer chromatography, *Anal. Chim. Acta*, 830: 1–10.

21. Newsome, T.E. and Olesik, S.V. 2014. Silica-based nanofibers for electrospun ultra-thin layer chromatography, *J. Chromatogr. A*, 1364: 261–270.

22. Bezuidenhout, L.W. and Brett, M.J. 2008. Ultrathin layer chromatography on nanostructured thin films, *J. Chromatogr. A*, 1183: 179–185.

23. Jim, S.R., Taschuk, M.T., Morlock, G.E., Bezuidenhout, L.W., Schwack, W., and Brett, M.J. 2010. Engineered anisotropic microstructures for ultrathin-layer chromatography, *Anal. Chem.*, 82: 5349–5356.

24. Oko, A.J., Jim, S.R., Taschuk, M.T., and Brett, M.J. 2011. Analyte migration in anisotropic nanostructured ultrathin-layer chromatography media, *J. Chromatogr. A*, 1218: 2661–2667.

25. Hall, J.Z., Taschuk, M.T., and Brett, M.J. 2012. Polarity-adjustable reversed phase ultrathin-layer chromatography, *J. Chromatogr. A*, 1266: 168–174.

26. Jim, S.R., Foroughi-Abari, A., Krause, K.M., Li, P., Kupsta, M., Taschuk, M.T., Cadien, K.C., and Brett, M.J. 2013. Ultrathin-layer chromatography nanostructures modified by atomic layer deposition, *J. Chromatogr. A*, 1299: 118–125.

27. Wannenmacher, J., Jim, S.R., Taschuk, M.T., Brett, M.J., and Morlock, G.E. 2013. Ultrathin-layer chromatography on $SiO_2$, Al2O3, $TiO_2$, and $ZrO_2$ nanostructured thin films, *J. Chromatogr. A*, 1318: 234–243.

28. Kirchert, S., Wang, Z., Taschuk, M.T., Jim, S.R., Brett, M.J., and Morlock, G.E. 2013. Inkjet application, chromatography, and mass spectrometry of sugars on nanostructured thin films, *Anal. Bioanal. Chem.*, 405: 7195–7203.

29. Song, J., Jensen, D.S., Hutchison, D.N., Turner, B., Wood, T., Dadson, A., Vail, M.A., Linford, M.R., Vanfleet, R.R., and Davis, R.C. 2011. Carbon-nanotube-templated microfabrication of porous silicon-carbon materials with application to chemical separations, *Adv. Funct. Mater.*, 21: 1132–1139.

30. Jensen, D.S., Kanyal, S.S., Gupta, V., Vail, M.A., Dadson, A.E., Engelhard, M., Vanfleet, R., Davis, R.C., and Linford, M.R. 2012. Stable, microfabricated thin layer chromatography plates without volume distortion on patterned, carbon and $Al_2O_3$-primed carbon nanotube forests, *J. Chromatogr. A*, 1257: 195–203.

31. Jensen, D.S., Kanyal, S.S., Madaan, N., Hancock, J.M., Dadson, A.E., Vail, M.A., Vanfleet, R. et al. 2013. Multi-instrument characterization of the surfaces and materials in microfabricated, carbon nanotube-templated thin layer chromatography plates. An analogy to 'The Blind Men and the Elephant', *Surf. Interface Anal.*, 45: 1273–1282.

32. Kanyal, S.S., Jensen, D.S., Miles, A.J., Dadson, A.E., Vail, M.A., Olsen, R., Scorza, F. et al. 2013. Effects of catalyst thickness on the fabrication and performance of carbon nanotube-templated thin layer chromatography plates, *J. Vac. Sci. Technol. B*, 31: 031203-1-8.

33. Jensen, D.S., Kanyal, S.S., Madaan, N., Miles, A.J., Davis, R.C., Vanfleet, R., Vail, M.A., Dadson, A.E., and Linford, M.R. 2013. Ozone priming of patterned carbon nanotube forests for subsequent atomic layer deposition-like deposition of $SiO_2$ for the preparation of microfabricated thin layer chromatography plates, *J. Vac. Sci. Technol. B*, 31: 031803.

34. Kanyal, S.S., Jensen, D.S., Dadson, A.E., Vanfleet, R.R., Davis, R.C., and Linford, M.R. 2014. Atomic layer deposition of aluminum-free silica onto patterned carbon nanotube forests in the preparation of microfabricated thin-layer chromatography plates, *J. Planar Chromatogr.*, 27: 151–156.

35. Zhang, Z., Ratnayaka, S.N., and Wirth, M.J. 2011. Protein UTLC–MALDI–MS using thin films of submicrometer silica particles, *J. Chromatogr. A*, 1218: 7196–7202.

36. Costantini, F., Domenici, F., Mura, F., Scipinotti, R., Sennato, S., Manetti, C., and Bordi, F. 2013. A new nanostructured stationary phase for ultra-thin layer chromatography: A brush-gel polymer film, *Nanosci. Nanotechnol. Lett.*, 5: 1155–1163.

37. Desmet, G. and Baron, G.V. 1999. On the possibility of shear-driven chromatography, *J. Chromatogr. A*, 855: 57–70.

38. Desmet, G., Vervoort, N., Clicq, D., and Baron, G.V. 2001. Experimental demonstration of the possibility to perform shear-driven chromatographic separations in microchannels, *J. Chromatogr. A*, 924: 111–122.

39. de Malsche, W., Clicq, D., Eghbali, H., Fekete, V., Gardeniers, H., and Desmet, G. 2006. An automated injection system for sub-micron sized channels used in shear-driven-chromatography, *Lab Chip*, 6: 1322–1327.

40. Fekete, V., Clicq, D., de Malsche, W., Gardeniers, H., and Desmet, G. 2007. State of the art of shear driven chromatography. Advantages and limitations, *J. Chromatogr. A*, 1149: 2–11.

41. de Bruyne, S., de Malsche, W., Fekete, V., Thienpont, H., Ottevaere, H., Gardeniers, H., and Desmet, G. 2013. Exploring the speed limits of liquid chromatography using shear-driven flows through 45 and 85 nm deep nano-channels, *Analyst*, 138: 6127–6133.
42. de Malsche, W., Eghbali, H., Clicq, D., Vangelooven, J., Gardeniers, H., and Desmet, G. 2007. Pressure-driven reverse-phase liquid chromatography separations in ordered nonporous pillar array columns, *Anal. Chem.*, 79: 5915–5926.
43. Detobel, F., de Bruyne, S., Vangelooven, J., de Malsche, W., Aerts, T., Terryn, H., Gardeniers, H., Eeltink, S., and Desmet, G. 2010. Fabrication and chromatographic performance of porous-shell pillar-array columns, *Anal. Chem.*, 82: 7208–7217.
44. Op de Beeck, Jeff, de Malsche, W., Tezcan, D.S., de Moor, P., and Desmet, G. 2012. Impact of the limitations of state-of-the-art micro-fabrication processes on the performance of pillar array columns for liquid chromatography, *J. Chromatogr. A*, 1239: 35–48.
45. Kirchner, T.B., Hatab, N.A., Lavrik, N.V., and Sepaniak, M.J. 2013. Highly ordered silicon pillar arrays as platforms for planar chromatography, *Anal. Chem.*, 85: 11802–11808.
46. Hayen, H. and Volmer, D.A. 2005. Rapid identification of siderophores by combined thin-layer chromatography–matrix-assisted laser desorption–ionization mass spectrometry, *Rapid Commun. Mass Spectrom.*, 19: 711–720.
47. Luftmann, H. 2004. A simple device for the extraction of TLC spots: Direct coupling with an electrospray mass spectrometer, *Anal. Bioanal. Chem.*, 378: 964–968.
48. Häbe, T.T. and Morlock, G.E. 2015. Quantitative surface scanning by direct analysis in real time mass spectrometry, *Rapid Commun. Mass Spectrom.*, 29: 474–484.
49. Mennickent, S., de Diego, M., and Vega, M. 2013. Ultrathin-layer chromatography (UTLC), *Chromatographia*, 76: 1233–1238.
50. Patel, R.B., Gopani, M.C., and Patel, M.R. 2013. UTLC: An advanced technique in planar chromatography, *Chromatographia*, 76: 1225–1231.
51. Morlock, G.E. 2015. Miniaturized planar chromatography using office peripherals— Office chromatography, *J. Chromatogr. A*, 1382: 87–96.
52. Häbe, T.T. and Morlock, G.E. 2015. Office chromatography: Precise printing of sample solutions on miniaturized thin-layer phases and utilization for scanning Direct Analysis in Real Time mass spectrometry, *J. Chromatogr. A*, in print.

# Section II

## Practical Applications of Planar Chromatography-Mass Spectrometry Methodology

# 10 Strategies of Coupling Planar Chromatography to HPLC–MS

*Claudia Oellig and Wolfgang Schwack*

## CONTENTS

## 10.1 STRATEGIES OF COUPLING PLANAR CHROMATOGRAPHY TO HIGH-PERFORMANCE LIQUID CHROMATOGRAPHY– MASS SPECTROMETRY

Coupling of planar chromatography to mass spectrometry (MS) integrating an additional chromatographic separation step by high-performance liquid chromatography (HPLC) is a special technique of linking high-performance thin-layer chromatography (HPTLC) to MS. The integration of HPLC offers a second, orthogonal dimension concerning selectivity, as HPTLC is almost performed on normal-phase silica gel plates and HPLC usually on reversed-phase C18 columns. By this strategy, the separation efficiency of "only" HPTLC can be outperformed and the high versatility of HPTLC can clearly be shown [1]. Concerning the MS detection process, various ion sources such as electrospray ionization (ESI), atmospheric pressure chemical ionization, or atmospheric pressure photo ionization can be used, depending on the analytes under focus. In food analysis, ESI is by far the most used ionization technique in nearly each field of application for polar, semipolar, and even quite nonpolar analytes.

During the last 10 years, hyphenating the open planar system with MS has mainly focused on elution-based techniques and interfaces, leading to the development of the semiautomated TLC–MS interface (CAMAG), which today is frequently in use (see Chapter 3). The TLC–MS interface is universal and versatile, and not restricted to special TLC carrier materials, layer types, analytes, or elution solvents [1–3]. For the outlined coupling strategies of HPTLC through HPLC to MS, the TLC–MS interface is an integral part of the system, offering the easy, simple, and rapid zone elution from the planar thin-layer. Without doubt, it is the essential tool for a reliably repeatable elution process, which is the prerequisite for quantitative analysis.

### 10.1.1 ONLINE AND OFFLINE HIGH-PERFORMANCE THIN-LAYER CHROMATOGRAPHY–HIGH-PERFORMANCE LIQUID CHROMATOGRAPHY–MASS SPECTROMETRY COUPLING

Beside the conventional use of the TLC–MS interface, performing the direct connection to the MS by a capillary from the outlet line of the interface to the MS, a further very promising option to couple planar thin-layers to MS is realized by integrating an HPLC column between the thin-layer plate (directly after the TLC–MS interface) and the MS (Figure 10.1a).

Thus, the eluted HPTLC zone is directly transferred onto the column, when a monolithic column is necessary to prevent high back pressure and elution-head leakages. Alternatively, the target zones are consecutively eluted from the plate into autosampler vials to subsequently perform HPLC–MS or GC–MS analysis (Figure 10.1b). This alternative is more time efficient for routine analysis, until a fully automated TLC–MS interface is available, because the HPLC–MS or GC–MS analysis of eluates in autosampler vials is done automatically.

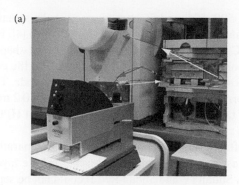
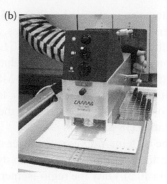

**FIGURE 10.1** (a) Online HPTLC–HPLC–MS; the dark arrow shows inlet line from the HPLC pump to the TLC–MS interface; the light arrows mark the outlet line from the interface to a monolithic column and to the MS and (b) offline HPTLC–HPLC–MS; elution of the target zones into vials to be placed into the autosampler of the HPLC–MS system.

## 10.2 SEPARATION OF LAYER MODIFICATIONS BY HIGH-PERFORMANCE THIN-LAYER CHROMATOGRAPHY–HIGH-PERFORMANCE LIQUID CHROMATOGRAPHY–MASS SPECTROMETRY

### 10.2.1 DETERMINATION OF BANNED FAT-SOLUBLE AZO DYES IN SPICES ON CAFFEINE-IMPREGNATED SILICA GEL PLATES

In 2003, the Sudan I dye was detected in France in a shipment of hot chili from India. This was the first time of an alert via the European Rapid Alert System for Food and Feed (RASFF). During the following years, unauthorized fat-soluble azo dyes were detected in more and more products, and efficient screening assays for differently challenging matrices were required.

Because HPTLC allows a rapid and matrix-robust screening for many samples, it was the best chance to screen for banned azo dyes. As dyes strongly absorb visible light, a good capability of visible detection is generally given. Coupling of HPTLC to MS offers an additional and improved detection possibility to verify positive findings, beside the conventionally performed comparison with UV/V is library spectra. Therefore, a rapid and reliable HPTLC method was developed in 2009 for the identification and quantitation of the most relevant azo dyes. The method included the novel online HPTLC–HPLC–MS coupling strategy, which was performed for the first time in this application, and was tested on powders of spices and spice mixes like chili, curry, and paprika [4].

After the addition of an internal standard, samples were extracted with acetone/methanol. Without further cleanup, the separation was performed on caffeine-impregnated HPTLC plates NANO-SIL-PAH, 20 × 10 cm (Macherey-Nagel), developed with *i*-hexane/methyl ethyl ketone (5/1, v/v). Interfering fat-soluble natural dyes (carotenoids) were bleached by UV irradiation, followed by multi-wavelength densitometry performed at 390, 415, 500, 525, and 550 nm, respecting the spectral properties of the different azo dyes, and by spectra recording (320–600 nm) [4]. For the subsequent MS detection, the TLC–MS interface, equipped with the oval-shaped elution head, was used for zone elution, coupled through a Chromolith RP 18e column (50 × 4.6 mm, Merck) to the MS system operated in the positive ESI mode. The eluent consisted of methanol/0.1% formic acid (90/10, v/v) at a flow rate of 0.2 mL/min, used for both the elution of the target zone for 30 s and the subsequent HPLC separation (18 min).

The caffeine-impregnated layer offered far superior chromatographic separation of the most frequently found azo dyes than normal-phase or reversed-phase layers (Figure 10.2). Only the regio-isomers Sudan IV and Sudan Red B could not be separated, which, however, generally is a highly challenging task, even by HPLC–MS/MS [5].

During the TLC–MS experiments for confirmation purposes, the additional orthogonal separation selectivity of a short monolithic RP 18e column was used to separate the caffeine impregnation, also eluting from the silica layer, from the azo dyes. The column was integrated in the outlet capillary line of the TLC–MS interface, when a direct online HPTLC–HPLC–MS hyphenation was performed.

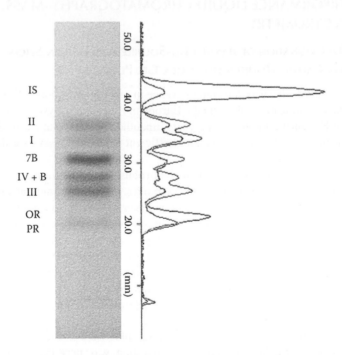

**FIGURE 10.2** Separation of azo dyes on caffeine-impregnated HPTLC plates and spectral scans at 500 nm (pink) and 415 nm (black). Sudan I (I), Sudan II (II), Sudan Red B (B), Sudan Orange G (OR), Sudan III (III), Sudan IV (IV), Sudan Red 7B (7B), Para red (PR), and 4-dimethylaminoazobenzene (IS). (Adapted from Pellissier, E. and Schwack, W. 2009. *CAMAG Bibliogr. Service CBS*, 103: 13–15.)

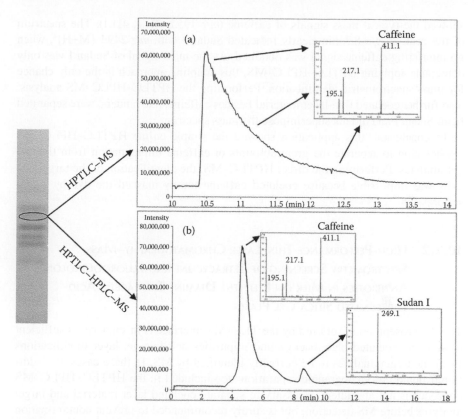

**FIGURE 10.3** Comparison of mass spectra obtained from online HPTLC–MS and HPTLC–HPLC–MS analysis: (a) HPTLC–MS chronogram and mass spectrum of the suspected zone of Sudan I and (b) HPTLC–HPLC–MS chromatogram of the suspected zone of Sudan I and mass spectra of the chromatographically separated peaks on the monolithic RP 18e column, indicating caffeine and Sudan I.

By comparing the mass spectra of the Sudan I zone, obtained from both the online HPTLC–MS and the online HPTLC–HPLC–MS analysis (Figure 10.3), the cleanup effect by the integrated monolithic RP 18e column was directly visible. The HPTLC–MS mass spectrum of the suspected Sudan I zone only showed the mass signals of the layer impregnation with $m/z$ 195.1 [M+H]$^+$, $m/z$ 217.1 [M+Na]$^+$, and most intensive $m/z$ 411.1 [2M+Na]$^+$, representing caffeine (Figure 10.3a). The mass signals of the protonated molecule, the sodium adduct, and the dimer of Sudan I, which are obtained by TLC–MS from nonimpregnated silica gel plates, were not visible. This was caused by the strong ion suppression effect of huge amounts of coeluted caffeine on the signal intensity of Sudan I. Even after software-based background subtraction, using a spectrum from an analyte-free layer region, where only the caffeine impregnation was present, the mass signals of the Sudan I dye did not become apparent. Thus, the merit of the additionally integrated HPLC separation performing the online HPTLC–HPLC–MS is obvious (Figure 10.3b). The coeluted caffeine impregnation was fully separated from the target Sudan I. The mass spectrum of the peak at $R_t = 5$ min showed the typical mass signals of caffeine (*m/z* 195.1, 217.1, 411.1). The spectrum of the peak at $R_t = 8.7$ min clearly indicated Sudan I with *m/z* 249.1 [M+H]$^+$, when no interfering caffeine signal was obtained. As the mass signal of Sudan I was only detectable applying HPTLC–HPLC–MS, this coupling approach is the only chance for mass spectrometric identification. Performing the HPTLC–HPLC–MS analysis, also further coeluted thin-layer material besides caffeine, like binders, were separated from Sudan I and did not superimpose the mass spectrum.

In conclusion, this application showed the simple online HPTLC–HPLC–MS hyphenation to separate the great amounts of caffeine impregnation from the target analytes. Performing the direct HPTLC–MS, the identification of the target azo dyes was impossible because coeluted caffeine totally masked the dye by signal suppression.

### 10.2.2 HIGH-PERFORMANCE THIN-LAYER CHROMATOGRAPHY–MASS SPECTROMETRY SCREENING OF TETRACYCLINE AND FLUOROQUINOLONE ANTIBIOTICS IN MILK ON ETHYLENE DIAMINE TETRAACETIC ACID-IMPREGNATED SILICA GEL PLATES

The "microseparation" offered by the TLC–MS interface is in some cases sufficient to separate coeluted plate background impurities or silica gel layer modifications from the target analytes to be correctly identified by MS. In these cases, the additional liquid chromatographic separation step included in the HPTLC–HPLC–MS approach is not absolutely necessary to separate coeluted layer material and target analytes before MS detection, but is surely recommended to prevent contamination of the MS equipment and to receive reliable results. The successful workflow could be easily shown for the identification of antibiotics in milk. The monitoring of antibiotic residues in foodstuffs has attracted great public interest during the last decade, since the abuse of antibiotics causes serious problems for human health associated with food safety and the well-known and often reported bacterial resistances [6]. Various approaches of antibiotic analysis have been reported during the last years [7–12], generally using similar analysis steps: the extraction with organic solvents, the cleanup by solid phase extraction (SPE), a preconcentration step, and the subsequent separation and detection by HPLC–MS. All of these methods need big efforts to gather high sensitivity and reproducible results. Keeping this in mind, a fast and efficient screening method for tetracycline and fluoroquinolone antibiotics, frequently found in milk, was developed, applying HPTLC for an effective solid phase purification and the separation of the analytes in one step. Beside fluorescence detection for quantitation, the mass selective detection using the TLC–MS interface was established for confirmatory purposes [6].

The extraction of milk samples was done by the quick, easy, cheap, effective, rugged, and safe (QuEChERS) method [13], modified by adding disodium ethylenediaminetetraacetate dihydrate (Na$_2$-EDTA). Without any further cleanup, the extract was separated on HPTLC silica gel plates modified by Na$_2$-EDTA. The development was performed with chloroform/methanol/ammonium hydroxide solution (25%), 60/35/5 (v/v/v), followed by fluorescence densitometry (FLD) at 366 nm/<400 nm for tetracyclines, 280 nm/<320 nm for enrofloxacine and ciprofloxacine, and 300 nm/<400 nm for marbofloxacine. TLC–MS experiments were performed on a single quadrupole MS working in the positive ESI mode, when total ion current chronograms in full-scan mode were recorded from $m/z$ 200 to $m/z$ 700. The elution of the analyte zones was done with the oval-shaped elution head using acetonitrile/10 mM ammonium formate with 2% methanol (90/10, v/v) at a flow rate of 0.3 mL/min for 30 s [6].

Tetracyclines and fluoroquinolones form strong complexes with bivalent ions like calcium. Therefore, EDTA was added during milk extraction and EDTA-modified silica gel was selected as a layer material offering the best separation (free of tailing) of the target compounds and a significant fluorescence enhancement effect for a low limit of detection. The selected solvent system provided the complete separation of the seven antibiotics (Figure 10.4), when a 10% EDTA solution for the layer modification was verified as optimal for the best separation of TCs and FQs [6].

The additional HPTLC–MS analysis was very useful for the confirmation of the HPTLC–FLD screening results. Applying the TLC–MS interface, the target compounds were eluted from the modified silica gel layer and directly transferred into the ion source of the MS. Interfering ion suppression effects of the EDTA modification were omitted by a suitable elution solvent. Methanol in combination with ammonium formate resulted in strong ion suppression and contamination of the ion source, caused by coeluted EDTA. Since acetonitrile hardly dissolved EDTA salts, a mixture of acetonitrile/ammonium formate (9/1, v/v) was chosen as ionization efficiency and peak performance were optimal for this mixture. Figure 10.5 depicts the typical HPTLC–MS elution profile received for a target compound from the EDTA-modified silica gel layer.

The antibiotics were eluted from the plate first, which only took 0.25 min, exemplarily seen in the resulting mass spectrum of chlortetracycline with the monoisotopic signal at $m/z$ 479.1 [M+H]$^+$ and the chlorine isotope signal at $m/z$ 481.1 (Figure 10.5a). When the elution of the target compound was almost completed,

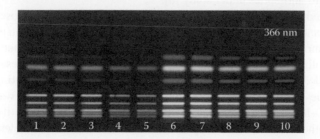

**FIGURE 10.4** Plate image of the HPTLC separation of target analytes on an EDTA-modified silica gel plate under UV 366 nm. Track assignments: (1) and (8) whole milk (3.5% fat) spiked at 100 and 200 µg/kg, (2) and (9) skimmed milk (1.5% fat) spiked at 100 and 200 µg/kg, (3) and (10) whole milk (bio, 3.5% fat) spiked at 100 and 200 µg/kg, (4) and (5) standards of 10 ng/zone (6) and 50 ng/zone (7). Standards, $hR_F$: OTC, 7; CTC, 11; TC, 17; DC, 23; CF, 38; MF, 49; EF, 58. (Reprinted from Chen, Y., and Schwack, W., *J. Chromatogr. A*, 1312, 143–151, 2013. Copyright 2013, with permission from Elsevier.)

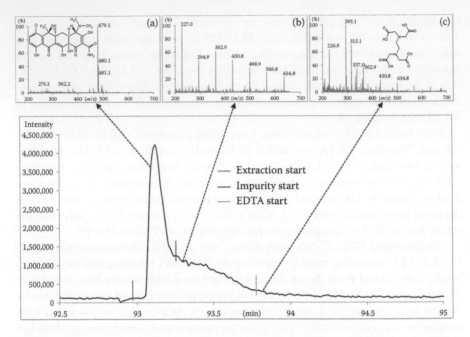

**FIGURE 10.5** HPTLC–MS total ion current chronogram in the ESI positive mode of a target compound (chlortetracyline) from the EDTA-modified silica gel plate. Mass spectra were extracted at the top of the peak (a), the beginning of the shoulder (b), and at the tail (c). (Reprinted from Chen, Y., and Schwack, W., *J. Chromatogr. A*, 1312, 143–151, 2013. Copyright 2013, with permission from Elsevier.)

silica gel impurities eluted in the time range of 0.25–0.65 min, characterized by a signal at $m/z$ 227 and a series of masses differing by 68 amu (Figure 10.5b). At the end of the elution process, EDTA partly entered the MS, verified by mass signals at $m/z$ 293.1 $[M+H]^+$ and $m/z$ 315.1 $[M+Na]^+$ (Figure 10.5c). The elution profile was identical for all antibiotics under study [6].

The adapted and optimized TLC–MS eluent offered a slight microseparation of the analytes and impurities, first by the elution step itself (as acetonitrile only dissolved low amounts of EDTA) and second by the specific eluent properties and the interaction with the investigated analytes generating a separation represented by the "elution profile." Thus, a slight separation of the target compounds eluting first from plate impurities and the most prominent interfering compound EDTA was achieved. This HPTLC–MS approach offered the possibility to sensitively identify the target substance without an additional separation step by HPLC. Nevertheless, the high amount of EDTA and further coeluted substances strongly contaminated the MS. A possible strategy to avoid this contamination could be to stop the elution process directly after exceeding the peak maximum of the total ion chronogram (elution profile), when a nearly full elution of the target analyte was performed. For an unknown compound, however, this might cause nondetection if it elutes later in the hump of the elution profile. In this context, the HPTLC–HPLC–MS coupling would be the best technique as well, offering more reliable results as the analytes will be fully separated from EDTA and further impurities, without losing analytes. Nevertheless, it was shown for this application that the HPTLC–HPLC–MS approach is not always strictly necessary to receive good results. This is especially true because tetracycline and fluoroquinolone antibiotics are best detected in the ESI positive mode, when the suppression effects of EDTA are not as strong as in the ESI negative mode because EDTA is more likely to produce [M–H]⁻ ions. Consequently, if analytes require the ESI negative mode, the HPTLC–HPLC–MS technique will be necessary to prevent strong ion suppression effects by the very high EDTA presence as compared to the analytes of interest.

## 10.3 HIGH-PERFORMANCE THIN-LAYER CHROMATOGRAPHY FOR CLEANUP

A great advantage of HPTLC is the easy localization and visibility of target analytes and matrix components. The combination of cleanup and determination was already shown for numerous examples. For instance, the quite resistant synthetic sweetener sucralose was determined in river water and sewage effluents [14,15]. An optimized separation system in combination with a selective and sensitive postchromatographic derivatization was applied for the separation of sucralose from coextracted matrix and the quantitation down to 100 ng/L [14,15]. Other applications used the HPTLC separation for cleanup instead of cartridge solid phase extraction (cSPE). Cleanup using TLC was performed as preparative TLC [16], when the whole plate width was used for the separation of multi-component extracts. A single zone of interest was scraped off the layer, subsequently extracted and analyzed using different detection methods. Several examples are presented in the literature, as for pesticide residue analysis by HPTLC [17,18] and GC–ECD [19], and for the determination of PAHs in marine samples [20] or sewage sludge [21] by GC–MS.

Otherwise, applying small bands allows the cleanup of multiple samples in parallel on a single plate. This technique was applied for the determination of PAHs in aerosol samples using GC isotope ratio MS to identify the source of contamination [22], as the $\delta^{13}C$ values differed depending on the locality from where the samples were collected. As a further application using TLC as the efficient cleanup step, the separation of PAHs from coextracted matrix components in vegetable oil samples was described, followed by GC–MS determination [23]. This example shows the high performance of TLC for this application field, as extraction and cleanup for fatty matrices is known to be very challenging. Another application did not use solvents to extract the scraped-off zones from the layer material, but rather applied thermal desorption. Thereby, the identification by GC–MS was possible down to 20 ng/spot for PAHs, naphthalenes, and several pesticides [24].

### 10.3.1 High-Throughput Planar Solid Phase Extraction and High-Performance Liquid Chromatography–Mass Spectrometry for Pesticide Residue Analysis

Using HPTLC, a new and efficient cleanup method was recently developed for pesticide residue analysis. The technique was established for extracts of fruit and vegetables [25] and was further adapted for tea [26]. The method, named high-throughput planar solid phase extraction (HTpSPE), transferred the cSPE concept on planar thin-layers and thereby offered a fast and easy cleanup in the microscale. Using the highly automated instrumental HPTLC devices, with the TLC–MS interface as an integral part of the method for the detection by MS, an effective technique for reliable results in pesticide residue analysis was established.

The HTpSPE concept used a twofold development, whereafter pesticides were focused in a sharp zone and fully separated from the coextracted matrix compounds. For the following mass selective detection, the TLC–MS interface was applied to elute the analytes from the target zone. To achieve an additional chromatographic selectivity, an HPLC column was integrated for separation of the target analyte mixture, when different coupling strategies were applied. On the one hand, the TLC–MS interface was directly connected to the HPLC–MS, using a monolithic RP 18e column (Figure 10.1a). This online HTpSPE–HPLC–MS strategy resulted in the highest sensitivity for the target analytes (Figure 10.6). Alternatively, the offline HTpSPE–HPLC–MS approach was established when all analyte zones of a plate were successively collected in autosampler vials followed by HPLC–MS measurements (Figure 10.1b). The advantage of this offline HTpSPE–HPLC–MS strategy is the high time efficiency as all target zones were eluted with the TLC–MS interface one after the other and were afterward injected and measured automatically. Unfortunately, a fourfold dilution was obtained during the TLC–MS elution in autosampler vials, and also only an aliquot of the eluate could be injected and thus measured by HPLC–MS. This resulted in lower signal intensities, and hence higher detection limits, clearly shown in Figure 10.6. The pesticide signals in the total ion current chromatogram (TIC) of a standard mixture by online HTpSPE–HPLC–MS are much more intensive than those obtained by the offline HTpSPE–HPLC–MS approach for the same amounts of pesticides present in the target zone.

The higher sensitivity obtained for the online HTpSPE–HPLC–MS approach was a great advantage of this hyphenation, but until a fully automated TLC–MS interface is available, the online HTpSPE–HPLC–MS coupling model is not attractive

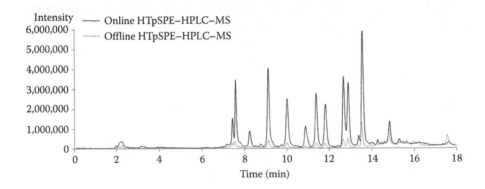

**FIGURE 10.6** Total ion current chromatograms of a pesticide mixture (0.2–1.2 mg/kg, depending on the pesticide) in the ESI positive mode, using online (black chromatogram) and offline (gray chromatogram) HTpSPE–HPLC–MS.

because each HPLC–MS run has to be started manually. Consequently, the more time-efficient offline HTpSPE–HPLC–MS approach was established for the planar cleanup technique, when the main drawback of lower sensitivity may partly be compensated by more sensitive mass spectrometers. Higher injection volumes, however, affecting the separation, are not recommended. Including a concentration step would only be time-consuming and may additionally cause the loss of pesticides.

### 10.3.1.1 High-Throughput Planar Solid Phase Extraction and High-Performance Liquid Chromatography–Mass Spectrometry for Pesticide Residue Analysis in Fruit and Vegetables

To ensure the compliance with the maximum residue limits of pesticides in food and feed, robust analytical techniques with sensitive and selective techniques are required. The most serious problems in pesticide residue analysis are caused by the huge amount of coextracted matrix compounds. The well-known matrix effects in GC–MS and HPLC–MS often appear in the form of signal suppression, retention time shifting, or inexact quantitation in general. A reliable way to prevent matrix effects in pesticide residue analysis is an efficient and effective cleanup of extracts. The HTpSPE–HPLC–MS concept allows a rapid cleanup by HTpSPE for a full separation of pesticides from coextracted matrix compounds followed by HPLC–MS analysis.

Sample extraction was performed according to the QuEChERS method [13]. Two internal standards were applied, tris(1,3-dichloroisopropyl)phosphate (TDCPP) for quantitation and Sudan II as a visible marker to locate the target analyte zone. The homogenized sample (10 g) was extracted with 10-mL acetonitrile by vigorously shaking for 1 min. For phase separation and regulating the pH, sodium chloride, magnesium sulfate, and citrate buffer salts were added, followed by shaking for another minute and centrifugation at 4000 rpm. The supernatant was directly used for HTpSPE on TLC aluminum foils silica gel 60 $NH_2$ $F_{254}$s without an additional cleanup. Before sample application, the layer was dipped 2 cm deep in formic acid solution (2% in acetonitrile) and dried in a stream of warm air. Extracts (50 µL) were area (3.0 × 4.0 mm) applied, and development was first performed with acetonitrile to a migration distance of 75 mm. After drying the foil, the second development was done with acetone to a migration distance of 45 mm in the backward direction. For the following HPLC–MS analysis, the elution of the target analyte zones into autosampler vials was performed with TLC–MS interface using acetonitrile/10 mM ammonium formate (1/1, v/v) at a flow rate of 0.2 mL/min for 60 s. The subsequent separation of the pesticides was performed on a Chromolith Performance RP 18e (100 mm × 3.0 mm, Merck) with the corresponding precolumn using a gradient elution within 18 min. A single quadrupole MS was applied in the full-scan measurement mode for identification and in the selected ion monitoring (SIM) mode for quantitation [25]. The manifold detection options in planar chromatography made the successful cleanup directly visible (Figure 10.7).

Almost the complete matrix including organic acids, sugars, and plant phenols remained at the application position and was fully separated from the pesticides, which are focused in the target analyte zone, visible under white light and UV 366 nm. Fatty acids were also completely removed by HTpSPE, displayed for oleic

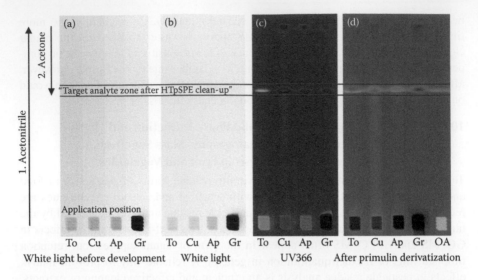

**FIGURE 10.7** Separation of matrix and pesticides on TLC aluminum foils silica gel 60 $NH_2$ $F_{254}$s (tomatoes (To), cucumbers (Cu), apples (Ap), and red grapes (Gr); oleic acid (OA) was applied as a fatty acid example): before development under white light (a), after twofold development under white light (b), UV 366 nm (c), and UV 366 nm after derivatization with primuline (d). (Reprinted from Oellig, C., and Schwack, W., *J. Chromatogr. A*, 1218, 6540–6547, 2011. Copyright 2011, with permission from Elsevier.)

acid after primuline derivatization, which especially is responsible for prominent matrix effects in GC–MS analysis.

Following this HTpSPE cleanup, the target zone (pesticides) was easily eluted by the TLC–MS interface into autosampler vials, performing the offline HTpSPE–HPLC–MS coupling technique. Figure 10.8 shows the complete workflow for a spiked apple extract including the HTpSPE cleanup, the TLC–MS elution, and the following HPLC–MS analysis, which was performed in the full-scan mode to assess the cleanup effect and for identification of the target analytes by the resulting mass spectra.

The obtained chromatograms of blank and spiked extracts clearly showed the cleanup effect of HTpSPE compared to common dSPE with primary secondary amine (PSA) (Figure 10.9). The blank QuEChERS raw extracts of tomatoes exemplarily present an immense matrix load across the entire chromatogram with matrix signals particularly between 7 and 9 min (polar compounds) and from 13 min on (nonpolar substances), when broad humps and distinct chromatographic peaks were observed. After dSPE cleanup the matrix load was only marginally reduced, but after HTpPSE, the chromatograms were nearly free of matrix signals and interferences, when both polar and nonpolar substances were removed. Thus, matrix effects were completely eliminated. In spiked QuEChERS raw extracts, coelution of matrix substances and pesticides strongly occurred, which also remained after dSPE cleanup with PSA. Since chromatograms of spiked HTpSPE extracts are nearly identical to

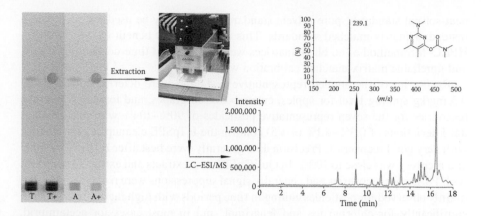

**FIGURE 10.8** Extraction of a target zone with the TLC–MS interface followed by HPLC–MS, total ion current chromatogram of an apple extract spiked with a mixture of pesticides of various substance classes (A+) and mass spectrum of the peak with $R_t$ = 9 min (pirimicarb, $m/z$ 239.1, [M+H]$^+$).

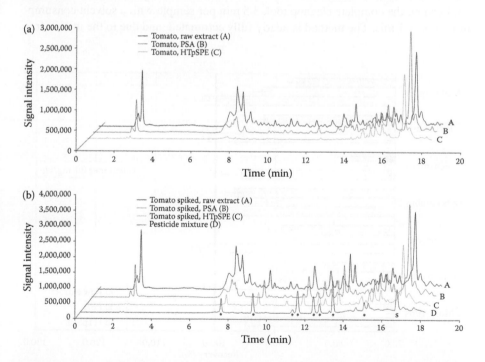

**FIGURE 10.9** Comparison of HPLC–MS full-scan total ion current chromatograms of tomato blank extracts (a) and extracts spiked with a pesticide mixture at 0.5 mg/kg and TDCPP (*) (b): QuEChERS raw extract after dSPE and after HTpSPE cleanup. (Reprinted from Oellig, C., and Schwack, W., *J. Chromatogr. A*, 1218, 6540–6547, 2011. Copyright 2011, with permission from Elsevier.)

neat solvent standards, pure solvent standards could easily be used for quantitation instead of matrix-matched standards. This is a particular benefit of the HTpSPE–HPLC–MS method as no blank matrices were needed, and time-consuming, costly, and unreliable matrix-matched calibration was avoided.

Recoveries of the applied representative pesticides were determined at 0.1 and 0.5 mg/kg spiking level for apples, cucumbers, red grapes, and tomatoes. Average recoveries for the seven representative pesticides of 90%–104% with relative standard deviations of 0.3%–4.1% ($n = 5$) confirm the HTpSPE cleanup as reproducible with very good recoveries. Precision data generally were best after HTpSPE cleanup and recovery was close to 100%. In QuEChERS raw extracts and extracts after dSPE with PSA, poor recoveries and generally signal suppressions were received. This was mainly observed for pesticides eluting in time periods with high matrix background, significantly for chlorpyrifos and fenarimol, and in most cases for acetamiprid. [25]. Detailed recovery values are exemplarily shown in Figure 10.10 for cucumber extracts at a spiking level of 0.1 mg/kg, illustrating the diverse results for the different cleanup methods.

In conclusion, HTpSPE offers a simultaneous sample cleanup of 20 extracts within 20-min developing time on a 20-cm plate. Including the automatic sample application, the complete cleanup took 3.5 min per sample with a solvent consumption of only 1 mL. The method is nearly fully automated, and due to the matrix-free

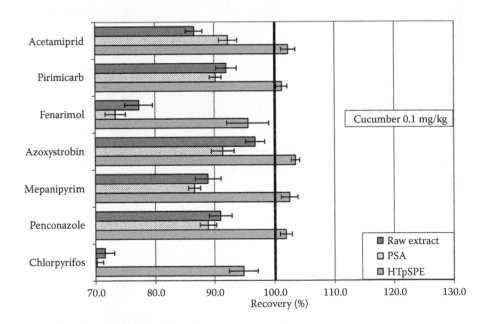

**FIGURE 10.10** HTpSPE–HPLC–MS recovery results from QuEChERS raw extracts, after dSPE cleanup with PSA, and after HTpSPE cleanup for seven representative pesticides spiked at 0.1 mg/kg ($n = 5$), pesticides ordered by increasing retention time. (Reprinted from Oellig, C., and Schwack, W., *J. Chromatogr. A*, 1218, 6540–6547, 2011. Copyright 2011, with permission from Elsevier.)

extracts, calibration could simply be done with pure solvent standards. Thus, HTpSPE is a cost-effective, reliable, and rapid alternative to commonly used cleanup techniques. The new HTpSPE–HPLC–MS approach was successfully proven with a pesticide mixture of various substance classes in different fruit and vegetable matrices. Compared to common dispersive SPE methods, sample extracts are much cleaner and matrix effects are almost completely eliminated. Average recoveries of the representative pesticides spiked in four different matrices were almost 100% with relative standard deviations lower than 4%.

### 10.3.1.2 High-Throughput Planar Solid Phase Extraction and High-Performance Liquid Chromatography–Mass Spectrometry for Pesticide Residue Analysis in Tea

Tea leaves naturally contain a great variety of components, and some specific compounds were additionally formed during the tea production. Thus, tea is a very complex and problematic sample for residue analysis requiring time-consuming and complicated sample treatment procedures. Hence, the HTpSPE cleanup concept was applied to the particularly challenging tea matrix. Using conventional methods, the extracts contained high amounts of coextracted matrix compounds. Beside significant quantities of polyphenols and chlorophylls, particularly the high amounts of coextracted caffeine resulted in strong matrix effects, both in HPLC–MS and in GC–MS. For the tea matrix, the formerly developed HTpSPE procedure on amino-modified silica layers for fruit and vegetables was not suitable to remove the high amounts of coextracted substances, especially caffeine. Additionally, the matrix load was generally too high for the capacity of the thin-layer. Therefore, tea samples were extracted with acetonitrile without an aqueous soaking step to reduce the matrix load. Nevertheless, a precleaning by dSPE was necessary before HTpSPE could be performed, when normal-phase silica gel was best suited for the separation of the target analytes from the tea matrix. This modified HTpSPE concept provided very clean tea extracts offering reproducible and exact validation results [26].

Dry black and green tea samples (2 g) were extracted with acetonitrile (10 mL) by homogenization (27,000 rpm) for 1 min. After centrifugation, the extracts were subjected to dSPE using PSA, C18, and $MgSO_4$ (acetonitrile-dSPE extracts). TDCPP for quantitation and Sudan II as visible marker for the analyte zone were used as internal standards. For HTpSPE, the acetonitrile-dSPE extracts (50 µL) were applied onto silica gel glass plates 60 $F_{254}$ (20 × 10 cm) as areas of 3 mm length and 16 mm height. A twofold development was done with acetonitrile/water (19/1, v/v) to a migration distance of 85 mm and in the backward direction with acetone/water (35/5, v/v) to a migration distance of 31 mm. Using the TLC–MS interface, the target analyte zones were eluted into autosampler vials with acetonitrile/10 mM ammonium formate (1/1, v/v) at a flow rate of 200 µL/min for 1 min. The HPLC–MS(/MS) analysis was performed on a Chromolith RP 18e column (100 × 3 mm) with a gradient consisting of acetonitrile and 10 mM ammonium formate [26].

Evaluating different layer materials and mobile phases, a twofold development on TLC silica gel was most successful for the separation of especially caffeine and chlorophyll from the target pesticides in tea samples. (Figure 10.11) The modified HTpSPE procedure for black and green tea resulted in colorless extracts free

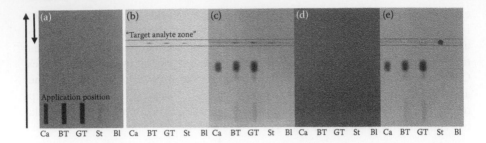

**FIGURE 10.11** Separation of acetonitrile-dSPE extracts of black tea (BT) and green tea (GT), and a pesticide mixture (St) on TLC silica gel plates before development under UV 254 nm (a), after the twofold development under white light (b), UV 254 nm (c), UV 366 nm (d), and UV 254 nm after extraction of the target zones by the TLC–MS interface (e). Caffeine (Ca) and a blank acetonitrile-dSPE extract (Bl) of the used dSPE materials were applied for comparison. (Reprinted from Oellig, C., and Schwack, W., *J. Chromatogr. A*, 1260, 42–53, 2012. Copyright 2012, with permission from Elsevier.)

of caffeine, tea phenols, and chlorophyll, impressively demonstrated by the various detection possibilities of HPTLC (Figure 10.12). The difference between the acetonitrile-HTpSPE and the QuEChERS-dSPE method was directly visible. Acetonitrile-HTpSPE extracts were much cleaner than extracts obtained by the commonly applied QuEChERS-dSPE method [13], with almost no residual coextracted substances.

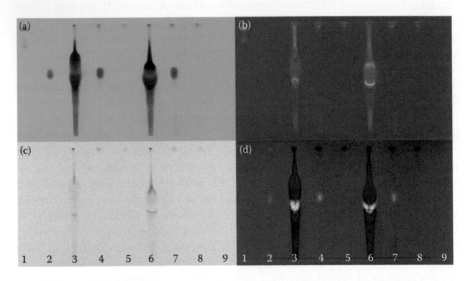

**FIGURE 10.12** Plate images of extracts of black (3, 4, 5) and green tea (6, 7, 8) after single development with acetonitrile at 254 nm (a), 366 nm (b), white light (c), and at 366 nm after derivatization with primuline (d): QuEChERS-dSPE extracts (3, 6), acetonitrile-dSPE extracts before (4, 7) and after HTpSPE (5, 8), pesticide mixture (each approximately 500 ng) (1), caffeine (10 µg) (2) and an extraction blank (9). (Reprinted from Oellig, C., and Schwack, W., *J. Chromatogr. A*, 1260, 42–53, 2012. Copyright 2012, with permission from Elsevier.)

After the twofold development (HTpSPE), the target zones—visible by Sudan II—were easily eluted by the TLC–MS interface into autosampler vials to perform the offline HTpSPE–HPLC–MS(/MS) analysis. The direct transfer of the eluates by the online HTpSPE–HPLC–MS(/MS) hyphenation was additionally possible, but due to the poor time efficiency not routinely applied. The cleanup effect of HTpSPE, especially attributed to the separation of caffeine, was easily demonstrated by HPLC–MS analysis in the full-scan mode (Figure 10.13).

Blank acetonitrile-HTpSPE extracts of black tea were almost free of caffeine and other coextracted substances, different from the QuEChERS-dSPE extracts presenting a high matrix load (Figure 10.13a). Spiked acetonitrile-HTpSPE extracts of black tea also provided almost matrix-free chromatograms without matrix inter-ferences (Figure 10.13b), which were nearly identical to a chromatogram of a pure pesticide solvent standard. The results for green tea were almost the same as those for black tea. The merit of this method mainly is the elimination of caffeine inter-ferences, which are especially responsible not only for difficulties in HPLC–MS analysis but also for great problems in GC–MS by masking or hiding early eluting pesticides [26].

The quantitative performance of the HTpSPE cleanup for black and green tea samples was proven for seven representative pesticides. Mean recoveries of

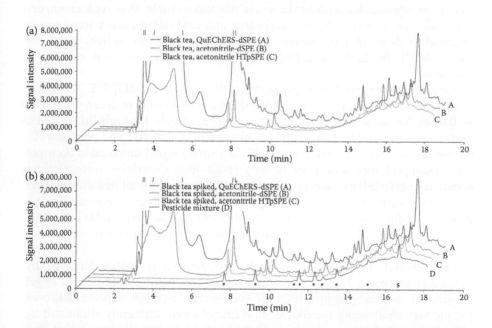

**FIGURE 10.13** HPLC–MS full-scan total ion current chromatograms of black tea extracts: QuEChERS-dSPE extracts (A), acetonitrile-dSPE extracts before (B) and after HTpSPE (C); (a) blank extracts, (b) extracts spiked with pesticides at 1 mg/kg and TDCPP (*), Sudan II (s). (Reprinted from Oellig, C., and Schwack, W., *J. Chromatogr. A*, 1260, 42–53, 2012. Copyright 2012, with permission from Elsevier.)

## TABLE 10.1
## Mean Recoveries by HPLC–MS/MS of Acetonitrile-HTpSPE Extracts of Black and Green Tea at 0.1 and 0.01 mg/kg Spiking Level

| Spiking Level | 0.1 mg/kg | | | | 0.01 mg/kg | | | |
|---|---|---|---|---|---|---|---|---|
| LC–MS/MS (n = 4) | Recovery (%) | | %RSD | | Recovery (%) | | %RSD | |
| Tea Type | Black | Green | Black | Green | Black | Green | Black | Green |
| Acetamiprid | 73 | 72 | 4.7 | 2.3 | 73 | 77 | 3.8 | 3.4 |
| Azoxystrobin | 111 | 108 | 3.8 | 3.7 | 114 | 105 | 3.7 | 3.2 |
| Chorpyrifos | 87 | 106 | 1.8 | 3.1 | 101 | 102 | 3.7 | 2.7 |
| Fenarimol | 95 | 94 | 3.6 | 2.4 | 106 | 94 | 0.8 | 1.6 |
| Mepanipyrim | 103 | 99 | 2.4 | 2.9 | 104 | 100 | 2.5 | 1.7 |
| Penconazole | 78 | 88 | 1.1 | 3 | 87 | 87 | 2.7 | 0.7 |
| Pirimicarb | 95 | 96 | 4.3 | 3.2 | 102 | 103 | 2.1 | 4 |

72%–111% at 0.1 and 0.01 mg/kg spiking levels provided successful results with low relative standard deviations of 0.7%–4.7%, thus approving the HTpSPE cleanup as reproducible without the loss of pesticides (Table 10.1). As acetonitrile-HTpPSE extracts were almost matrix-free and calibration curves were nearly identical to those of pure solvent standards, neat pesticide solvent standards could simply be used for calibration instead of matrix-matched calibration standards.

Comparing the validation parameters, the acetonitrile-HTpSPE technique clearly outperformed the QuEChERS-dSPE method. Results of green tea spiked at 0.01 mg/kg showed high signal enhancement effects for QuEChERS-dSPE extracts (Figure 10.14). Especially for pirimicarb, fenarimol, and penconazole, recoveries were significantly above 100%, but strong signal suppression occurred for acetamiprid with recoveries of only about 40%. Contrarily, recoveries for acetonitrile-HTpSPE extracts provided near-100% values for all pesticides expect acetamiprid suffering from a slight signal suppression effect. The precision data were successful as well and showed the sufficient and well repeatable extraction efficiency of the HTpSPE cleanup with almost no remaining matrix compounds and matrix effects [26].

In conclusion, HTpSPE was developed as a cost-effective, rapid, and nearly fully automated alternative to common cleanup techniques such as dSPE, cSPE, or gel permeation chromatography (GPC) for multi-residue analysis of pesticides, even for the very challenging matrix tea. Interferences were efficiently eliminated by HTpSPE, which fully separated coextracted matrix compounds from target analytes. Twelve sample extracts could be cleaned on a $20 \times 10$ cm plate in parallel at one go, when the total cleanup only took about 6 min/sample with a very low solvent consumption of 1 mL/sample. The offline HTpSPE–HPLC–MS/MS analysis provided highly successful validation parameters for representative pesticides,

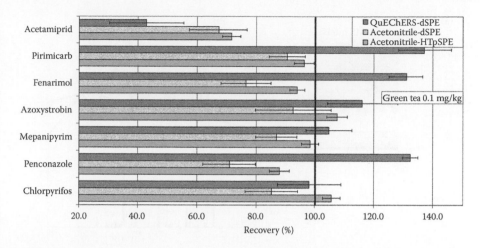

**FIGURE 10.14** Recoveries determined by HPLC–MS/MS of QuEChERS-dSPE, acetonitrile-dSPE, and acetonitrile-HTpSPE extracts for seven pesticides spiked at 0.1 mg/kg to green tea (*n* = 4). (Reprinted from Oellig, C., and Schwack, W., *J. Chromatogr. A*, 1260, 42–53, 2012. Copyright 2012, with permission from Elsevier.)

calibrated against pure solvent standards, when a high sensitivity is thereby additionally ensured [26].

### 10.3.2 HIGH-THROUGHPUT PLANAR SOLID PHASE EXTRACTION COUPLED TO MICROLITER-FLOW INJECTION ANALYSIS–TIME-OF-FLIGHT MASS SPECTROMETRY FOR A FAST PESTICIDE SCREENING

Universal screening methods have gained increasing importance in pesticide residue analysis because the number of pesticides, metabolites, and degradation products that have to be checked to protect the consumer are constantly growing. The so-called nontarget analysis for the detection and identification of an unlimited number of not predefined substances is therefore getting more and more important in residue analysis.

Therefore, a new HPTLC–MS coupling strategy was developed for a fast pesticide screening in residue analysis of food [27]. HTpSPE was thereby combined with a high-resolution MS (HRMS) through a microliter-flow injection analysis (μL-FIA) without a liquid chromatographic separation, which directly transferred the sample extracts to the time-of-flight MS (TOFMS). After injection, the complete sample information was obtained within a few minutes as a single FIA peak, when the detection of all pesticides was enabled at the same time in a single high-resolution mass spectrum. The method was developed for apples, cucumbers, red grapes, and tomatoes with very successful recovery and precision values for the applied pesticides calculated against pure solvent standards, which was only possible for the very clean HTpSPE extracts.

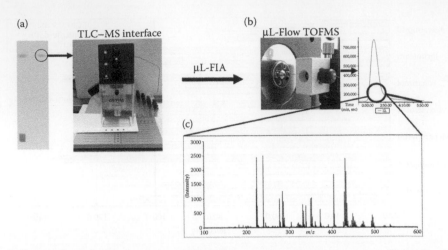

**FIGURE 10.15** Workflow scheme of HTpSPE–μL-FIA–TOFMS screening analysis: (a) elution of the target analytes from the thin-layer after HTpSPE by the TLC–MS interface; (b) FIA of the extracts using the μL-flow TOFMS system; (c) the full-scan mass spectrum obtained from the complete FIA peak. (Reprinted from Oellig, C., and Schwack, W., *J. Chromatogr. A*, 1351, 1–11, 2014. Copyright 2014, with permission from Elsevier.)

Sample extraction and HTpSPE followed the procedure presented in Section 10.3.1.1 for fruit and vegetables. For μL-FIA–TOFMS analysis, acetonitrile/water (1/1, v/v) was applied including 0.05% formic acid at a capillary flow rate of 2 μL/min. The eluent included 5% mass calibration solution to perform the mass axis calibration of the system. High-resolution mass spectra were recorded in the full-scan mode, and the quantitation of pesticides was done using the signal-to-noise ratios of the exact mass signals, normalized to TDCPP, when pure solvent standards were applied for comparison [27].

The concept of HTpSPE–μL-FIA–TOFMS is sketched in Figure 10.15. First, the target zone was eluted into autosampler vials, performed by the TLC–MS interface (Figure 10.15a). Subsequently, the offline HTpSPE–μL-FIA–TOFMS coupling was done by a μFlow-LC, which injected and transferred the extracts directly to the HRMS without a liquid chromatographic separation. Thus, the entire sample information was obtained in a single, focused FIA peak of the chronogram (Figure 10.15b). The mass spectrum, which was received from the full-scan data covering the entire FIA peak, contained the mass information of the whole sample (Figure 10.15c), which is why a rapid pesticide screening was possible. Depending on this chromatography-free analysis workflow, very clean and matrix-free sample extracts without matrix interferences were strongly required to achieve reliable results. As only HTpSPE meets these cleanness requirements, such a fast and easy μL-FIA–TOFMS approach was not successfully established before [27].

The cleanup efficiency of HTpSPE was easily demonstrated by the single mass spectrum covering the entire sample FIA peak. After mass calibration and background subtraction, the mass spectrum could be evaluated using the spectrum

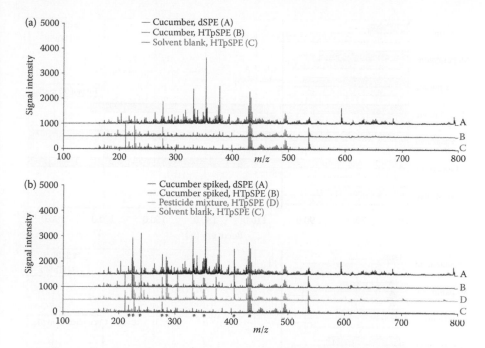

**FIGURE 10.16** μL-FIA–TOFMS mass spectra of the entire FIA peak of cucumber blank extracts including the ISTDs (a), and cucumber extracts spiked with pesticides (b); QuEChERS dSPE extracts (A) and HTpSPE extracts (B). Track (D) depicts a pesticide (*) solvent standard mixture of seven representative pesticides, including the ISTDs Sudan II and TDCPP, after HTpSPE. Track (C) refers to a solvent blank after HTpSPE including the ISTDs, displaying the layer background signals. (Reprinted from Oellig, C., and Schwack, W., *J. Chromatogr. A*, 1351, 1–11, 2014. Copyright 2014, with permission from Elsevier.)

course. To verify the difference between HTpSPE and dSPE, the mass spectra of blank and spiked QuEChERS extracts of cucumber were compared as an example (Figure 10.16). Blank dSPE extracts expectedly showed high amounts of coextracted matrix, with interfering signals across the whole *m/z* range. The highest intensity of interfering signals was obtained between *m/z* 200 and *m/z* 400, with a high overall intensity level as well as distinct *m/z* signals. On the other hand, HTpSPE extracts only showed marginal interfering signals, almost all coextracted matrix compounds were eliminated. In spiked extracts after dSPE, mass signals of coextracted matrix overlapped with mass signals of nearly all spiked target analytes. Contrarily, spiked extracts after HTpSPE were practically matrix-free and the obtained mass spectra were almost identical with the mass spectrum of a pure pesticide solvent standard. Thus, quantitation will be easily possible using the mass intensities of a neat pesticide solvent standard. The same successful HTpSPE–μL-FIA–TOFMS results concerning the cleanup efficiency were obtained for apples, red grapes, and tomatoes [27].

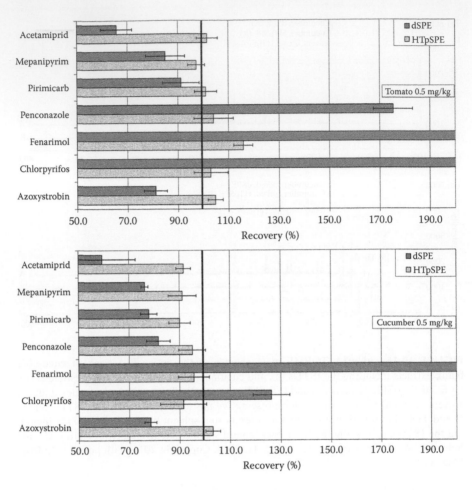

**FIGURE 10.17** Recoveries of the μL-FIA–TOFMS approach after dSPE and HTpSPE for seven pesticides spiked at 0.5 mg/kg into QuEChERS raw extracts of tomato and cucumber (postextraction spiking, $n = 5$). (Reprinted from Oellig, C., and Schwack, W., *J. Chromatogr. A*, 1351, 1–11, 2014. Copyright 2014, with permission from Elsevier.)

Quantitatively, the cleanup effect and performance of μL-FIA–TOFMS was verified by recovery values (Figure 10.17), comparing the mass signal intensities of spiked extracts and a pesticide solvent standard. After dSPE, recovery and precision data of μL-FIA–TOFMS for spiked tomato and cucumber extracts (0.5 mg/kg) strongly varied. Extremely high signal enhancement was observed for chlorpyrifos and fenarimol and to some extent for penconazole, which was due to intensive matrix mass signals with similar *m/z* values. On the other hand, a clear signal suppression occurred for acetamiprid. After HTpSPE, average recoveries for all pesticides were between 86% and 116%, successfully indicating no pesticide losses during HTpSPE or inexact measurements by μL-FIA–TOFMS. The precision data with relative standard deviations of 1.3%–10% also reflected the reproducible HTpSPE cleanup with the sufficient elution efficiency by the TLC–MS interface. Hence, HTpSPE clearly showed superior results concerning every tested validation parameter than dSPE. The reliable performance of HTpSPE–µL-FIA–TOFMS for pesticide residue analysis of fruit and vegetables could be outlined [27].

A database-dependent target and nontarget screening for the µL-FIA–TOFMS mass data offered a fast and easy search for pesticides in extracts of fruits and vegetables. The list of exact masses of the mass spectrum covering the entire FIA peak was compared with a pesticide database list containing the exact masses of about 250 pesticides. Based on specific searching criteria, an ACCESS query either provided a list of all target pesticides in the sample by a positive comparison (target oriented), or a list of all exact masses (substances) in the sample without the mass entries of the database by a negative comparison, last of which offered a real nontarget screening. Applying the target screening for spiked QuEChERS extracts after dSPE, up to 16 false-positives were obtained, and up to four spiked pesticides could not be identified correctly, each value depending on the matrix (Figure 10.18). For spiked QuEChERS extracts after HTpSPE, the database-dependent target screening provided successful results. Almost all spiked pesticides were detected and correctly identified, while only a very low number of false-positive findings occurred for tomato and cucumber extracts.

HTpSPE–µL-FIA–TOFMS provided reliable results for several real sample extracts as well. The pesticides that were identified using the database-dependent target screening were quite identical compared to those detected by a target HPLC–MS/MS analysis of QuEChERS dSPE extracts (Table 10.2). Regarding the low sensitivity of the applied TOFMS system, especially toward boscalid, a high degree of correspondency in detected pesticides in samples from the market was obtained. This emphasized the successful and robust direct offline HTpSPE–HRMS hyphenation approach with the TLC–MS interface as an integral part of the method for a rapid pesticide screening, and verified the concept to be excellently capable for reliable routine residue analysis.

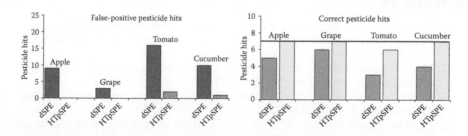

**FIGURE 10.18** Pesticides found by the database-dependent target screening search. False-positive pesticide hits and correct pesticide hits in spiked sample extracts for QuEChERS dSPE extracts and HTpSPE extracts ($n = 2$). (Reprinted from Oellig, C., and Schwack, W., *J. Chromatogr. A*, 1351, 1–11, 2014. Copyright 2014, with permission from Elsevier.)

**TABLE 10.2**

**Real Samples: HPLC–MS/MS Target Analysis (QuEChERS dSPE Extracts, Matrix-Matched Calibration) Compared to μL-FIA–TOFMS Analysis (HTpSPE Extracts) Using the Database-Dependent Target Screening**

| Sample | Pesticide | HPLC–MS/MS (mg/kg) | μL-FIA–TOFMS (S/N) |
|---|---|---|---|
| Banana | Thiabendazole | 0.76 | 2004 |
| | Imazalil | 0.73 | 1090 |
| | Bifenthrin | <0.01 | n.d. |
| | Chlorpyrifos | <0.01 | n.d. |
| Blackberry | Cyprodinil | 0.86 | 2347 |
| | Lambda-cyhalothrin | 0.01 | n.d. |
| | Thiacloprid | 0.01 | n.d. |
| Currant | Cyprodinil | 0.47 | 1373 |
| | Boscalid | 0.37 | n.d. |
| | Pyraclostrobin | 0.14 | 124 |
| | Trifloxystrobin | 0.06 | 121 |
| Savoy cabbage | Azoxystrobin | 1.3 | 1770 |
| | Difenoconazole | 0.39 | 317 |
| | Pymetrozine | 0.2 | n.d. |
| | Cyfluthrin | 0.09 | n.d. |
| | Indoxacarb | 0.03 | n.d. |
| | Thiacloprid | <0.01 | n.d. |
| | Dimethomorph | <0.01 | n.d. |

*Source:* Reprinted from Oellig, C., and Schwack, W., *J. Chromatogr. A*, 1351, 1–11, 2014. Copyright 2014, with permission from Elsevier.

*Note:* Instead of quantitation, signal-to-noise ratios (S/N) were calculated for TOFMS analysis.

## REFERENCES

1. Morlock, G. 2012. High-performance thin-layer chromatography–mass spectrometry for analysis of small molecules, In: *Mass Spectrometry Handbook*, 1st ed., M.S. Lee, (Ed.), John Wiley & Sons, New York, Chapter 49.
2. Morlock, G. and Schwack, W. 2010. Coupling of planar chromatography to mass spectrometry, *Trends Anal. Chem.*, 29: 1157–1171.
3. Morlock, G. and Schwack, W. 2010. Hyphenations in planar chromatography, *J. Chromatogr. A*, 1217: 6600–6609.
4. Pellissier, E. and Schwack, W. 2009. Determination of unauthorised fat-soluble azo dyes in spices by HPTLC, *CAMAG Bibliogr. Service CBS*, 103: 13–15.
5. Sun, H.W, Wang, F.C., and Ai, L.F. 2007. Determination of banned 10 azo-dyes in hot chili products by gel permeation chromatography–liquid chromatography–electrospray ionization–tandem mass spectrometry, *J. Chromatogr. A*, 1164: 120–128.
6. Chen, Y. and Schwack, W. 2013. Planar chromatography mediated screening of tetracycline and fluoroquinolone antibiotics in milk by fluorescence and mass selective detection, *J. Chromatogr. A*, 1312: 143–151.

7. Moreno-Bondi, M.C., Marazuela, M.D., Herranz, S., and Rodriguez E. 2009. An overview of sample preparation procedures for LC–MS multiclass antibiotic determination in environmental and food samples, *Anal. Bioanal. Chem.*, 395: 921–946.
8. Chafer-Pericas, C., Maquieira, A., and Puchades, R. 2010. Fast screening methods to detect antibiotic residues in food samples, *Trends Anal. Chem.*, 29: 1038–1049.
9. Reig, M. and Toldra, M. 2007. Veterinary drug residues in meat: Concerns and rapid methods for detection, *Meat Sci.*, 78: 60–67.
10. Canada-Canada, M., Munoz de la Pena, A., and Espinosa-Mansilla, A. 2009. Analysis of antibiotics in fish samples, *Anal. Bioanal. Chem.*, 395: 987–1008.
11. Stolker, A.A.M. and Brinkman, U.A.T. 2005. Analytical strategies for residue analysis of veterinary drugs and growth-promoting agents in food-producing animals, *J. Chromatogr. A*, 1067: 15–53.
12. Patel, Y.P., Shah, N., Bhoir, I.C., and Sundaresan, M. 1998. Simultaneous determination of five antibiotics by ion-pair high-performance liquid chromatography, *J. Chromatogr. A*, 828: 287–290.
13. Anastassiades, M., Lehotay, S.J., Stajnbaher D., and Schenck, F. 2003. Fast and easy multiresidue method employing acetonitrile extraction/partitioning and dispersive solid-phase extraction for the determination of pesticide residues in produce, *J. AOAC Int.*, 86: 412–431.
14. Schwack, W. 2015. Environmental applications, In: *Instrumental Thin-Layer Chromatography*, 1st ed., C. Poole, Ed., Elsevier, Amsterdam, Netherlands, Chapter 16.
15. Morlock, G.E., Schuele, L., and Grashorn, S. 2011. Development of a quantitative high-performance thin-layer chromatographic method for sucralose in sewage effluent, surface water, and drinking water, *J. Chromatogr. A*, 1218: 2745–2753.
16. Kowalska, T. and Sherma, J. (Eds.) 2006. *Preparative Layer Chromatography*, CRC Press/Taylor & Francis, Boca Raton, FL.
17. Tuzimski, T. and Soczewinski, E. 2004. Use of database of plots of pesticide retention (RF) against mobile-phase compositions for fractionation of a mixture of pesticides by micropreparative thin-layer chromatography, *Chromatographia*, 59: 121–128.
18. Tuzimski, T. 2005. Two-stage fractionation of a mixture of 10 pesticides by TLC and HPLC, *J. Liq. Chromatogr. Relat. Technol.*, 28: 463–476.
19. Sukul, P. 1994. Extraction and clean up procedures for the analysis of permethrin, cypermethrin, deltamethrin and fenvalerate in crops by GLC-ECD, *Toxicol. Environ. Chem.*, 44: 217–223.
20. Filipkowska, A., Lubecki, L., and Kowalewska, G. 2005. Polycyclic aromatic hydrocarbon analysis in different matrices of the marine environment, *Anal. Chim. Acta*, 547: 243–254.
21. Tyrpien, K., Bodzek, D., and Janoszka, B. 1995. Application of thin layer chromatography for isolation of polycyclic aromatic hydrocarbons from sewage sludges, *Acta Chromatogr.*, 4: 102–108.
22. Liu, X., Bi, X., Mai, B., Sheng, G., and Fu, J. 2005. Separation of PAHs in aerosol by thin layer chromatography for compound-specific stable carbon isotope analysis, *Talanta*, 66: 487–494.
23. Diletti, G., Scortichini, G., Scarpone, R., Gatti, G., Torreti, L., and Migliorati, G. 2005. Isotope dilution determination of polycyclic aromatic hydrocarbons in olive pomace oil by gas chromatography–mass spectrometry, *J. Chromatogr. A*, 1062: 247–254.
24 Chen, X. and Smart, R.B. 1992. Direct analysis of thin-layer chromatography spots by thermal extraction-gas chromatography–mass spectroscopy, *J. Chromatogr. Sci.*, 30: 192–196.
25. Oellig, C. and Schwack, W. 2011. Planar solid phase extraction: A new clean-up concept in multi-residue analysis of pesticides by liquid chromatography–mass spectrometry, *J. Chromatogr. A*, 1218: 6540–6547.

26. Oellig, C. and Schwack, W. 2012. Planar solid phase extraction clean-up for pesticide residue analysis in tea by liquid chromatography–mass spectrometry, *J. Chromatogr. A*, 1260: 42–53.
27. Oellig, C. and Schwack, W. 2014. Planar solid phase extraction clean-up and microliter-flow injection analysis-time-of-flight mass spectrometry for multi-residue screening of pesticides in food, *J. Chromatogr. A*, 1351: 1–11.

# 11 Drug Analysis by TLC–DESI MS

*Anna Bodzoń-Kułakowska, Przemysław Mielczarek, Piotr Suder, and Jerzy Silberring*

## CONTENTS

## 11.1 INTRODUCTION

Mass spectrometer equipped with desorption electrospray (DESI) ion source is capable of detection and identification of different substances from the surface. Moreover, the information about spatial distribution of those substances is retained. Connection of this technique with TLC not only allows for the measurement of retention times for separated chemicals (spatial distribution), but also for their unambiguous identification, based on the molecular weight of certain substances and their fragmentation spectra. Additionally, because DESI works under ambient conditions, there is no need to apply a high vacuum system for the sample introduction. Moreover, samples analyzed by DESI practically do not require any kind of preparation (e.g., covering with matrix prior to MALDI analysis), thus connection of those two techniques is relatively easy. Certainly, not all the substances, due to their chemical features, may be detected with this technique. Only compounds, which are able to ionize in this type of ion source, may be analyzed.

Combination of DESI MS with TLC separation was proposed for the first time by Van Berkel et al. [1]. In their study, apart from showing the possibility of such connection, the authors demonstrated practical application of this method during analyses of the FD&C dyes (food dyes) and a mixture of aspirin, acetaminophen, and caffeine from a tablet of *Extra Strength Excedrin*. In the following year, this system was further upgraded and improved by automating the process of analysis [2]. It was then used to separate the Goldenseal (*Hydrastis canadensis*) and related alkaloids from several commercial dietary supplements [3]. In the following section, we describe several practical aspects of DESI analysis of drugs separated on a TLC plate.

## 11.2   MATERIALS AND METHODS

The DESI ion source (OMNIspray, Prosolia, Indianapolis, IN), used for the experiments, was controlled by the Omnispray 2D software (Prosolia, Indianapolis, IN). The ion source was connected to an AmaZon ETD mass spectrometer (Bruker Daltonics, Bremen, Germany) working under the TrapControl program (ver. 7.0, Bruker Daltonics, Bremen, Germany). Signals received from both instruments were coordinated by the HyStar program (ver. 3.2, Bruker Daltonics, Bremen, Germany). Data visualization and evaluation was performed with the aid of the BioMap freeware (ver. 3.x, Novartis, Basel, Switzerland), and the DataAnalysis program (ver. 3.2, Bruker Daltonics, Bremen, Germany).

For optimization purposes, $3 \times 2$ μL of 1 mg mL$^{-1}$ standard solutions of amphetamine, methamphetamine, para-methoxy-$N$-methylamphetamine (PMMA), and benzydamine (BAM) were spotted in regular intervals, on the surface of a silica gel TLC plate (Fluka 99573) with glass support. This plate was used for optimization of the analysis. Then, the substances were administered on the TLC plate and developed in acetone:ammonia 0.1%.

Geometric parameters of the source were as follows: the distance between capillaries was set to 5 mm; the nebulization capillary height over the sample was 2 mm; nebulization capillary angle was 58°; MS inlet height over the sample was 1 mm; and nebulizing gas pressure (nitrogen) was 11 atm.

During optimization of the procedure we have tested 100% methanol; 70% methanol: 30% water with 0.1% formic acid (FA); 100% methanol with 0.1% FA; 100% acetonitrile; 100% ethanol; and 70% methanol: 30% acetonitrile, as DESI solvents sprayed on the TLC plate surface. Finally, 100% methanol with a flow rate of 3 μL min$^{-1}$ was used as an optimal solvent, providing best results. Other mass spectrometer acquisition settings were as follows: mass spectra scan range: 70–500 $m/z$; ion accumulation time: 200 ms; heated capillary temperature: 280°C; voltage between capillaries: 3200 V. Positively charged ion acquisition mode was applied.

## 11.3   CHOOSING THE BEST THIN-LAYER CHROMATOGRAPHIC PLATE AND ITS PREPARATION FOR THE MEASUREMENT

In the case of combining DESI ion source with TLC separation technique for its analysis, it is advisable to use good quality TLC plates. During the ionization process, the stationary phase might be detached from the plate surface and, in extreme cases, may clog the MS inlet. TLC plates with aluminum support seem to be more prone to such process than are those with glass support.

As DESI works under ambient conditions, preparation of the TLC plate is usually limited to its firm attachment to the moving table by the aid of double-sided adhesive tape. Another crucial step is to find the exact starting position for the analysis. To achieve this, it is advisable to mark the point near the start of the separation lane with an easily ionizable substance. A small dot of Rhodamine B (MW = 442) from a red marker pen is frequently used for this purpose. Such a dot is clearly visible on the surface of a TLC plate and it produces a very intensive signal on the MS spectrum when the nebulizing capillary is moving exactly above the spot. In such a way, the starting point for the measurements can be precisely indicated.

## 11.4 GEOMETRY OF THE ION SOURCE

Intensity of the signal depends on the optimal configuration of the DESI ion source. This includes proper optimization of the pressure of the nebulizing gas, solvent flow rate, and capillary voltage. Additionally, one should pay attention to the proper alignment of all parts of a DESI ion source [4]. This includes nebulization capillary angle, nebulization capillary height over the scanned surface, distance between nebulization capillary and MS inlet, and nebulization capillary and MS inlet geometry (Figure 11.1).

In the case of TLC analysis, the parameters from Table 11.1 might be considered as a starting point for optimization. Careful manipulation of those parameters might lead to better results with more intense signals for the desired substances (Table 11.1).

## 11.5 DESORPTION ELECTROSPRAY IONIZATION SOLVENTS

Choosing an optimal solvent for TLC plate analysis is also very important. Solvent in the DESI source is delivered to the analyzed surface via nebulizing capillary, as a

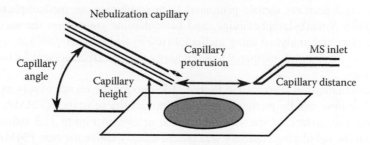

**FIGURE 11.1**   Typical DESI ion source.

**TABLE 11.1**
**Typical Parameters of DESI Ion Source Geometry**

| Parameters | Positive-Ion Mode | Negative-Ion Mode |
| --- | --- | --- |
| Capillary protrusion | 0.5 mm | 0.5 mm |
| Gas pressure | 11 atm | 11 atm |
| Solvent flow | 2–3 µL min⁻¹ | 2–3 µL min⁻¹ |
| Capillary voltage | 3000 V | 4500 V |
| Nebulization capillary angle | 58° | 60° |
| Nebulization capillary height | 3.0 mm | 3.0 mm |
| Capillary distance | 5.0 mm | 5.0 mm |
| MS inlet height | 0–1 mm | 0–1 mm |

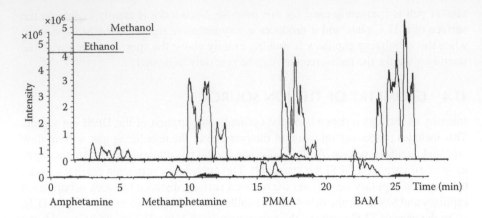

**FIGURE 11.2**   Different solvents (methanol and ethanol) used for analysis of amphetamine, methamphetamine, PMMA, and BAM.

spray of tiny, charged droplets. Those droplets form a thin, wet layer on the surface, leading to dissolving the analytes present on the surface. Then, subsequent droplets of the same solvent are responsible for producing so-called secondary droplets, which consist of dissolved analyte that is delivered to the mass spectrometer.

Figure 11.2 presents signals generated from amphetamine, methamphetamine, paramethoxy-*N*-methylamphetamine, and benzydamine spotted on the surface of the TLC plate and analyzed using methanol (100%) and ethanol (96%) as solvents. As shown in Figure 11.2, methanol was obviously the best DESI solvent for this type of chemicals.

The chromatogram presented in Figure 11.3 supports the choice of solvent. Here, we may see how rapidly methanol is able to extract the substance (PMMA in this case) from the surface of the TLC plate. The arrows in Figure 11.3 indicate the time when the nebulizing capillary was placed exactly above the new PMMA spot. Intensity of the signal drops down quite rapidly, which demonstrates that the substance is quickly eluted from the spot.

## 11.6   SINGLE LINE, SEVERAL LINES, TANDEM MASS SPECTROMETRY

After optimizing all parameters, the TLC plate can be analyzed in two ways. The simplest and fastest way is to measure a single line, which goes exactly across the place where the substances were spotted, to the end of the distance where the eluent traveled. Such analysis is very fast, and usually takes approximately 10–15 min. The total analysis time depends on the scanning rate (usually $100~\mu m \cdot s^{-1}$) and the length of the path (usually up to 8–10 cm). To obtain very good representation of the spot on the surface, the measurement of several nearby lines may be performed. Additionally, MS/MS spectra can be obtained to confirm the identity of the substance (Figure 11.4).

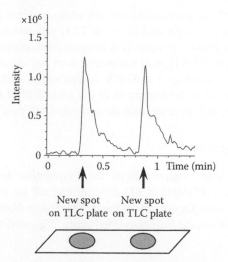

FIGURE 11.3 Extracted ion chromatogram for 181 *m/z*. Analysis of PMMA from two different spots on the TLC plate.

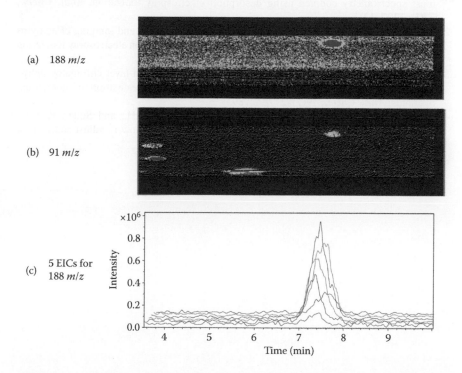

FIGURE 11.4 Different ways of results visualization. (a) Detailed visualization of the plate with seligiline (160 lines for the whole plate, about 30 lines for seligiline); (b) characteristic fragment (91—tropylium cation) of seligiline, PMMA, methamphetamine, and amphetamine separated on the same plate (data presented using a BioMap software); and (c) 6 lines representing seligiline (extracted ion chromatograms for *m/z* 188, data presented using a DataAnaysis software).

Summarizing, DESI due to its ability to work under ambient conditions allows for convenient connection of simple and low-cost TLC separation and highly specific MS analysis. Of the currently popular MS imaging techniques, DESI seems to be the most comprehensive. This type of ion source does not cause extensive fragmentation of the sample as in the case of SIMS. Additionally, since there is no need to use any kind of matrix or high vacuum, as in the case of MALDI, the molecules of low molecular weight, such as drugs and their metabolites, may be easily analyzed.

## ACKNOWLEDGMENTS

The authors acknowledge support from the Foundation for Polish Science— POMOST Programme (POMOST/2011-3/1) cofinanced by the European Union within European Regional Development Fund, The Polish National Science Center 2012/07/B/NZ4/01468 and the EuroNanoMed grant, 5/EuroNanoMed/2012.

## REFERENCES

1. Van Berkel, G.J., Ford, M.J., and Deibel, M.A. 2005. Thin-layer chromatography and mass spectrometry coupled using desorption electrospray ionization. *Anal. Chem.*, 77(5): 1207–1215.
2. Van Berkel, G.J. and Kertesz, V. 2006. Automated sampling and imaging of analytes separated on thin-layer chromatography plates using desorption electrospray ionization mass spectrometry. *Anal. Chem.*, 78(14): 4938–4944.
3. Van Berkel, G.J., Tomkins, B.A., and Kertesz, V. 2007. Thin-layer chromatography–desorption electrospray ionization mass spectrometry: Investigation of goldenseal alkaloids. *Anal. Chem.*, 79(7): 2778–2789.
4. Bodzon-Kulakowska, A., Drabik, A., Ner, J., Kotlinska, J.H., and Suder, P. 2014. Desorption electrospray ionisation (DESI) for beginners—How to adjust settings for tissue imaging. *Rapid Commun. Mass Spectrom.*, 28(1): 1–9.

# 12 Application of TLC and Plasma-Based Ambient MS in Bioanalytical Sciences

Marek Smoluch, Przemysław Mielczarek,
Michał Cegłowski, Grzegorz Schroeder,
and Jerzy Silberring

## CONTENTS

## 12.1 INTRODUCTION

Plasma-based ambient ionization mass spectrometry techniques, such as DART (direct analysis in real time), FAPA (flowing atmospheric pressure afterglow), DBDI (dielectric barrier discharge ionization), ASAP (atmospheric solids analysis probe), DAPCI (desorption atmospheric pressure chemical ionization), and some others, are gaining growing interest as they do not require time-consuming sample preparation, are rapid, and work under ambient experimental conditions. An additional advantage is also a possibility for samples analysis in gas, liquid, or solid forms. These techniques can be applied in a wide range of applications, such as warfare agents' detection, chemical reactions control, mass spectrometry imaging, identification of polymers, food safety monitoring, drug and pharmaceutical analysis, medical diagnostics, forensic research, biochemical analyses, etc.

Plasma-based ambient MS methods have been used to detect compounds directly from TLC plates. Several applications have been described in this chapter. The majority of them applies to DART, but suitability of DBDI and FAPA sources have also been demonstrated.

## 12.2  APPLICATIONS

First coupling of planar chromatography with DART was reported in 2006 [1]. The thin-layer plate was cut and introduced to the source, as shown in Figure 12.1. The optimized position of the TLC plate allowed obtaining the best signal-to-noise ratio. This setup was capable of detecting nanogram amounts of isopropylthioxanthone deposited on the TLC plate. For qualitative purposes, such coupling was well suited, although quantification was problematic. Good results were achieved by additional application of stable isotope-labeled standards. In this work, TLC–DART was compared to a plunger-based extraction device for TLC–ESI, thus bringing comparable results in terms of repeatability and analytical response.

Phytochemicals in the extract of herbal medicines were analyzed by TLC–DART [2]. Decursin and decursinol from *Angelica gigantis* radix, alkaloid compounds of rutaecarpine and evodiamine from *Evodiae fructus*, and lignin molecules of gomisin A, N, and schisandrin from *Schisandrae fructus* were separated and identified from the TLC plates. The TLC–DART coupling provided specific information on the major components of crude plant drugs on TLC, directly in real time. This application proved the usefulness of this technique for the efficient and reliable quality control of botanical drugs and herbal medicinal products.

The lack of quantitation limits the use of DART in many fields. A new system was proposed, which possesses an option for quantitative analyses [3]. This group demonstrated the analysis of a total extract of *Schisandra chinensis* fruit on a TLC plate. Three major lignin compounds were identified and quantitated. UV densitometry, TLC–DART–MS, and HPLC–UV were compared as detection methods. For DART analysis, the width of a TLC plate was cut to a narrow slice of 3 mm. The developed

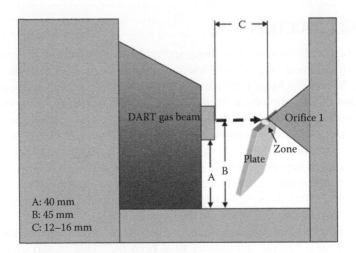

**FIGURE 12.1**  Scheme for manual positioning of the HPTLC plate into the DART gas beam; signal response was best at a distance of approximately 1 mm aside orifice 1, and an angle of approximately 160° vertical to the gas flow. (Reprinted from Morlock, G., and Ueda, Y., *J. Chromatogr. A*, 1143, 243–51, 2007. Copyright 2007. With permission.)

TLC plate on the carrier was directly introduced into a DART ion source by physical impulsion from a syringe pump. This system was shown to be a powerful analytical tool for efficient quantitation of natural products from crude drugs.

The TLC–DART coupling was also employed in forensic sciences [4]. TLC with visual detection is commonly applied in many forensic laboratories when analyzing unknown drugs or mixtures. Detection is usually confirmed by the application of GC–MS. This confirmation step usually takes some time to complete, mainly due to additional extraction and derivatization procedures. Combination of TLC with DART markedly shortens the time required for confirmation of the results. TLC–DART is equivalent to GC–MS in terms of sensitivity and selectivity. Both techniques were compared by analysis of several pharmaceutical drugs, such as codeine/acetaminophen, hydrocodone/acetaminophen, or oxycodone/acetaminophen. Another application of TLC–DART in forensic sciences was shown [5]. Authors applied the separation on TLC plate prior to DART detection in order to identify the active ingredients of drugs. Direct analysis of such compounds might be difficult, due to the complex mass spectrum obtained from unseparated mixture. Utilizing TLC prior to sample introduction provides a simple, low-cost solution prior to acquisition of mass spectra of the purified drug preparation. Simplified mass spectra (after TLC separation) were obtained for 91 preparations and were uploaded to an in-house drug standard library. Some new features of DART and its coupling to TLC were shown by Chernetsova et al. [6]. This group demonstrated, for the first time, the feature of this source for desorption at an angle. Until now, to analyze the TLC plate by DART, the plate had to be cut and placed as shown in Figure 12.1. A new approach allowed for scanning the surface, including TLC plates (Figure 12.2). For the optimal conditions for desorption/ionization, the proper positioning of the samples (TLC plate) is crucial. To achieve this goal, a simple approach for the visualization of the DART stream on a surface was implied, based on the chemical reaction on a filter paper or TLC plate on heating. A novel system utilizing TLC and plasma-assisted multiwavelength laser desorption ionization MS (PAMLDI–MS) for

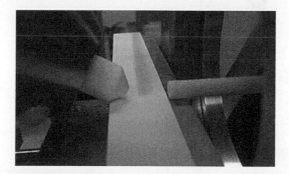

**FIGURE 12.2**  Experimental setup with the DART ion source with desorption at an angle (DART SVP-A). (From Chernetsova, E.S., Revelsky, A.I., and Morlock, G.E., *Rapid Commun. Mass Spectrom.*, 25, 2275–82, 2011. Copyright Wiley-VCH Verlag GmbH & Co. KGaA. Reproduced with permission.)

separation and identification of low-molecular-weight compounds was demonstrated [7]. The schematic diagram of the setup, which involves an automated 3D platform for optimization of the geometry of the setup, is shown in Figure 12.3. The results indicate that the laser desorption was wavelength-dependent, which additionally improves the system in terms of specificity. The detection level of 5 ng mm$^{-2}$ was obtained for dye mixtures, drug standards, and tea extract separated on the normal-phase silica gel. TLC is a very popular technique to monitor reactions in synthetic chemistry. Srbek et al. [8] demonstrated the analyses of several substances, directly identified on TLC plates by DART. In this case, pure substance solutions were spotted onto TLC plates and directly analyzed by DART without separation. The TLC plate served as a sample carrier only. Recently, a novel study on the differentiation of natural products using HPTLC and DART using multivariate data analysis was shown [9]. The chemometric evaluation of HPTLC and DART data brought vital, complementary information. This approach allowed for categorization of 91 propolis samples, with high level of confidence, based on their phenolic compound profiles. This approach could be considered fully complementary, as it provides information on polarity, functional groups, and spectral properties of marker compounds (HPTLC), as well as on the possible elemental formulae of principal components of a complex mixture (DART–MS). The TLC and DART coupling was also used to analyze organophosphorus insecticides in fatty foods [10]. Authors demonstrated that TLC–DART coupling is more useful for the analysis of polar and nonpolar pesticides, as compared to GC–MS and GC–MS/MS, which are more susceptible to matrix effects. The detection limits for the compounds tested were in the range of nano- to picograms. The TLC was also coupled to a DBDI source, as shown in Figure 12.4 [11]. The sample detection was improved by the application of a heating element located underneath the TLC plate. Heating caused an increased volatility

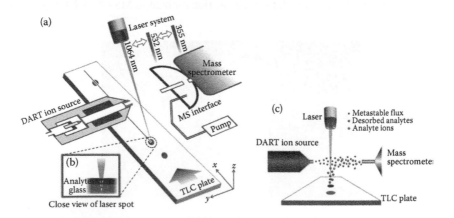

**FIGURE 12.3**  (a) Schematic illustration of the TLC/PAMLDI–MS setup. (b) Close view of the relative position of the laser focal point and the plane of the TLC surface. (c) Proposed desorption/ionization process. (Reprinted with permission from Zhang, J. et al., *Anal. Chem.*, 84, 1496–503, 2012. Copyright 2012 American Chemical Society.)

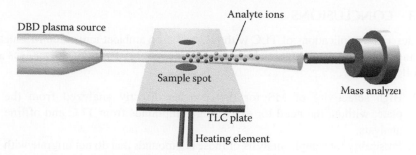

**FIGURE 12.4** Schematic diagram of DBD–TLC coupling. (Adapted from Cegłowski, M. et al., *PLoS One*, 9, e106088, 2014.)

of the compounds, and allowed obtaining better quality spectra, thus enhancing the detection limit of the method (100 ng spot⁻¹). This setup was applied for the separation and analyses of six pyrazole derivatives. The proof of principle was also shown for TLC–FAPA coupling. In this case, exactly the same setup as demonstrated in Figure 12.4 was applied, but the DBDI source was exchanged with FAPA. For this coupling, the separation of three active components of Saridon analgesic (composed of paracetamol, caffeine, and prophyphenazone) was shown (Figure 12.5).

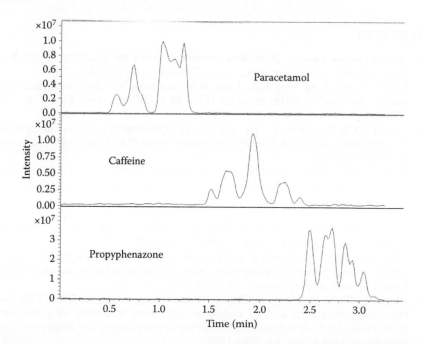

**FIGURE 12.5** TLC–FAPA extracted ion chromatograms for three active components of Saridon: paracetamol, caffeine, and propyphenazone were consecutively detected from TLC plate after moving the TLC plate over the heating element.

## 12.3 CONCLUSIONS

All described applications of TLC with plasma-based ambient ionization MS methods indicate an immense potential of this type of coupling. The main advantages are as follows:

1. High selectivity of MS for the samples directly analyzed from the plate, without the need for extracting compounds from TLC and offline analysis.
2. Possibility for sample analysis of those compounds that do not migrate with the mobile phase (advantage over HPLC–MS technique).
3. No limitations in the choice of eluent.
4. High sensitivity.
5. Fast sample identification when utilizing online coupling.
6. Low costs and simplicity.

The main drawbacks of TLC and plasma-based ambient MS techniques are difficulties with quantitation and still limited number of applications.

## ACKNOWLEDGMENTS

The authors acknowledge support from the EuroNanoMed grant, 5/EuroNanoMed/ 2012.

## REFERENCES

1. Morlock, G. and Ueda, Y. 2007. New coupling of planar chromatography with direct analysis in real time mass spectrometry, *J. Chromatogr. A*, 1143: 243–251.
2. Kim, H.J., Jee, E.H., Ahn, K.S., Choi, H.S., and Jang, Y.P. 2010. Identification of marker compounds in herbal drugs on TLC with DART–MS, *Arch. Pharm. Res.*, 33: 1355–1359.
3. Kim, H.J., Oh, M.S., Hong, J., and Jang Y.P. 2011. Quantitative analysis of major dibenzocyclooctane lignans in *Schisandrae fructus* by online TLC–DART–MS, *Phytochem. Anal.*, 22: 258–262.
4. Howlett, S.E. and Steiner, R.R. 2011. Validation of thin layer chromatography with AccuTOF-DART™ detection for forensic drug analysis, *J. Forensic Sci.*, 56: 1261–1267.
5. Wood, J.L. and Steiner, R.R. 2011. Purification of pharmaceutical preparations using thin-layer chromatography to obtain mass spectra with direct analysis in real time and accurate mass spectrometry, *Drug Test Anal.*, 3: 345–351.
6. Chernetsova, E.S., Revelsky, A.I., and Morlock, G.E. 2011. Some new features of direct analysis in real time mass spectrometry utilizing the desorption at an angle option, *Rapid Commun. Mass Spectrom.*, 25: 2275–2282.
7. Zhang, J., Zhou, Z., Yang, J., Zhang, W., Bai, Y., and Liu, H. 2012. Thin layer chromatography/plasma assisted multiwavelength laser desorption ionization mass spectrometry for facile separation and selective identification of low molecular weight compounds, *Anal. Chem.*, 84: 1496–1503.
8. Srbek, J., Klejdus, B., Douša, M., Břicháč, J., Stasiak, P., Reitmajer, J., and Nováková, L. 2014. Direct analysis in real time—High resolution mass spectrometry as a valuable tool for the pharmaceutical drug development, *Talanta*, 130: 518–526.

9. Morlock, G.E., Ristivojevic, P., and Chernetsova, E.S. 2014. Combined multivariate data analysis of high-performance thin-layer chromatography fingerprints and direct analysis in real time mass spectra for profiling of natural products like propolis, *J. Chromatogr. A*, 1328: 104–112.

10. Kiguchi, O., Oka, K., Tamada, M., Kobayashi, T., and Onodera, J. 2014. Thin-layer chromatography/direct analysis in real time time-of-flight mass spectrometry and iso-tope dilution to analyze organophosphorus insecticides in fatty foods, *J. Chromatogr. A*, 1370: 246–254.

11. Cegłowski, M., Smoluch, M., Babij, M., Gotszalk, T., Silberring, J., and Schroeder, G. 2014. Dielectric barrier discharge ionization in characterization of organic compounds separated on thin-layer chromatography plates, *PLoS One*, 9: e106088.

# 13 TLC/MALDI MS for the Analysis of Lipids

*Jürgen Schiller, Beate Fuchs, Rosmarie Süß,*
*Yulia Popkova, Hans Griesinger, Katerina*
*Matheis, Michaela Oberle, and Michael Schulz*

## CONTENTS

## 13.1 INTRODUCTION

Thin-layer chromatography (TLC) and its refined version, high-performance thin-layer chromatography (HPTLC), are established separation techniques in synthetic organic chemistry and natural product chemistry, whereby lipids in particular are traditionally investigated by TLC [1–4]. Nonmodified silica gel is used in the majority of cases [2], so we will discuss here exclusively this type of stationary phase.

The separation of even complex lipid mixtures is not a major problem for modern (1D or 2D) HPTLC and phospholipids can be easily separated due to the different polarities of their headgroups. However, the unequivocal identification of a dedicated lipid with specific acyl (or alkyl and alkenyl) residues is more challenging when TLC alone is used. It is the aim of this chapter to provide evidence that this problem may be overcome when TLC separation is combined with mass spectrometric (MS) detection. We will focus on glycerophospholipids (GPL). These molecules possess a significant biological relevance and should confirm our claim as they are characterized by considerable structural variability. This is also true for glyco-(sphingo)-lipids. However, these species will be discussed here only superficially, as glycolipids will be discussed in more detail elsewhere (see Chapter 18).

## 13.2   IMPORTANT GLYCEROPHOSPHOLIPIDS

As a comprehensive survey of all physiologically relevant lipids [5] would exceed the size of this chapter by far, a few comments regarding the most important structural aspects of lipids have to be made. GPL represent important constituents of cellular and subcellular membranes and are generated by the esterification of glycerol with two (normally different) fatty acids in *sn*-1 and *sn*-2 position. When the free hydroxyl group of this diacylglycerol (DAG) is additionally esterified with phosphoric acid, phosphatidic acid (PA) is generated. Although the *in vivo* concentration of PA is normally very small, PA can be considered as the "educt" of all other GPL because the phosphate is bivalent and can be additionally modified with different molecules such as choline or ethanolamine [6]. Thus, GPL are characterized by a phosphorylated, polar headgroup, and several apolar acyl residues.

### 13.2.1   Differences in the Headgroups

Some of the most important headgroups of GPL are shown in Figure 13.1. The headgroup is essential for the analysis of GPL for two reasons: on one hand, the polarity of a GPL (i.e., the structure of the headgroup) determines the separation quality achievable by (normal phase) TLC. On the other hand, the structure of the headgroup determines the charge of the entire GPL, and this is essential regarding MS detection: the phosphate group is easily protonated while the quaternary ammonia of the phosphatidylcholine retains its positive charge under all conditions. Thus, phosphatidylcholines are most sensitively detectable as positive ions and this may even lead to the suppression of other, less sensitively detectable lipids [7].

### 13.2.2   The Fatty Acyl Composition and the Linkage Type

A special terminology [8] is used to denote the lipid structure and one selected example will be given to illustrate this approach: POPC, for instance, indicates that a PC contains a palmitoyl residue ("P") in the first and an oleoyl residue ("O") in the second position. The same molecule may also be termed PC 16:0/18:1. In this "*x:y*" nomenclature, "*x*" indicates the number of carbon atoms and "*y*" indicates the number of double bonds in one chain. No information at all is provided by this nomenclature about the position of the double bonds. We will also not discuss this aspect here to a major extent because the determination of the double bond positions of fatty acids is regularly done by GC/MS and/or silver ion chromatography—and these techniques are beyond the scope of this chapter [9].

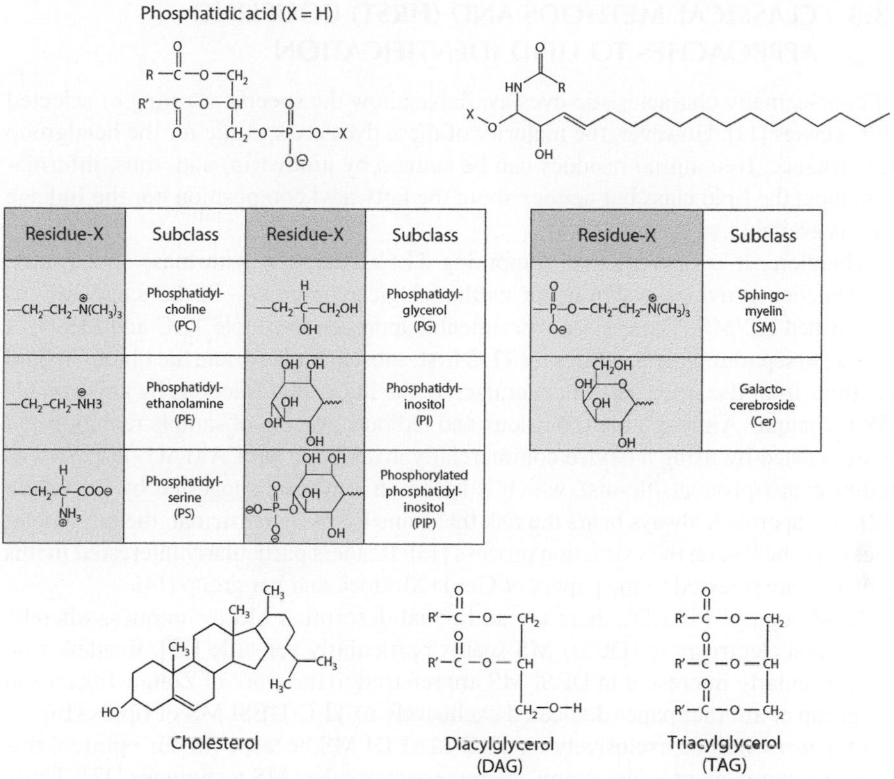

**FIGURE 13.1** Survey of lipids occurring in cellular membranes. The head group structures of the relevant phospholipids (derived from PA shown at the top) are shown in the left table, whereas the structures of selected sphingosin-derived lipids are shown at the right. Please note that only PC and PE represent neutral (zwitterionic) phospholipids, while all others are acidic phospholipids. $R$ and $R'$ represent varying fatty acyl residues. At the bottom, some apolar lipids (regularly present in cellular extracts) are additionally shown.

Another problem is that isomers cannot be so easily differentiated by MS; for instance, a given GPL with $2 \times 18{:}1$ possesses exactly the same molecular weight as a GPL with 18:0/18:2. This problem in many cases is not addressed and "GPL 36:2" is simply provided instead; that is, both residues are combined.

Another point is that there is often confusion regarding the terms "GPC" and "PC." "PC" should be used when there are exclusively ester linkages, while "GPC" is the more general term and includes ether linkages as well [8]. Therefore, the linkage type (alkyl, acyl, or alkenyl) further contributes to the diversity of lipids and "ether" lipids may represent a significant moiety in many lipid mixtures. Alkenyl ether lipids ("plasmalogens") are nowadays of particular interest because they are assumed to represent important antioxidants because the alkenyl ether is very oxidation sensitive. Fortunately, plasmalogens can be easily identified: they are extremely sensitive toward even traces of acids and already the surface of a normal phase TLC plate is sufficiently acidic to induce hydrolysis of the plasmalogen into an aldehyde and the corresponding lysolipid [10].

## 13.3   CLASSICAL METHODS AND (FIRST) COUPLING APPROACHES TO LIPID IDENTIFICATION

Of course, many characteristic dyes available allow the specific staining of selected GPL classes [11]. However, the majority of these dyes are specific for the headgroup (for instance, free amino residues can be stained by ninhydrin) and, thus, information about the lipid class but neither about the fatty acyl composition nor the linkage type is available.

Therefore, it is obvious that combining TLC separation with mass spectrometric detection provides a significant methodological progress—in the same way as established LC/MS. The easiest experimental approach to couple TLC and MS is, of course, to separate lipid mixtures by TLC first, subsequently reelute the obtained lipid fractions from the silica gel, and characterize the individual fractions by any suitable MS technique. Although the (laborious and tedious) process of sample reelution can be automated by using a device commercially available from CAMAG (http://www. camag.com/v/products/tlc-ms), which is based on a method suggested by Luftmann [12], this approach always bears the risk that some lipids (in particular, the more polar ones) may be lost on the extraction process [13]. Readers particularly interested in this approach are referred to the papers of Gerda Morlock and her group [14].

In addition to MALDI, there are additional desorption MS techniques, whereby desorption electrospray (DESI) MS seems particularly versatile [15]. Readers who are particularly interested in DESI MS are referred to the work of Zoltan Takats and his group or another paper dedicated exclusively to TLC/DESI MS of lipids [16].

Our focus will be exclusively on TLC/MALDI MS because (in our opinion) this coupling approach provides many advantages over other MS techniques [17]. Those advantages are as follows:

1. MALDI MS tolerates impurities (as well as high salt concentrations) to a significant extent. Thus, potential impurities from the TLC plate (such as binding agents) only play a minor role.
2. The spatial resolution is determined by the laser spot size, which usually has a diameter of about 50 μm when a UV laser is used. Thus, even poorly resolved TLC spots can be well characterized.
3. As MALDI MS generates preferentially singly charged ions, this makes interpretation of the spectra quite simple.
4. Very little pretreatments are necessary. For instance, there is no need for applying dyes.
5. Automation of measurements is possible; this provides significant high-throughput capacity.

## 13.4   MALDI MS IDENTIFICATION DIRECTLY FROM THE TLC PLATE

MALDI MS represents a desorption technique [18] and, thus, allows MS measurements directly from sample surfaces. Limited by the laser spot size, spatially resolved mass information of the molecules on the TLC plate could be obtained. This "MALDI imaging" [19] attracts significant interest—at least since the available software and laser repetition rates were improved in the last years. Main research efforts are particularly in the biomedical sector, where MALDI imaging is widely used for tissue screening [19].

A comprehensive discussion of the basics of MALDI MS is clearly outside the scope of this chapter. Readers interested in the methodological aspects of MALDI or the fundamentals of the related ionization process should consult the excellent book by Hillenkamp and Jasna-Katalinić [20] or the review by Knochenmuss [21], respectively.

To summarize briefly, the most important aspect regarding successful MALDI MS is the embedding of the analyte with the most appropriate "matrix" for optimum ionization performance. Therefore, the careful selection of the matrix is extremely important: using UV MALDI (the majority of commercially available MALDI devices are equipped with a UV laser), we recommend 2,5-dihydroxybenzoic acid (DHB) for positive ion detection and 9-aminoacridine (9-AA) for negative ions. A survey of further useful MALDI matrices is available in Reference 22. Matrices are often specialized for different experimental issues and the combined use of DHB and 9-AA is often quite helpful because

1. DHB ($pK \approx 2.9$) is an excellent positive ion matrix, but is not the matrix of choice for recording negative ion spectra: the intense background (DHB cluster ions) in the negative ion mode [23] increases the complexity of the spectra considerably.

2. In contrast, 9-AA ($pK \approx 10$) is an excellent matrix to detect negative ions and is capable of detecting phospholipids such as PC in the positive ion mode. Unfortunately, some lipids such as triacylglycerols and cholesterol are not detectable in the presence of 9-AA. Charged functional groups (or the addition of auxiliary substances such as sodium acetate [24]) are apparently necessary for these molecules to become detectable in the presence of 9-AA.

When the (lipid) spot of interest is analyzed directly in the presence of the silica gel on the TLC plate, two requirements must be fulfilled: (1) the matrix must be applied onto the TLC plate in a sufficient excess (a higher matrix excess in comparison to conventional MALDI targets is needed) [25] and (2) the analyte must be extracted from "the inner" of the silica layer to the surface. This is achieved by the evaporation of the solvent and necessary because UV irradiation does not penetrate deeply (<5 μm) into the silica layer. One might argue that this causes problems because the depth of an analyte in the silica gel depends on the $R_F$ value: the larger the migration distance, the deeper the analyte is located in the silica gel. However, thus far we were not able to detect major sensitivity differences in dependence on the $R_F$ values of the individual lipids.

Of course, major "delocalization" of the analyte during (or because of) the addition of the matrix solution must be avoided. Otherwise, this would significantly compromise the quality of the chromatographic separation. These important prerequisites were already discussed in detail in Reference 26.

In a nutshell, the deposition of the MALDI matrix onto the TLC plate is a very important step of successful TLC/MALDI measurements [27]. There are different methods of matrix application [3] available and the most useful methods for combined TLC/MS are as follows:

1. *Matrix droplets applied onto the region of interest.* If only a small area of the TLC plate is of interest (for instance, to identify a defined spot), the addition of some small droplets of the matrix solution onto the (previously marked) spots of interest by a pipette or a syringe is a good approach. It is strongly recommended to use a solvent (such as water) or solvent mixture with a significant surface tension because this results in a small drop size [25].

2. *Spraying the matrix solution onto the TLC plate* (e.g., by using electrospray equipment). Instruments based on this approach are nowadays commercially available (for instance, from SunChrom or Bruker Daltonics) and widely used in the context of MS imaging. Although such devices work excellently when small areas have to be coated with matrix, larger areas are normally coated rather inhomogeneously: the matrix concentration is normally smaller at the edges in comparison to the center. Another disadvantage is the plugging of the spray mechanism when very concentrated matrix solutions are needed.

3. *Dipping the entire plate into the matrix solution.* This process is a bit laborious because several dipping and drying steps are required, but it is, in our opinion, the method of choice to evenly cover the entire TLC plate with matrix. This technique has been successfully applied with DHB as matrix, but it seems that thus far there were no experiments with other matrix compounds. A detailed description of this approach is available as an application note from the Bruker Daltonics webpage (www.bruker.com). The matrix solution should be as concentrated as possible while the contact time between the TLC plate and the matrix solution should be very short to avoid blurring of the spots.

After application of the matrix, the TLC plate is loaded directly into the MALDI device. The most obvious and simple approach is to fix the TLC plate with conductive adhesive tape onto a standard MALDI target (although a dedicated TLC adapter is now also available from Bruker Daltonics). To avoid charging effects in the MALDI source by residual charged particles on the surface and to enable successful ion desorption, an electrically conductive surface is needed. Therefore, the use of TLC glass plates is absolutely discouraged, whereas alumina TLC plates are perfect for this application. Such plates are commercially available with different stationary phases.

## 13.5 SELECTED GLYCEROPHOSPHOLIPID THIN-LAYER CHROMATOGRAPHY–MATRIX-ASSISTED LASER DESORPTION IONIZATION DATA

Recording MALDI-TOF mass spectra of "small molecules" is still challenging: although some methods were suggested to overcome (or at least to reduce) the problem of analyte and matrix overlap, this is still a major problem [28]. Therefore, thus far there were no attempts to characterize free fatty acids and their oxidation products by TLC/MALDI but the available data are nearly exclusively dedicated to phospholipids and glycolipids. Since glycolipids will be comprehensively discussed in the "carbohydrate" chapter of this book (Chapter 18), we will focus here on the analysis of phospholipids.

There are two different approaches for the MALDI MS characterization of TLC-separated PLs. Both methods have their specific advantages and drawbacks and, thus, the choice of the method will depend on the available equipment.

### 13.5.1 INFRARED MATRIX-ASSISTED LASER DESORPTION IONIZATION

The first method is based on the use of an IR laser. Even if the mechanism of IR MALDI is less well-understood [21] in comparison to UV MALDI, IR MALDI confers two important advantages:

1. Hydroxyl groups are strongly absorbing at the IR wavelength (typically 2.94 μm). Therefore, glycerol (which is stable under high vacuum conditions, i.e., it does not evaporate) is a typical IR MALDI matrix. Since glycerol is a liquid, the matrix/analyte mixture is more homogeneous in comparison to the cocrystals typically obtained with UV MALDI matrices such as DHB or cinnamic acid derivates. This improves the shot-to-shot reproducibility.
2. IR radiation leads to a more significant ablation [29] of the analyte in comparison to a UV laser. This confers the advantage that even analytes in deeper layers of the silica can be successfully analyzed. Thus, bringing the analyte to the surface is less important.

Rohlfing and coworkers [30] investigated different phospholipids after separation on a silica layer (chloroform/methanol/2-propanol/triethylamine/0.25% KCl [30:9:25:18:6 v/v/v/v] as eluent system) by using an IR laser and glycerol as matrix. Additionally, these authors [30] have also used an orthogonal (not an axial) MALDI MS device. This instrument configuration has the advantage that the process of ion formation is completely independent from the ion separation and detection step [31]. This leads to a significantly improved mass accuracy because irregularities of the TLC plate can be compensated.

All investigated phospholipid mixtures (PC, PE, PG, PA, CL, and SM) could be easily separated by TLC and unequivocally characterized by subsequent MALDI MS. The achieved sensitivity was between 10 and 150 pmol depending on the analyte acidity, the $R_F$ value, and the ion polarity. The achievable lateral resolution was on the order of the laser focus diameter (about $220 \times 300$ μm). This was sufficient to differentiate PL species of different acyl chain compositions within a given HPTLC spot and, thus, to provide evidence that the lipid distribution within one TLC spot is inhomogeneous. Analyte diffusion (due to the addition of glycerol to the HPTLC plate) was found to be of minor importance. Although quantitative data analysis is still the weak point of MALDI MS, these authors [30] have also shown that the

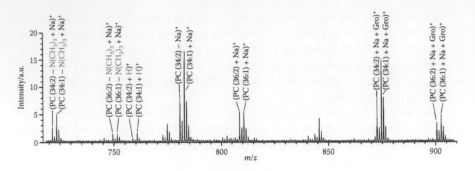

**FIGURE 13.2**   HPTLC/IR–MALDI–TOF mass spectra acquired directly from the PC fraction on a glycerol-wetted TLC plate in positive ion mode. (Reprinted with permission from Rohlfing, A. et al., *Anal. Chem.*, 79, 5793–5808, 2007. Copyright 2007. American Chemical Society.)

relative concentrations of selected PL species can be determined directly on the TLC plate. However, it should be noted that at conditions of IR MALDI quite unusual adducts (for instance, with glycerol, which is not seen at UV MALDI MS) are generated. This is illustrated in Figure 13.2 where the positive ion IR MALDI mass spectrum of one selected PC band is shown ("Gro" denotes ions containing glycerol).

### 13.5.2   ULTRAVIOLET MATRIX-ASSISTED LASER DESORPTION IONIZATION

Another approach that was used nearly at the same time as the IR MALDI investigation [30] of PL relied on a nitrogen UV laser ($\lambda = 337$ nm) and standard DHB as matrix. As one example of physiological interest, an organic extract from hen egg yolk [32] was used because it is easily obtained and contains many different lipid species in significantly different amounts [33]. Phospholipids were separated on silica gel by using $CHCl_3$, ethanol, water, and triethylamine (35:35:7:35, v/v/v/v). A special adapter target (now commercially available from Bruker Daltonics) was used for the introduction of the TLC plate into the MALDI MS device and helped to compensate the height of the TLC plate when attached to the target. Using this approach, resolutions of about 3000 and mass accuracies of about 100 ppm could be achieved. This is poor in comparison to the work mentioned above where an orthogonal TOF MS was used [30], but still sufficient to discriminate lipids differing in just one double bond (2 Da difference).

However, it must be explicitly noted that isobaric ions cannot be discriminated at these conditions: for instance, the differentiation of the sodium adduct of PC 16:0/18:1 (*m/z* 782.5676) and the proton adduct of PC 16:0/20:4 (*m/z* 782.5699) would require a mass accuracy of about 3 ppm, which is not achievable by this simple approach. Fortunately, this is not absolutely necessary because both ions can be easily differentiated in the presence of an excess of $Cs^+$ ions as it has been recently demonstrated [34].

The TLC lane of the egg yolk extract and some selected positive ion MALDI TOF mass spectra are shown in Figure 13.3 to illustrate the achievable spectral

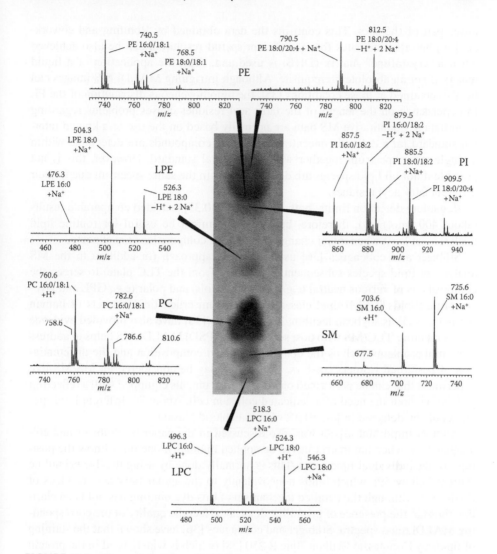

**FIGURE 13.3** Expanded region of a TLC-separated egg yolk extract and the corresponding positive ion MALDI-TOF mass spectra recorded directly from the indicated positions on the TLC plate. Only selected mass ranges are shown for clarity and assignments are provided directly in the individual traces. Please note that the PE fraction provides different spectra, depending on the position where the laser hits the PE spot. The only marked fragmentation is the loss of the headgroup of SM ($m/z$ = 677.5). (Reprinted with modifications from Fuchs, B. et al., *J. Planar Chromatogr.*, 22, 35–42, 2009. With permission from Akademiai Kiado.)

quality [35]. Two aspects are obvious: (1) even minor amounts of rare PL (such as phosphatidylinositol [PI], which makes up only 0.5% of all egg yolk PL) [33] can be detected and (2) the lower and the upper part of the PE spot are characterized by different mass spectra: PEs with longer fatty acyl (in particular arachidonoyl [20:4]) residues are detected in the upper and PEs with shorter fatty acyl residues in the lower part of the spot. This confirms the data obtained by Rohlfing and cowork-ers [30] but also indicates that a sufficient spatial resolution can be also achieved when a "crystalline" matrix (DHB) is used and, thus, the application of a liquid matrix is not an absolute prerequisite. Although intriguing MALDI MS images can be also obtained at these conditions [35], the inhomogeneous distribution of the PL in dependence on the length of the fatty acyl residues causes problems regarding quantitation: quantitative MS data are normally based on the use of a known inter-nal standard (at a defined concentration) and all compounds are detectable within a single mass spectrum together with the internal standard. However, this is not possible if not all lipid species are detectable within the same spectrum due to their different fatty acyl residues.

Regarding detection limits, both approaches [30,33] provided comparable results (about 400 pmol) and, therefore, both methods might be useful for routine lipid analysis—at least when major changes of the lipid compositions are expected.

Stübiger and colleagues [36] used a similar approach (in addition to the MS analysis of lipid species subsequent to reelution from the TLC plate) to screen the compositions of various neutral (e.g., triacylglycerols) and polar (e.g., GPL and glyc-erosphingolipids [GSL]) lipid classes derived from crude lipid extracts of human plasma as well as soybean lecithin. These authors [36] have also provided evidence that combining TLC/MS with post source decay (PSD) MALDI MS helps to address structural problems such as the detailed fatty acyl composition and the differentia-tion of positional isomers ($sn$-1 vs. $sn$-2). PSD may be considered an MS/MS-like experiment that can be performed on all TOF instruments equipped with a reflectron [20] but without the need of a dedicated collision cell. About 70 different lipid spe-cies could be detected in just 50 µL of human blood plasma.

Another important aspect was also discussed in the paper by Stübiger and col-leagues [36]: when the matrix has to be applied manually, one must know the posi-tions of the individual lipid spots. This is normally done by using the dye primuline (Direct Yellow 59), which binds noncovalently to the apolar fatty acyl residues of lipids [37]. Although the detailed mechanism of this dye binding has not been clari-fied thus far, the presence of primuline does not affect the quality of the correspond-ing MALDI mass spectra. Stübiger and colleagues [36] have shown that the staining of lipids by Coomassie Brilliant Blue R-250 [38] (which is widely used in the protein field) can also be used to stain lipids prior to MS analysis.

An automated routine to record MALDI mass spectra from a TLC plate is now also available and was already successfully applied to investigate the (phospho) lipid composition of human mesenchymal stem cells and human erythrocytes [39]: evidence was provided that MS detection is much more sensitive in comparison to typical staining techniques, that is, some lipids could be exclusively detected by MS while the primuline staining monitored exclusively the more abundant lipids.

Many important diseases are accompanied by inflammation and this leads to an increased content of lipid oxidation products. There is evidence that such products can be analyzed by TLC/MALDI MS [40] and this is illustrated in Figure 13.4. However, even if some oxidation products can be easily detected by this approach, it must be explicitly stated that some important lipid oxidation products (for instance, lipid hydroperoxides) are not detectable by MALDI MS—or only with very low

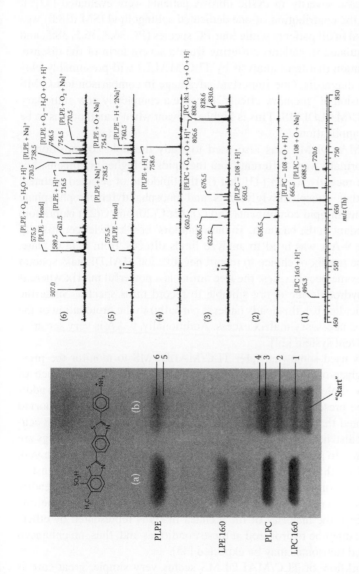

**FIGURE 13.4** Positive ion MALDI-TOF mass spectra of the individual fractions of an air-oxidized mixture of PLPC and PLPE. The developed TLC plate from which the spectra were recorded is shown on the left. Lane (a) represents a PLPC–PLPE–LPC 16:0–LPE 16:0 mixture as control while lane (b) represents the sample of air-oxidized PLPC–PLPE. Positions of the acquired mass spectra right off the TLC plate are labeled by numbers. Ions are labeled according to their m/z ratios and the most prominent peaks are structurally assigned. The structure of the most abundant ion (m/z = 454.1) from the primuline dye is also indicated (left top). Due to the presence of the sulfonic acid residue, primuline is detectable only with very low sensitivity as positive ion. The reasons of the dark background in lane (b) are thus far unknown. (From Bischoff, A. et al., *Acta Chromatogr.*, 23, 365–375, 2011. With permission.)

sensitivities. This is probably due to the tendency of these compounds to be decomposed at conditions of laser irradiation [41].

Of course, there were already some papers dealing with (pre)clinical applications of combined TLC/MALDI analysis. For instance, typical PL signatures associated with respiratory disease severity in cystic fibrosis patients were evaluated [42]: it could be shown that the contribution of one dedicated sphingolipid (SM d18:0) was significantly increased in all patients while four PC species (PC 36:3, 36:5, 38:5, and 38:6) were down regulated in patients suffering from a severe form of the disease. This is a clear indication that lipid analysis by TLC/MALDI will presumably play an increasing role in diagnosis. One important advantage in comparison to LC/MS is the complete exclusion of "memory effects" because a completely new stationary phase is used on TLC/MALDI MS. This is highly relevant when a method has to be certified for clinical applications.

Combined TLC/MALDI MS was also used to study the lipid composition of bacteria, which is normally very different from the lipids of higher organisms. For instance, it has been recently shown [43] that (1) the lipidome of selected archaeal bacteria contains ether phosphatidylglycerols and phosphatidylglycerophosphate methyl esters as the main lipid components and (2) that C(20) and C(25) isopranoid chains are very abundant in the bacteria. To these authors' best knowledge, this was the first work where 9-AA was used to analyze lipids directly from a TLC plate. Although 9-AA is the matrix of choice to record negative ion MALDI mass spectra [24], 9-AA also has some peculiarities: the free amine is a powerful matrix whereas the corresponding hydrochloride is not suitable to record mass spectra. Since the silica gel surface is acidic [10], this leads (at least partially) to the protonation of the 9-AA and reduces the necessary matrix excess. Additionally, 9-AA is very sensitive to changes of the solvent system [24].

The same authors used somewhat later TLC/MALDI MS to monitor the presence of diphytanylglycerol analogues of PI and PG as well as the presence of N-acetylglucosamine-diphytanylglycerol phosphate in selected bacteria [44]. In addition, evidence for the presence of ether lipids of the cardiolipin type was reported [44]. It should be noted that these ether lipids are not only of interest from an academic viewpoint but also have an important application background: many drugs are entrapped in liposomes to improve their incorporation into the target cells. Egg yolk PC is typically used for this purpose because it is easily available and inexpensive. However, the egg yolk contains nearly exclusively diacyl lipids, which are readily digested by enzymes such as phospholipase $A_2$ ($PLA_2$), leading to a reduced lifetime of the liposomes. Since the majority of the archaea lipids is represented by ethers but not esters, they cannot be hydrolyzed at these conditions and, thus, an enhanced stability of the related liposomes may be expected [45].

Although the workflow of TLC/MALDI MS seems very simple, great care is necessary to obtain reproducible data. There is no need to say that the purity of the applied reagents and particularly the solvents is very important. However, the type of TLC plates used is also very important: it has been shown recently that the thickness of the TLC layer has a tremendous impact on the quality of the MALDI mass spectra [46]. This fact is illustrated in Figure 13.5. It is obvious that the analyte peaks are barely detectable at the highest thickness (200 μm) because the spectra

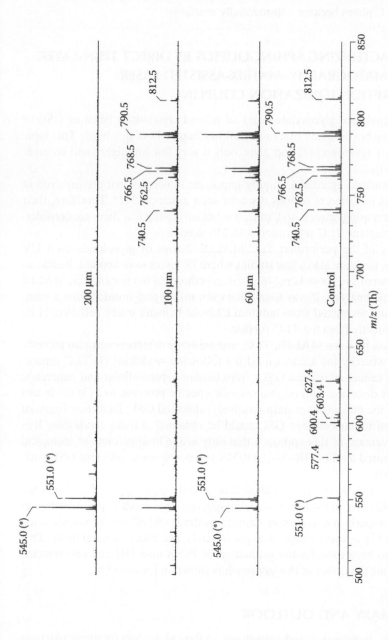

**FIGURE 13.5** Positive ion MALDI-TOF mass spectra of hen egg yolk PE recorded directly from TLC plates with different thicknesses of the stationary phase. The thickness of the used HPTLC plates is indicated in the figure. Spectra labeled with "Control" correspond to the PE mixture desorbed directly from a conventional stainless steel MALDI target. Only selected mass spectra are shown. Note that reasonable peak intensities can be exclusively achieved in the case of a reduced silica gel thickness, but not if 200-μm plates are used. (From Griesinger, H. et al., *Anal. Biochem.*, 451, 45–47, 2014. With permission.)

are dominated by matrix peaks (marked by asterisks). When the thickness of the silica gel layer is decreased, spectral quality is increased and the expected analyte signals are detectable. This is presumably caused by the fact that the analytes are closer at the surface when "thinner" silica gel layers are used [46]. In the meantime, "MS-grade" TLC plates became commercially available.

## 13.6   CHARACTERIZING SPHINGOLIPIDS BY DIRECT THIN-LAYER CHROMATOGRAPHY–MATRIX-ASSISTED LASER DESORPTION IONIZATION COUPLING

Many sphingolipids are glycosylated and all related compounds (such as GSL or gangliosides) will be discussed in more detail in Chapter 18 of this book. This topic has been recently reviewed [47] and, thus, only a very few highlights will be mentioned here shortly.

GSL are nowadays regarded as highly important molecules that are involved in the pathogenesis of different serious diseases such as cancer [47]. Therefore, their analysis is of increasing interest and, thus, it is not surprising that there are considerable efforts to combine TLC separation with MS detection.

The majority of the performed TLC/MALDI studies of glycolipids used UV lasers. However, there are also a few studies where IR lasers were applied. Beside an IR laser, Dreisewerd and coworkers [48] used an orthogonal but not an axial MALDI MS for glycolipid analysis. It was found that even minor gangliosides from a complex lipid mixture (extracted from cultured Chinese hamster ovary cells) could be characterized directly from the TLC surface.

A combination between MALDI, TLC, and antibody detection was also recently suggested [49] whereby the authors used the following workflow: (1) TLC separation of putative cancer-associated GSLs from human hepatocellular and pancreatic tumors, (2) their detection with oligosaccharide-specific proteins, and (3) the *in situ* MS analysis of the previously protein-(antibody)-detected GSL. Detection limits of less than 1 ng of immunostained GSL could be obtained at these conditions. It is a particular advantage of this approach that only crude lipid extracts of biological sources are required for TLC/IR–MALDI/MS and no laborious previous GSL purification is needed.

A TLC-Blot-MALDI-Imaging method was recently also suggested [50] to visualize whole lipids and individual molecular species. This method provides higher sensitivity in comparison to common staining methods and allows for visualization of all lipids within a linear range of approximately one order of magnitude. This method has also been used for the evaluation of PL in tuna [51] and one selected image to illustrate the power of this approach is shown in Figure 13.6.

## 13.7   SUMMARY AND OUTLOOK

TLC is a simple, inexpensive, and convenient analytical method for many (particularly small) organic molecules. As $R_F$ values are not very reliable and staining techniques are often not very specific, identifying the individual compounds by their

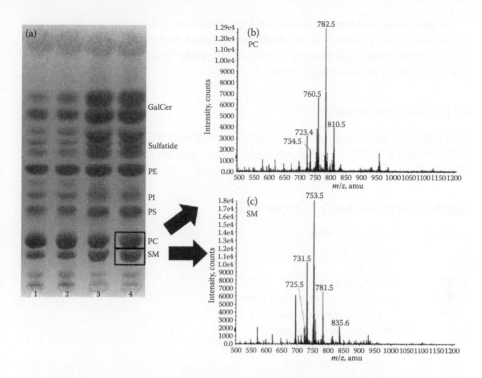

**FIGURE 13.6** (a) Thin-layer chromatogram stained with primuline. Lanes (1–4) contain human brain lipid extracted from gray matter of inferior frontal gyrus (lane 1), gray matter of hippocampus (lane 2), white matter of inferior frontal gyrus (lane 3), and white matter of hippocampus (lane 4). The MS spectra of PC (b) and SM (c) allowed to directly analyze the blotted PVDF membrane. (From Goto-Inoue, N. et al., *J. Chromatogr. A*, 1216, 7096–7101, 2009. With permission.)

molecular weights represents a powerful approach. In combination with LC, MS analysis is widely established, but thus far there are much less attempts to combine TLC with MS. There were already different reports about the successful combining of TLC with MS "spray" desorption techniques such as DESI MS [52]. It was one aim of this chapter to show that the combination of TLC and MALDI is also a powerful, but underestimated, methodological couple.

The most important advantages of TLC MALDI are (1) the easy combination (in the simplest way the TLC plate is fixed directly to the MALDI target) and (2) the simple MALDI mass spectra because (in contrast to ESI MS) exclusively singly charged ions are generated.

As far as these authors can say, TLC MALDI MS is the method of choice when a screening of the lipid compositions of unknown mixtures is sufficient. However, if quantitative (absolute) data of the concentrations of the different lipid species is necessary, extraction-based approaches should be preferentially used because data can be more easily quantified when the use of internal standards is possible. These aspects have been recently reviewed [53,54].

Despite these problems, however, we hope the illustrated examples confirmed the significant future potential of the direct combination between TLC and MALDI in the lipid field. This is particularly important as certain lipid species are increasingly considered to be of therapeutic value.

## ACKNOWLEDGMENTS

This study was supported by the German Research Council (DFG Schi 476/12-1, SFB 1052/B6, and FU 771/1-2). The advice of Detlev Suckau and Martin Schürenberg (Bruker Daltonics) is also gratefully acknowledged.

## ABBREVIATIONS AND ACRONYMS

| | |
|---|---|
| 9-AA | 9-aminoacridine |
| CL | cardiolipin |
| Da | Dalton |
| DAG | diacylglycerol |
| DESI | desorption electrospray ionization |
| DHB | 2,5-dihydroxybenzoic acid |
| ESI | electrospray ionization |
| GPC | glycerophosphatidylcholine |
| GPL | glycerophospholipids |
| GSL | glycosphingolipids |
| HP | high performance |
| IR | infrared |
| $\lambda$ | wavelength |
| LC | liquid chromatography |
| LDI | laser desorption ionization |
| LPC | lyso-phosphatidylcholine |
| LPE | lyso-phosphatidylethanolamine |
| MALDI | matrix-assisted laser desorption and ionization |
| MS | mass spectrometry |
| $m/z$ | mass over charge |
| PA | phosphatidic acid |
| PC | phosphatidylcholine |
| PE | phosphatidylethanolamine |
| PG | phosphatidylglycerol |
| PI | phosphatidylinositol |
| PL | phospholipid |
| $PLA_2$ | phospholipase $A_2$ |
| ppm | parts per million |
| PS | phosphatidylserine |
| PVDF | polyvinylidene difluoride |
| $R_F$ | retardation factor |
| SA | sinapinic acid |
| SM | sphingomyelin |

| S/N | signal to noise |
|-----|-----------------|
| TAG | triacylglycerol |
| THA | 2,4,6-trihydroxyacetophenone |
| TLC | thin-layer chromatography |
| TOF | time-of-flight |
| UV | ultraviolet |

## REFERENCES

1. Fried, B. 2005. Lipids, In: *Handbook of Thin-Layer Chromatography*, 3rd ed., Sherma, J. and Fried, B., Eds., Marcel Dekker, Basel, Chapter 22, pp. 826–875.
2. Fuchs, B., Süss, R., Teuber, K., Eibisch, M., and Schiller, J. 2011. Lipid analysis by thin-layer chromatography—A review of the current state, *J. Chromatogr. A*, 1218: 2754–2774.
3. Fuchs, B., Süß, R., Nimptsch, A., and Schiller, J. 2009. Matrix-assisted laser desorption and ionization time-of-flight mass spectrometry (MALDI-TOF MS) directly combined with thin-layer chromatography (TLC)—A review of the current state, *Chromatographia*, 69: 95–105.
4. Touchstone, J.C. 1995. Thin-layer chromatographic procedures for lipid separation, *J. Chromatogr. B*, 671: 169–195.
5. Leray, C. Ed. 2013. *Introduction to Lipidomics—From Bacteria to Man*, CRC Press, Boca Raton, FL.
6. Fuchs, B. and Schiller, J. 2009. Application of MALDI-TOF mass spectrometry in lipidomics, *Eur. J. Lipid Sci. Technol.*, 111: 83–98.
7. Eibisch, M., Fuchs, B., Schiller, J., Süß, R., and Teuber, K. 2011. Analysis of phospholipid mixtures from biological tissues by matrix-assisted laser desorption and ionization time-of-flight mass spectrometry (MALDI-TOF MS): A laboratory experiment. *J. Chem. Educat.*, 88: 503–507.
8. Liebisch, G., Vizcaíno, J.A., Köfeler, H., Trötzmüller, M., Griffiths, W.J., Schmitz, G., Spener, F., and Wakelam, M.J. 2013. Shorthand notation for lipid structures derived from mass spectrometry, *J. Lipid Res.*, 54: 1523–1530.
9. Brenna, J.T. 2013. Fatty acid analysis by high resolution gas chromatography and mass spectrometry for clinical and experimental applications, *Curr. Opin. Clin. Nutr. Metab. Care*, 16: 548–554.
10. Schiller, J., Müller, K., Süss, R., Arnhold, J., Gey, C., Herrmann, A., Lessig, J., Arnold, K., and Müller, P. 2003. Analysis of the lipid composition of bull spermatozoa by MALDI-TOF mass spectrometry—A cautionary note. *Chem. Phys. Lipids*, 126: 85–94.
11. Wang, Y., Krull, I.S., Liu, C., and Orr, J.D. 2003. Derivatization of phospholipids, *J. Chromatogr. B*, 793: 3–14.
12. Luftmann, H. 2004. A simple device for the extraction of TLC spots: Direct coupling with an electrospray mass spectrometer, *Anal. Bioanal. Chem.*, 378: 964–968.
13. Teuber, K., Riemer, T., and Schiller, J. 2010. Thin-layer chromatography combined with MALDI–TOF–MS and $^{31}$P-NMR to study possible selective bindings of phospholipids to silica gel. *Anal. Bioanal. Chem.*, 398: 2833–2842.
14. Morlock, G. and Sherma, J. 2009. New and improved liquid chromatographic methods for food analysis, *J. AOAC Int.*, 92: 689–690.
15. Paglia, G., Ifa, D.R., Wu, C., Corso, G., and Cooks, R.G. 2010. Desorption electrospray ionization mass spectrometry analysis of lipids after two-dimensional high-performance thin-layer chromatography partial separation, *Anal. Chem.*, 82: 1744–1750.

16. Seng, J.A., Ellis, S.R., Hughes, J.R., Maccarone, A.T., Truscott, R.J., Blanksby, S.J., and Mitchell, T.W. 2014. Characterisation of sphingolipids in the human lens by thin layer chromatography-desorption electrospray ionisation mass spectrometry, *Biochim. Biophys. Acta*, 1841: 1285–1291.

17. Schiller, J., Süss, R., Arnhold, J., Fuchs, B., Lessig, J., Müller, M., Petković, M., Spalteholz, H., Zschörnig, O., and Arnold, K. 2004. Matrix-assisted laser desorption and ionization time-of-flight (MALDI-TOF) mass spectrometry in lipid and phospholipid research. *Prog. Lipid Res.*, 43: 449–488.

18. Ellis, S.R., Brown, S.H., In Het Panhuis, M., Blanksby, S.J., and Mitchell, T.W. 2013. Surface analysis of lipids by mass spectrometry: More than just imaging, *Prog. Lipid Res.*, 52: 329–353.

19. Gode, D. and Volmer, D.A. 2013. Lipid imaging by mass spectrometry—A review, *Analyst*, 138: 1289–1315.

20. Hillenkamp, F. and Peter-Katalinić, J. 2014. *MALDI MS—A Practical Guide to Instrumentation, Methods, and Applications*, 2nd ed., Wiley-Blackwell, Weinheim, Germany.

21. Knochenmuss, R. 2006. Ion formation mechanisms in UV–MALDI, *Analyst*, 131: 966–986.

22. Fuchs, B. and Schiller, J. 2009. Recent developments of useful MALDI matrices for the mass spectrometric characterization of apolar compounds. *Curr. Org. Chem.*, 13: 1664–1681.

23. Schiller, J., Süss, R., Fuchs, B., Müller, M., Petković, M., Zschörnig, O., and Waschipky, H. 2007. The suitability of different DHB isomers as matrices for the MALDI-TOF MS analysis of phospholipids: Which isomer for what purpose? *Eur. Biophys. J.*, 36: 517–527.

24. Sun, G., Yang, K., Zhao, Z., Guan, S., Han, X., and Gross, R.W. 2008. Matrix-assisted laser desorption/ionization time-of-flight mass spectrometric analysis of cellular glycerophospholipids enabled by multiplexed solvent dependent analyte-matrix interactions. *Anal. Chem.*, 80: 7576–7585.

25. Nakamura, K., Suzuki, Y., Goto-Inoue, N., Yoshida-Noro, C., and Suzuki, A. 2006. Structural characterization of neutral glycosphingolipids by thin-layer chromatography coupled to matrix-assisted laser desorption/ionization quadrupole ion trap time-of-flight MS/MS, *Anal. Chem.*, 78: 5736–5743.

26. Mehl, J.T., Gusev, A.I., and Hercules, D.M. 1997. Coupling protocol for thin layer chromatography matrix-assisted laser desorption ionization, *Chromatographia*, 46: 358–364.

27. Wilson, I.D. 1999. The state of the art in thin-layer chromatography–mass spectrometry: A critical appraisal, *J. Chromatogr. A*, 856: 429–442.

28. Bergman, N., Shevchenko, D., and Bergquist, J. 2014. Approaches for the analysis of low molecular weight compounds with laser desorption/ionization techniques and mass spectrometry, *Anal. Bioanal. Chem.*, 406: 49–61.

29. Fan, X. and Murray, K.K. 2010. Wavelength and time-resolved imaging of material ejection in infrared matrix-assisted laser desorption, *J. Phys. Chem. A*, 114: 1492–1497.

30. Rohlfing, A., Müthing, J., Pohlentz, G., Distler, U., Peter-Katalinić, J., Berkenkamp, S., and Dreisewerd, K. 2007. IR–MALDI–MS analysis of HPTLC-separated phospholipid mixtures directly from the TLC plate, *Anal. Chem.*, 79: 5793–5808.

31. Guilhaus, M., Selby, D., and Mlynski, V. 2000. Orthogonal acceleration time-of-flight mass spectrometry, *Mass Spectrom. Rev.*, 19: 65–107.

32. Schiller, J., Süss, R., Fuchs, B., Müller, M., Zschörnig, O., and Arnold, K. 2007. MALDI-TOF MS in lipidomics, *Front. Biosci.*, 12: 2568–2579.

33. Fuchs, B., Schiller, J., Süss, R., Schürenberg, M., and Suckau, D. 2007. A direct and simple method of coupling matrix-assisted laser desorption and ionization time-of-flight mass spectrometry (MALDI-TOF MS) to thin-layer chromatography (TLC) for the analysis of phospholipids from egg yolk, *Anal. Bioanal. Chem.*, 389: 827–834.

34. Schiller, J., Süss, R., Petković, M., Hilbert, N., Müller, M., Zschörnig, O., Arnhold, J., and Arnold, K. 2001. CsCl as an auxiliary reagent for the analysis of phosphatidylcholine mixtures by matrix-assisted laser desorption and ionization time-of-flight mass spectrometry (MALDI-TOF MS), *Chem. Phys. Lipids*, 113: 123–131.
35. Fuchs, B., Schiller, J., Süß, R., Nimptsch, A., Schürenberg, M., and Suckau, D. 2009. Capabilities and disadvantages of combined matrix-assisted laser desorption/ionization time-of-flight mass spectrometry (MALDI-TOF MS) and high-performance thin-layer chromatography (HPTLC): Analysis of egg yolk lipids, *J. Planar Chromatogr.*, 22: 35–42.
36. Stübiger, G., Pittenauer, E., Belgacem, O., Rehulka, P., Widhalm, K., and Allmaier, G. 2009. Analysis of human plasma lipids and soybean lecithin by means of high-performance thin-layer chromatography and matrix-assisted laser desorption/ionization mass spectrometry, *Rapid Commun. Mass Spectrom.*, 23: 2711–2723.
37. White, T., Bursten, S., Federighi, D., Lewis, R.A., and Nudelman, E. 1998. High-resolution separation and quantification of neutral lipid and phospholipid species in mammalian cells and sera by multi-one-dimensional thin-layer chromatography, *Anal. Biochem.*, 258: 109–117.
38. Yao, J.K. and Rastetter, G.M. 1985. Microanalysis of complex tissue lipids by high-performance thin-layer chromatography, *Anal. Biochem.*, 150: 111–116.
39. Fuchs, B., Schiller, J., Süss, R., Zscharnack, M., Bader, A., Müller, P., Schürenberg, M., Becker, M., and Suckau, D. 2008. Analysis of stem cell lipids by off-line HPTLC-MALDI-TOF MS, *Anal. Bioanal. Chem.*, 392: 849–860.
40. Bischoff, A., Eibisch, M., Fuchs, B., Süß, R., Schürenberg, M., Suckau, D., and Schiller, J. 2011. A simple TLC/MALDI method to monitor oxidation products of phosphatidyl-cholines and -ethanolamines, *Acta Chromatogr.*, 23: 365–375.
41. Fuchs, B. 2014. Mass spectrometry and inflammation-MS methods to study oxidation and enzyme-induced changes of phospholipids. *Anal. Bioanal. Chem.*, 406: 1291–1306.
42. Guerrera, I.C., Astarita, G., Jais, J.P., Sands, D., Nowakowska, A., Colas, J. Sermet-Gaudelus, I. et al. 2009. A novel lipidomic strategy reveals plasma phospholipid signatures associated with respiratory disease severity in cystic fibrosis patients, *PLoS One*, 4: e7735.
43. Angelini, R., Corral, P., Lopalco, P., Ventosa, A., and Corcelli, A. 2012. Novel ether lipid cardiolipins in archaeal membranes of extreme haloalkaliphiles, *Biochim. Biophys. Acta*, 1818: 1365–1373.
44. Lobasso, S., Lopalco, P., Angelini, R., Vitale, R., Huber, H., Müller, V., and Corcelli, A. 2012. Coupled TLC and MALDI-TOF/MS analyses of the lipid extract of the hyper-thermophilic archaeon *Pyrococcus furiosus*, *Archaea*, 2012: 957852.
45. Benvegnu, T., Lemiègre, L., and Cammas-Marion, S. 2009. New generation of liposomes called archaeosomes based on natural or synthetic archaeal lipids as innovative formulations for drug delivery, *Recent Pat. Drug Deliv. Formul.*, 3: 206–220.
46. Griesinger, H., Fuchs, B., Süß, R., Matheis, K., Schulz, M., and Schiller, J. 2014. Stationary phase thickness determines the quality of thin-layer chromatography/matrix-assisted laser desorption and ionization mass spectra of lipids, *Anal. Biochem.*, 451: 45–47.
47. Meisen, I., Mormann, M., and Müthing, J. 2011. Thin-layer chromatography, overlay technique and mass spectrometry: A versatile triad advancing glycosphingolipidomics, *Biochim. Biophys. Acta*, 1811: 875–896.
48. Dreisewerd, K., Müthing, J., Rohlfing, A., Meisen, I., Vukelić, Z., Peter-Katalinić, J., Hillenkamp, F., and Berkenkamp, S. 2005. Analysis of gangliosides directly from thin-layer chromatography plates by infrared matrix-assisted laser desorption/ionization orthogonal time-of-flight mass spectrometry with a glycerol matrix, *Anal. Chem.*, 77: 4098–4107.

49. Kouzel, I.U., Pirkl, A., Pohlentz, G., Soltwisch, J., Dreisewerd, K., Karch, H., and Müthing, J. 2014. Progress in detection and structural characterization of glycosphingolipids in crude lipid extracts by enzymatic phospholipid disintegration combined with thin-layer chromatography immunodetection and IR-MALDI mass spectrometry, *Anal. Chem.*, 86: 1215–1222.

50. Goto-Inoue, N., Hayasaka, T., Taki, T., Gonzalez, T.V., and Setou, M. 2009. A new lipidomics approach by thin-layer chromatography-blot-matrix-assisted laser desorption/ionization imaging mass spectrometry for analyzing detailed patterns of phospholipid molecular species, *J. Chromatogr. A*, 1216: 7096–7101.

51. Zaima, N., Goto-Inoue, N., Adachi, K., and Setou, M. 2011. Selective analysis of lipids by thin-layer chromatography blot matrix-assisted laser desorption/ionization imaging mass spectrometry, *J. Oleo Sci.*, 60: 93–98.

52. Van Berkel, G.J., Ford, M.J., and Deibel, M.A. 2005. Thin-layer chromatography and mass spectrometry coupled using desorption electrospray ionization, *Anal. Chem.*, 77: 1207–1215.

53. Morlock, G. and Schwack, W. 2010. Hyphenations in planar chromatography, *J. Chromatogr. A*, 1217: 6600–6609.

54. Morlock, G.E. 2014. Background mass signals in TLC/HPTLC–ESI–MS and practical advices for use of the TLC–MS interface, *J. Liq. Chromatogr. Relat. Technol.*, 37: 2892–2914.

# 14 Application of TLC–MS to Drug Photodegradation Studies

*Urszula Hubicka, Jan Krzek,* *Anna Maślanka,*
*and Barbara Żuromska-Witek*

## CONTENTS

## 14.1 INTRODUCTION

The first law of photochemistry states that only light which is absorbed by a system can bring about a photochemical change, and the second (Stark–Einstein's law of photochemistry) states that for each photon of light absorbed by a chemical system, only one molecule is activated for a photochemical reaction. Molecules possessing suitable chromophores (moieties capable of absorbing ultraviolet [UV] or visible light in the range of 290–700 nm such as those with the extended conjugation of double bonds or aromatic rings) may be activated photochemically by UV or visible radiation. Consequently, these photoactivated molecules may alter biological systems and if the exposure is sufficient, may elicit harmful effects, including phototoxicity (e.g., erythema/edema, pigmentary alterations, and visual impairment/

---

* Professor Krzek passed away on February 1st, 2015.

ocular damage), photoallergy, or photocarcinogenicity. Especially, there are specific chemical classes of pharmaceuticals, such as the fluoroquinolone antibiotics, which have been associated with a manifestation/exacerbation of these effects [1]. The photostability of active pharmaceutical ingredients (APIs) and drug products (DPs) may impact the potency, shelf life, handling, and packaging of the product. A photounstable API may be problematic to isolate or to formulate, complex to pack for shipping, or difficult to dose (e.g., infusion), and it is an indicator for photosafety concerns that may require further investigation [2]. Therefore, stability testing of the drug substances and the final preparation is important and recommended by International Conference on Harmonization (ICH) guidelines [3].

ICH Q1B describes tests for drug photostability determination—forced degradation studies [2–3]. Forced degradation is a degradation of a new drug substance and a drug product at conditions more severe than accelerated conditions. It is required to demonstrate the specificity of stability-indicating methods and also provides insight into degradation pathways and degradation products of the drug substance and helps in the elucidation of the structure of the degradation products. Forced degradation studies show the chemical behavior of the molecule, which in turn helps in the development of formulation and package. A minimal list of stress factors suggested for forced degradation studies must include acid and base hydrolysis, thermal degradation, photolysis, and oxidation, and may include freeze–thaw cycles and shear. The design of photolysis studies is left to the applicant's discretion, although Q1B specifies the light source, outputs, and exposure levels [4].

The photostability testing of drug substances must be evaluated to demonstrate that light exposure does not result in an unacceptable change. Some recommended conditions for photostability testing are described in ICH guidelines. Photostability studies are performed to generate primary degradants of drug substance by exposure to combining visible and UV light, xenon or metal halide lamp, or to both the cool white fluorescent and near UV lamp. Drug substance and drug product samples should be exposed to light for a minimum of 1.2 million lux hours and an integrated near UV energy of not less than 200 Wh/m$^2$. The most commonly accepted wavelength of light is in the range of 300–800 nm to cause the photolytic degradation. During examination an appropriate control of temperature should be maintained including a dark control in the same environment. Samples may be exposed side by side with a validated chemical actinometric system to ensure the specified light dose, or for the appropriate time when conditions have been monitored using calibrated radiometers/lux meters [3–4].

This chapter describes the thin-layer chromatography–mass spectrometric methods (TLC–MS) helpful for the development of a stability-indicating method.

## 14.2   BETAHISTINE

Betahistine, N-methyl-2-(pyridin-2-yl)ethanamine, pyridine derivative of the side chain at position 2 is a synthetic analog of histamine, used as the hydrochloride in the treatment of Meniere disease.

The TLC method was used to separate the photodegradation products and derivatization of betahistine with dansyl chloride [5] (Figure 14.1).

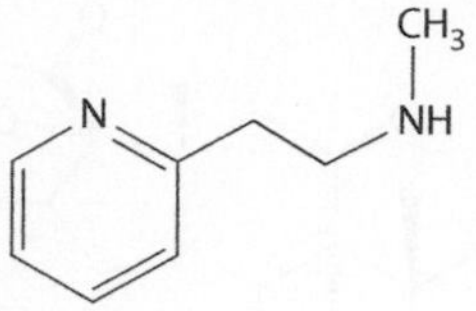

**FIGURE 14.1**   Structure of betahistine.

*Sample preparation:* A sample film of betahistine powder of approximately 0.1 mm thickness in a glass dish was exposed to UV light for a maximum of 24 h. The distance between lamp and sample was 5 cm.

*Irradiation conditions:* The UV lamp used for photostress testing was 125 cm long and placed in the laminar flow cabinet.

*Stationary phase:* TLC silica gel plates with nonfluorescent background.

*Mobile phase:* Acetonitrile:dichloromethane (1:9 v/v).

*Preparation of samples for GC–MS analysis:* About 50 mg of UV-degraded betahistine was dissolved in 10 mL of acetonitrile and derivatized with dansyl chloride solution (1 part of betahistine solution and 20 parts of dansyl chloride solution and left for 20 min at 55°C). Dansyl chloride solution was prepared by dissolving 10 mg of reagent in 10 mL of acetonitrile. 5 mL of UV degraded and derivatized betahistine solution was spotted onto TLC plates. Migration distance of the mobile phase was not less than 15 cm. The bands were located by viewing under UV lamp at 245 and 366 nm, and were scratched, extracted in acetonitrile, and identified by GC–MS.

*GC–MS analysis:* GC–MS analyses were carried out on GC–MS Clarus 500 Gas Chromatograph, Clarus 500 Mass Spectrometer with software controller/integrator TurboMass. Elite 5MS GC capillary column 30 m × 0.25 mm × 0.5 μm (PerkinElmer, Shelton, CT) was used. Helium was the carrier gas with a 2 mL min$^{-1}$ flow, flow initial: 55.5 cm s$^{-1}$. MS scan from 50 to 650 amu.

The identification of the dansylated products obtained in UV were performed based on molecular ions [M+H]$^+$. The molecular ion at $m/z = 386.18$ amu can be attributed to the compound dansylatedbetahistine-$N$-oxide and the molecular ion at $m/z = 357.25$ amu was identified as O-dansylated β-pyridin-2-yl-ethanol.

## 14.3   BETAMETHASONE

Betamethasone, (8$S$,9$R$,10$S$,11$S$,13$S$,14$S$,16$S$,17$R$)-9-fluoro-11,17-dihydroxy-17-(2-hydroxyacetyl)-10,13,16-trimethyl-6,7,8,9,10,11,12,13,14,15,16,17-dodecahydro-$3H$-cyclopenta[$a$]phenanthren-3-one, is a potent corticosteroid with anti-inflammatory and immunosuppressive properties. The TLC method was used to separate the photodegradation products of betamethasone and betamethasone 17-valerate [6] (Figure 14.2).

*Sample preparation:* Solutions of betamethasone at various concentrations (10$^{-4}$ – 10$^{-3}$ M) in methanol were put into quartz cells and irradiated with 20 J cm$^{-2}$ UVB.

*Irradiation conditions:* The solution was irradiated with a Philips PL-S 9W/12 lamp, mainly emitting at 312 nm. The intensity of the radiation was 0.20 J cm$^{-2}$ min. Samples were maintained at room temperature during irradiation.

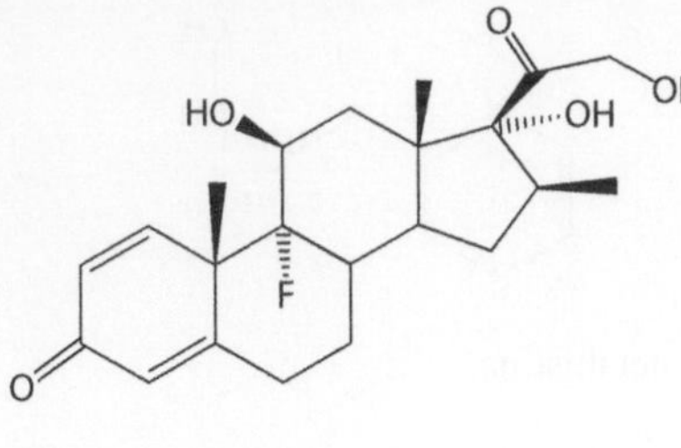

**FIGURE 14.2**   Structure of betamethasone.

*Stationary phase:* TLC silica gel plates.

*Mobile phase:* Chloroform:acetic acid (5:2 v/v).

*Preparation of samples for MS analysis*: The irradiated methanol solutions were concentrated and applied as bands to TLC plates. After development, the bands corresponding to the samples were scraped off, extracted with methanol, and taken to dryness. The residues were submitted to MS analysis.

*MS analysis:* MS analysis was carried out on an API–TOF Mariner spectrometer. The samples were dissolved in methanol to which either 1% HCOOH for positive-ion experiments or 0.5% $NH_4OH$ for negative-ion experiments was added.

The identification of the photodegradation products of betamethasone and betamethasone 17-valerate was performed on a basis of molecular ions [M+H]$^+$. Because of exposure to UVB, three photodegradation products of betamethasone were formed: photoproduct 1—$R_F$ value 0.43, a molecular ion at $m/z$ = 393 amu, photoproduct 2—$R_F$ value 0.60, a molecular ion at $m/z$ = 393 amu, and photoproduct 3—$R_F$ value 0.69, a molecular ion at $m/z$ = 333 amu.

Because of exposure to UVB, three photodegradation products of betamethasone17-valerate were also formed: photoproduct 3—$R_F$ value 0.69, a molecular ion at $m/z$ = 333 amu, photoproduct 4—$R_F$ value 0.41, a molecular ion at $m/z$ = 477 amu, and photoproduct 5—$R_F$ value 0.61, a molecular ion at $m/z$ = 477 amu. Their structures are shown in Table 14.1.

## 14.4   CARBAMAZEPINE

Carbamazepine, 5*H*-dibenzo[*b,f* ]azepine-5-carboxamide, is an anticonvulsant used to control grand mal and psychomotor or focal seizures. Preparative TLC method was used to isolate the products of carbamazepine decomposition [7] (Figure 14.3).

*Sample preparation:* 0.5 mmol of carbamazepine and 100 mmol hydrogen peroxide were dissolved in 500 mL of water. The solution was irradiated by UV light for 1 h.

*Irradiation conditions:* The solution was irradiated with a nominal 17-W low-pressure mercury monochromatic lamp emitting at 254 nm in a 0.420l photoreactor. The power output of the lamp was $2.7 \times 10^{-6}$ E s$^{-1}$.

*Stationary phase:* Preparative TLC silica gel plates.

*Mobile phase:* Toluene:chloroform: methanol (8:5:1 v/v/v).

*Preparation of samples for GC–MS analysis:* A solution of carbamazepine after irradiation was extracted with ethyl acetate (3 × 300 mL) and organic layers were

## TABLE 14.1
## Structures of the Photodegradation Products of Betamethasone and Betamethasone 17-Valerate

Photoproduct 1

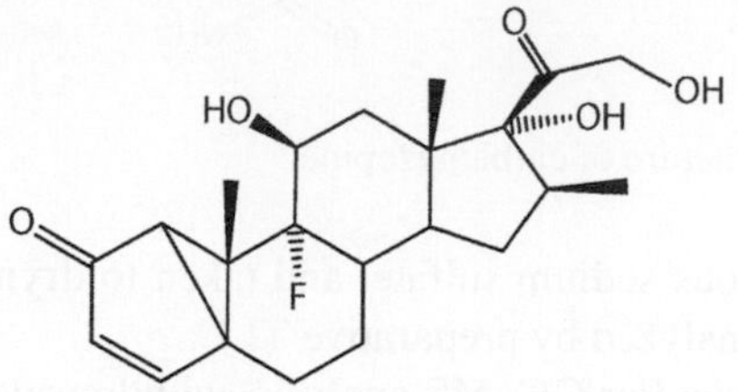

Photoproduct 2

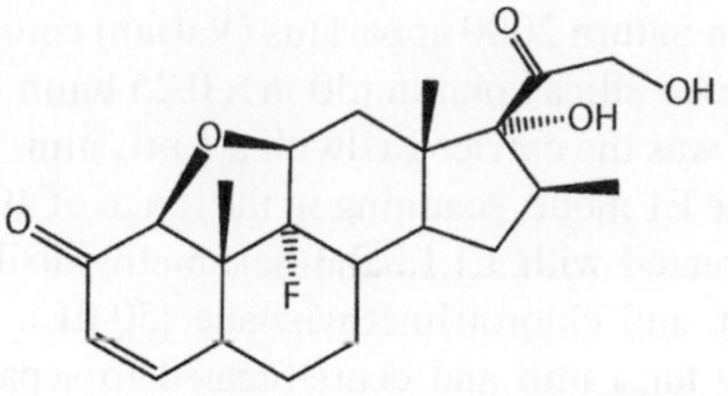

Photoproduct 3

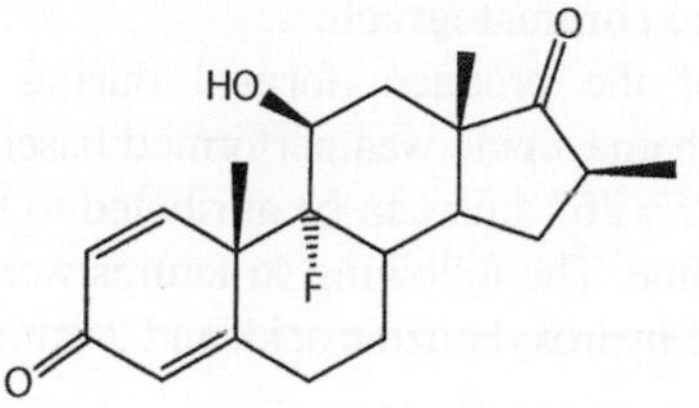

Photoproduct 4

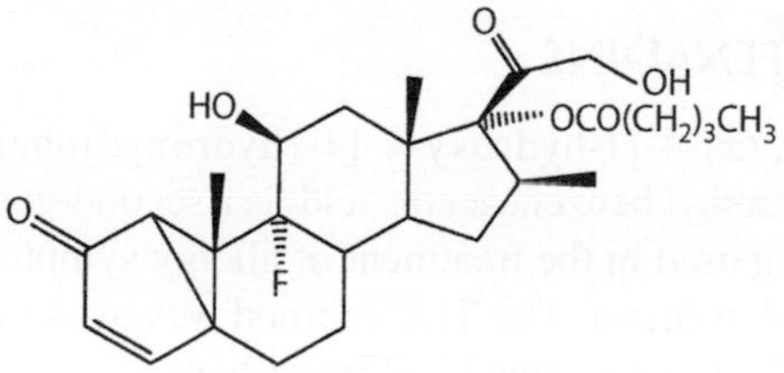

Photoproduct 5

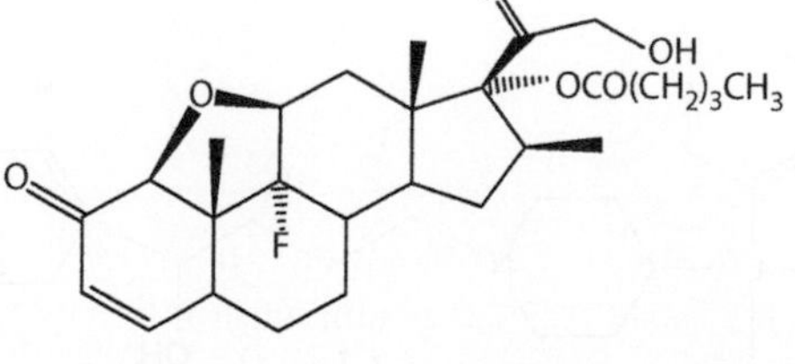

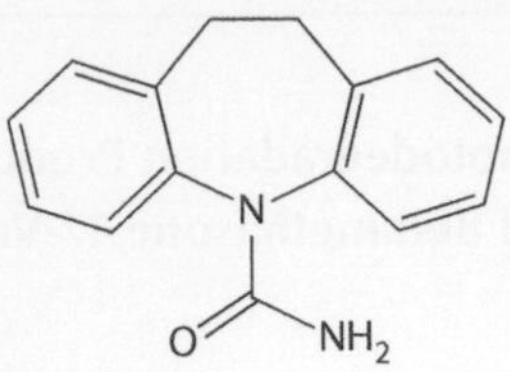

FIGURE. 14.3  Structure of carbamazepine.

dried over anhydrous sodium sulfate, and taken to dryness under vacuum at 25°C. The residue was analyzed by preparative TLC.

*GC–MS analysis:* For GC–MS analysis, withdrawals were lyophilized, the residue dissolved in methanol, and directly injected into a GC–MS instrument. Analyses were carried out on Saturn 2000 apparatus (Varian) equipped with an ion trap detector. A DB5-MS-fused silica column (30 m × 0.25 bmm ID, 0.25 μm film thickness) was used. Helium was the carrier gas with a 1 mL min$^{-1}$ flow rate. The MS detector was operated in the E1 mode, scanning in the range of 40–640 amu. When required, the residue was treated with 1,1,1,3,3,3-hexamethyldisilazane (200 μL), anhydrous pyridine (200 μL), and chlorotrimethylsilane (50 μL). The resulting mixture was shaken vigorously for 1 min and centrifugated to separate the precipitate formed prior to injection into the chromatograph.

The identification of the products formed during the photodegradation with oxidation process of carbamazepine was performed based on molecular ions [M+H]$^+$. The molecular ion at $m/z = 267$ amu can be attributed to the compounds 1-hydroxyacridine or 2-hydroxyacridine. The following structures were assigned to the other products: 2-hydroxyphenol, 2-hydroxybenzoic acid, and 2-aminobenzoic acid.

## 14.5   FEXOFENADINE

Fexofenadine, (±)-4-[1-hydroxy-4-[4-(hydroxydiphenylmethyl)-1-piperidinyl]-butyl]-α, α-dimethyl benzeneacetic acid, is a second-generation antihistamine pharmaceutical drug used in the treatment of allergy symptoms, such as hay fever, nasal congestion, and urticaria. The TLC method was used for isolated and purified photoproducts of the fexofenadine [8] (Figure 14.4).

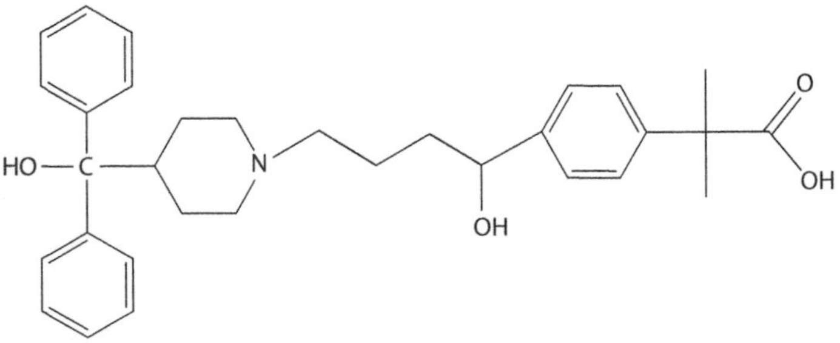

FIGURE 14.4  Structure of fexofenadine.

*Sample preparation:* Stock solution of fexofenadine hydrochloride in methanol (9.6 mg·mL$^{-1}$) pH 11.00 was prepared and irradiated for 18 h at 254 nm. The effect of light was studied exposing sample in 1-cm quartz cells.

*Irradiation conditions:* Two lamps were used for photostress testing: a UV fluorescent lamp, 15 W, emitting radiation at 254 nm, and a medium-pressure metal halide lamp. The temperature inside the chamber was below 30°C. The distance of the samples from the radiation source was 5 cm.

Stationary phase: Preparative TLC plates.

Mobile phase:

A—Methylene chloride:methanol (90:10 v/v)
B—Chloroform:methanol (80:20 v/v)
C—Chloroform:methanol (85:15 v/v)

*Preparation of samples for MS analysis:* After irradiation, the content of the quartz cells was collected in a vessel with an amount of 1 g of silica gel. This sample was used to separate the degradation products by column chromatography. The separation was carried out with chloroform and methanol gradient from (100:0 v/v) to (75:25 v/v). Two degradation products were isolated: DP-1 and DP-2. The fractions containing DP-1 were purified by preparative TLC using mobile phase A, and the fractions containing DP-2 were purified using mobile phase B. The TLC was performed with mobile phase C as eluent for both products.

*MS analysis:* Mass spectra were recorded on a VG Trio-2 mass spectrometer and high-resolution mass spectra were measured on a ZAB-SEQ4F mass spectrometer. The ionization method was electron impact at 70 eV.

The identification of the photodegradation products of fexofenadine obtained in UV was performed based on molecular ions [M+H]$^+$. The mass spectrum of DP-1 show the molecular ion at $m/z = 457$ amu, and the product was identified as the 4-[4-(hydroxydiphenyl-methyl)-1-piperidinyl]-1-(4-phenylisopropyl)butanol. The second product DP-2 ($m/z = 499$ amu) was identified as α,α,-dimethyl-4-[1-hydroxy-4-[4-(benzophenone)1-piperidinyl]buthyl]-benzene acetic acid.

## 14.6  FLUOROQUINOLONES

Fluoroquinolones are an important group of synthetic antibacterial agents exhibiting high activity against a broad spectrum of gram-negative and gram-positive bacteria and a large number of licensed products containing these antibiotics are available for use in animal husbandry. Fluoroquinolones are used in the treatment of systemic infections including urinary tract, respiratory, gastrointestinal, and skin infections. In the veterinary field, they are used not only for the treatment of diseases but also as feed additives to increase the animal mass. The mechanism of action of fluoroquinolones lies in inhibiting the activity of two bacterial enzymes—DNA gyrase (topoisomerase II) and topoisomerase IV, which regulate the spatial arrangement of DNA in bacterial cells. Inhibiting the activity of those enzymes by the formation of irreversible complex drug/enzyme/DNA disables DNA synthesis and leads to the bacterial cell death. Fluoroquinolones are a group of compounds that undergo photodegradation under UV light relatively easily. The degradation is diverse and depends on the conditions and structure of studied compounds [9–11].

## 14.6.1 Difloxacin

Difloxacin, 6-fluoro-1-(4-fluorophenyl)-7-(4-methylpiperazin-1-yl)-4-oxoquinoline-3-carboxylic acid, belongs to the second-generation class and is used in veterinary medicine. The TLC-densitometric method was developed for determination of difloxacin in the presence its photodegradation products [9] (Figure 14.5).

*Sample preparation:* 98.0 µg mL$^{-1}$ aqueous solution of difloxacin in methanol was measured off on quartz dishes of 4 cm diameter with the addition of water or of $CuSO_4$ $5H_2O$ water solution. The dishes were sealed with a quartz lid. For each sample, a dark control sample was prepared, which was protected with aluminum foil against irradiation.

*Irradiation conditions:* Irradiation was conducted in a climatic chamber at 20°C and 60% humidity using UVA radiation (320–400 nm) with maximum emission at 365 nm. The intensity of radiation was determined by means of radiometer, to be each time of 3.89 W/m$^2$. The distance of the samples from radiation source was 13 cm.

*Stationary phase:* TLC was performed on precoated TLC sheets of silica gel 60 with fluorescent indicator on aluminum 10 × 10 cm.

*Mobile phase:* Methylene chloride:methanol:2-propanol:ammonia 25% (4:4:5:2, v/v/v/v).

Twenty microliters of irradiated and control difloxacin solutions were applied using a Linomat V (CAMAG, Switzerland) sample applicator as 8-mm bands. Chromatograms were developed to a distance of 95 mm immediately after its preparation in a glass chromatographic chamber (18 × 9 × 18 cm in size). The plate was dried at room temperature for 30 min.

*Detection:* Registration of spots on chromatograms was achieved by means of a CAMAG TLC Scanner 3 with winCats 1.3.4 software at 294 nm in absorbance mode.

The method was validated for specificity, linearity, precision, recovery, the limit of detection, and limit of determination according to ICH guidelines. The linear regression analysis for the calibration curve presented a good linear correlation over the concentration range 1.18–2.35 µg per band. The limits of detection and quantification were, respectively, 0.01 and 0.03 µg per band.

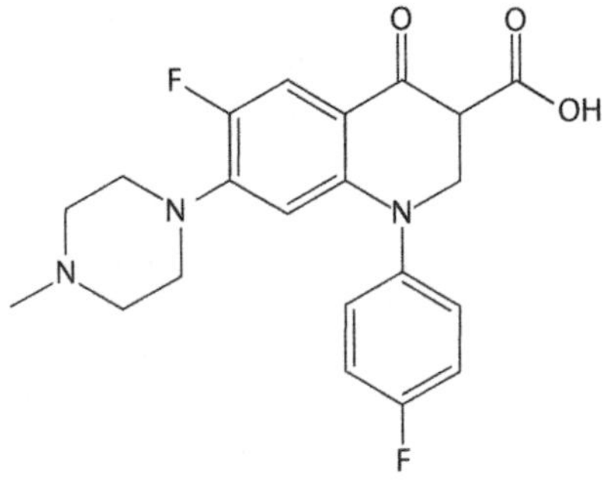

**FIGURE 14.5**　Structure of difloxacin.

Test solutions with and without metal ions were exposed to UVA radiation for 24, 48, 96, 120, and 168 h. Chromatograms recorded for dark control samples showed only single peak of difloxacin ($R_F \approx 0.43$). In chromatograms recorded after UVA exposure, three additional peaks of photodegradation products with retardation factors 0.25, 0.32, and 0.39 were observed beside the main peak of difloxacin. Degradation increased during the prolonged time of irradiation, reaching after 168 h 75.76% for samples without copper ions and 34.84% for samples with copper ions. The photodegradation process of difloxacin followed kinetics of the first order reaction for the substrate.

*Preparation of samples for UPLC–MS/MS analysis:* Extraction of the spots of difloxacin and its photodegradation products was made with TLC–MS interface (CAMAG, Switzerland) into vials with methanol.

*UPLC–MS/MS analysis:* 10 μL of each extract was injected onto a UPLC–ESI–MS/MS system. Chromatographic separations were carried out using the Acquity UPLC BEH (bridged ethyl hybrid) C18 column; 2.1 × 100 mm, and 1.7-μm particle size. The column was eluted under gradient from 95% of eluent A and 5% of eluent B to 100% of eluent B over 10.0 min, at a flow rate of 0.3 mL min⁻¹. Eluent A: water/formic acid (0.1%, v/v); eluent B: acetonitrile/formic acid (0.1%, v/v).

The identification of the products formed during the photodegradation process of difloxacin was performed based on molecular ions [M+H]⁺. The mass spectrum of spot with $R_F$ value 0.39 indicated a molecular ion at $m/z = 386.12$ amu, which can be attributed to the following compound: 6-fluoro-1-(4-fluorophenyl)-4-oxo-7-(piperazin-1-yl)-1,4-dihydroquinoline-3-carboxylic acid. The mass spectrum of spot with $R_F$ value 0.32 indicated a molecular ion at $m/z = 402.12$ amu, which can be attributed to the following compound: 6-fluoro-1-(4-fluorophenyl)-7-(3-hydroxypiperazin-1-yl)-4-oxo-1,4-dihydroquinoline-3-carboxylic acid. In the mass spectrum obtained for spot with $R_F$ value 0.25, two molecular ions at $m/z = 317.25$ amu and $m/z = 360.33$ amu were observed, which can be assigned to the following chemical compounds: 7-(2-aminoethylamino)-6-fluoro-1-(4-fluorophenyl)-4-oxo-1,4-dihydroquinoline-3-carboxylic acid and 7-amino-6-fluoro-1-(4-fluorophenyl)-4-oxo-1,4-dihydroquinoline-3-carboxylic acid.

### 14.6.2 Moxifloxacin

Moxifloxacin, 1-cyclopropyl-7-[(1S,6S)-2,8-diazabicyclo[4.3.0]nonan-8-yl]-6-fluoro-8-methoxy-4-oxoquinoline-3-carboxylic acid, is a fourth-generation synthetic fluoroquinolone antibacterial agent. Photostability of moxifloxacin studies after UVA irradiation in solutions and solid phase, with and without participation of Cu(II), Zn(II), Al(III), and Fe(III), were carried out by TLC-densitometric method and LC–MS/MS method [10] (Figure 14.6).

*Sample preparation for tests in solutions:* 60 μg mL⁻¹ water solution of moxifloxacin hydrochloride were measured off on quartz dishes of 4 cm diameter with the addition of water or of the appropriate water salt solution ($CuSO_4 \cdot 5H_2O$, $ZnSO_4 \cdot 7H_2O$, $Fe_2(SO_4)_3 \cdot H_2O$, $Al_2(SO_4)_3 \cdot 18H_2O$). The dishes were sealed with a quartz lid.

*Sample preparation for tests in solid phase:* Samples were prepared by measuring off 60-μg mL⁻¹ methanol solution of moxifloxacin hydrochloride with the addition of water or the appropriate salt aqueous solution on Petri dishes of 5 cm diameter.

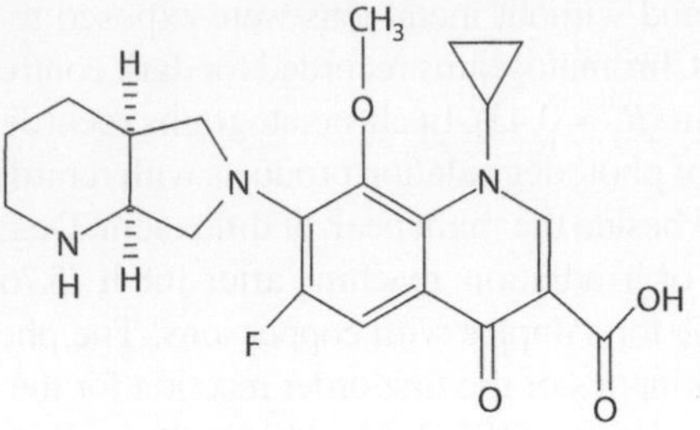

**FIGURE 14.6**   Structure of moxifloxacin.

Samples were mixed and evaporated in a water bath until dry matter was obtained. After irradiation, the content of individual dishes was dissolved in methanol.

For each sample, a dark control sample was prepared, which was protected with aluminum foil against irradiation.

*Irradiation conditions:* The same as previously described for difloxacin. The intensity of radiation was determined by means of a radiometer, to be each time of $5.09 \times 10^{-3}$ J cm$^{-2}$ min$^{-1}$.

*Stationary phase:* TLC was performed on precoated TLC sheets of silica gel 60 with fluorescent indicator on aluminum 13 × 12 cm.

*Mobile phase:* Methylene chloride:ethanol:toluene:*n*-butanol:ammonia 25%:water (6:6:2:3:1.8:0.3 v/v/v/v/v/v).

Twenty microliters of irradiated and control moxifloxacin solutions were applied using a Linomat V (CAMAG, Switzerland) sample applicator as 8-mm bands. Chromatograms were developed to a distance of 115 mm in a glass chromatographic chamber (18 × 9 × 18 cm in size). The plate was dried at room temperature for 30 min.

*Detection:* The identification of spots on chromatograms was achieved by means of a CAMAG TLC Scanner 3 with winCats 1.3.4 software at 294 nm.

The method was validated for specificity, linearity, precision, and recovery, the limit of detection and the limit of determination according to ICH guidelines. The method was characterized by a wide linear range, 0.03–1.50 µg per band. The limit of detection was *LOD* = 12 ng per band.

Exposure of moxifloxacin ($R_F \approx 0.27$) to UVA radiation in the absence of metal ions in solutions resulted in one additional peak ($R_F \approx 0.24$) originating from the degradation product. First changes giving evidence of moxifloxacin degradation were recorded after 24 h (2.48%). Degradation increased together with the time of irradiation, reaching 8.06% after 168 h.

Three products of photodegradation, with $R_F \approx 0.15$ (P-I), $R_F \approx 0.19$ (P-II), and $R_F \approx 0.24$ (P-III), were observed in the presence of Fe(III) ions. In the presence of Al(III), two degradation products P-II and P-III were detected. In the samples containing Cu(II) or Zn(II) ions, only one photoproduct P-III was observed in the chromatograms.

The highest concentration of photodegradation products after 168 h of irradiation was in the presence of Fe(III) (48.62%) and Cu(II) (15.87%), while the lowest was with Zn(II) (10.64%) and Al(III) (8.67%).

UVA irradiation of moxifloxacin without metal ions in solid phase resulted in three additional peaks originating from the products of degradation: P-I, P-II, and P-III. Moxifloxacin degradation was stronger in comparison to the studies in solutions, and after 3 h of irradiation was 29% and after 15 h was 60.66%.

In dark control samples, the presence of one additional peak with $R_F \approx 0.24$, which percentage amount was 2.24%, was observed.

The highest degradation, around 30%, was observed after 15 h exposition to UV radiation in the presence of Al(III). It was lower in the case of Zn(II) (~23%) and Cu(II) (~5%). Moxifloxacin did not decompose in the case of Fe(III).

It was confirmed that the photodegradation process occurs according to the kinetics of first-order reaction.

*LC–MS/MS analysis:* Liquid chromatography was performed using an Agilent 1100 LC system. Chromatographic separation was carried out with an XBridge C18 analytical column (30 mm × 2.1 mm, 3.5 μm).

Two solvent mixtures were used: Solvent A: acetonitrile/formic acid (0.01%) and Solvent B: $H_2O$/formic acid (0.01%). The following gradient was used: 0–5 min, 0%–100% A; 5–7 min, 100% A; 7–8 min, 100%–0% A; 8–20 min, 100% B. The flow rate was set at 600 μL min$^{-1}$. A sample volume of 20 μL was injected into the analytical column for compound analysis.

*Mass spectrometric conditions:* Mass spectrometric analyses were accomplished on Applied Biosystems MDS Sciex (Concord, Ontario, Canada) API 2000 triple quadrupole mass spectrometer equipped with an electrospray ionization (ESI) interface. ESI was performed in the positive ionization mode. Data acquisition and processing were accomplished using the Applied Biosystems Analyst version 1.4.2 software.

Protonated molecular ions of the main peak and peaks of degradation products in mass spectra can be attributed to the following compounds: moxifloxacin ($t_R$ = 2.21 min ) $m/z$ = 402.7 amu; P-II ($t_R$ = 2.11 min) $m/z$ = 416.3 amu 1-cyclopropyl-6-fluoro-8-methoxy-4-oxo-7-(2-oxo-octahydro-6*H*-pyrrolo[3,4-b]pyridine-6-yl)-1,4-dihydroquinoline-3-carboxylic acid; P-III ($t_R$ = 2.88 min) $m/z$ = 452.5 amu 7-[3-hydroxyamino-4-(2-carboxyethyl)pyrrolidin-1-yl]-1-cyclopropyl-6-fluoro-8-methoxy-4-oxo-1,4-dihydroquinoline-3-carboxylic, and P-I ($t_R$ = 2.47 min) $m/z$ = 293.5 amu 1-cyclopropyl-6-fluoro-7-amino-8-methoxy-4-oxo-1,4-dihydroquinoline-3-carboxylic acid. The above-mentioned products are formed as a result of oxidation of (4a*S*,7a*S*)-octahydro-6*H*-pyrrolo[3,4-b]pyridine-6-yl group present in position 7 of 1,4-dihydroquinoline moiety of moxifloxacin.

The structures of the photoproducts were further confirmed by $^1$H NMR analysis.

## 14.6.3 Sparfloxacin

Sparfloxacin, 5-amino-1-cyclopropyl-7-[(3*R*,5*S*)3,5-dimethylpiperazin-1-yl]-6,8-difluoro-4-oxo-quinolone-3-carboxylic acid, belongs to the third-generation class and is used in veterinary medicine. The TLC-densitometric method was developed for the determination of sparfloxacin in the presence of its photodegradation products. Nine products of photodegradation were identified by UPLC–MS/MS [11] (Figure 14.7).

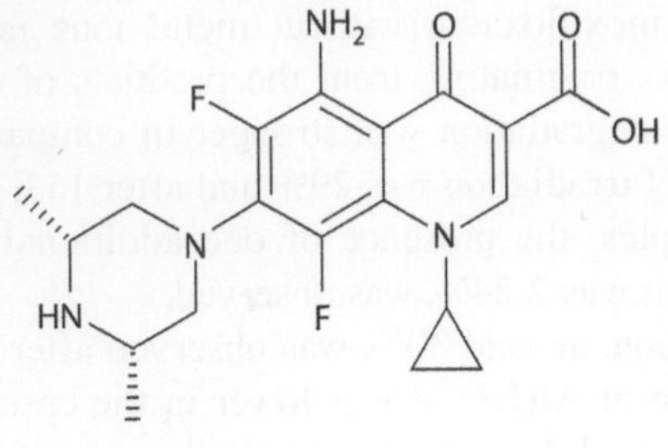

**FIGURE 14.7** Structure of sparfloxacin.

*Sample preparation:* 100.0 µg mL$^{-1}$ aqueous solution of sparfloxacin in methanol were measured off on quartz dishes of 4 cm diameter with addition of water or $ZnSO_4 \cdot 7H_2O$ aqueous solution. The dishes were sealed with a quartz lid. For each sample, a dark control sample was prepared, which was protected with aluminum foil against irradiation.

*Irradiation conditions:* The same as previously described for difloxacin. The intensity of radiation was determined by means of a radiometer, to be of 2.08 W m$^{-2}$ each time.

*Stationary phase:* TLC was performed on precoated TLC sheets of silica gel 60 with fluorescent indicator on aluminum 10 × 10 cm.

*Mobile phase:* Methylene chloride:methanol:2-propanol:ammonia 25% (4:4:5:2, v/v/v/v).

Twenty microliters of irradiated and control sparfloxacin solutions were applied using Linomat V (CAMAG, Switzerland) sample applicator as 8-mm bands. Chromatograms were developed to a distance of 95 mm in a glass chromatographic chamber (18 × 9 × 18 cm in size). The plate was dried at room temperature for 30 min.

*Detection:* Registration of spots on chromatograms was achieved by means of a CAMAG TLC Scanner 3 with winCats 1.3.4 software at 294 nm in absorbance mode.

The obtained values of retardation factors were as follows: for sparfloxacin $R_F \approx 0.42$, and for peaks of degradation products 0.16, 0.32, 0.48, and 0.55. The linear regression analysis for the calibration curve showed a good linear correlation over the concentration range 1.00–3.00 µg per band. The limits of detection and quantification were, respectively, 0.16 and 0.48 µg per band.

Chromatograms recorded for dark control samples showed only one peak with $R_F \approx 0.42$ corresponding to sparfloxacin. The first changes giving evidence of sparfloxacin photodegradation, reaching 9.19%, were recorded after 24 h for samples without metal ions. Whereas for samples containing zinc ions, the degradation process, reaching 1.71%, was observed after 3 h and reached 18.01% after 24 h. Degradation increased during prolonged irradiation, reaching 72.41% after 96 h for samples without metal ions and 80.94% for samples with zinc ions.

The photodegradation process of sparfloxacin followed the kinetics of a first-order reaction for the substrate.

*UPLC–MS/MS analysis:* UPLC–ESI–MS/MS separations were carried out using the Acquity UPLCBEH (bridged ethyl hybrid) C18 column; 2.1 × 100 mm and 1.7 µm particle size. The column was eluted under gradient conditions from 95%

to 0% of eluent A over 10 min, at a flow rate of 0.3 mL min$^{-1}$. Eluent A: 0.1% (v/v) formic acid in water; eluent B: 0.1% (v/v) formic acid in acetonitrile.

The identification of the products formed during the photodegradation process of sparfloxacin was performed based on molecular ions [M+H]$^+$ from UPLC–MS/MS analysis. On the UPLC chromatogram, five well-structured peaks were seen, having different intensities, whose percentage of the area was greater than 1%. In the case of TLC analysis, five different peaks with low intensity were identified. MS/MS analysis enables stating that for the particular peaks having $t_R$ values in UPLC and $R_F$ in TLC, the following molecular ions could be assigned: $m/z$ = 390.17 amu ($t_R$ = 1.99 min; $R_F$ = 0.16), 375.17 amu ($t_R$ = 3.12 min; $R_F$ = 0.32), 393.17 amu ($t_R$ = 3.20 min; $R_F$ = 0.42), 423.17 amu ($t_R$ = 3.38 min; $R_F$ = 0.48), 409.17 amu ($t_R$ = 3.42 min; $R_F$ = 0.55). Moreover, in the case of UPLC–MS/MS analysis, some signals with lower intensity were observed, which could be attributed to five additional photodegradation products with the following molecular ions ($m/z$): 404.14 amu ($t_R$ = 2.15 min), 402.13 amu ($t_R$ = 2.19 min), 388.15 amu ($t_R$ = 2.30 min), 389.19 amu ($t_R$ = 2.80 min), and 407.17 amu ($t_R$ = 3.08 min). Based on the UPLC–MS/MS investigation results, it is probable that there can be nine photodegradation products.

The probable path of the photodegradation process of sparfloxacin is presented in Figure 14.8.

## 14.7 FLUOXETINE

Fluoxetine, (RS)-N-methyl-3-phenyl-3-[4-(trifluoromethyl)phenoxy]propan-1-amine, is the first drug representing a group of selective serotonin reuptake inhibitors (SSRI) used in depression therapy. The activity mechanism of fluoxetine involves inhibition of serotonin reuptake (5-HT). Fluoxetine is used in therapy in the form of hydrochloride as a racemic mixture. Trifluoromethyl substituent is responsible for lipophilicity of the compound and its localization in *para* position of aromatic arrangement is responsible for the selectivity of serotonin uptake (Figure 14.9).

TLC-densitometric method was developed to monitor the effect of UVA radiation on fluoxetine stability in solid phase with and without the presence of selected metal ions [12].

*Sample preparation:* 2 mg mL$^{-1}$ fluoxetine solution in methanol with the addition of methanol or suitable metal salt solution (Al(III), Zn(II), Fe(III), Fe(II), Mn(II), and Ni(II) ions) were transferred on Petri dishes that are 5 cm in diameter. The samples were evaporated to the dry residue at a temperature of 40°C on a heating plate. During evaporation, the samples were protected against the light access. The irradiation was conducted in the presence of dark control samples. After the end of irradiation, the samples were dissolved in methanol.

*Irradiation conditions:* The same as previously described for difloxacin. The doses of UVA radiation were measured using a radiometer, obtaining the dose of 5.09 × 10$^{-3}$ J cm$^{-2}$ min$^{-1}$ each time.

*Stationary phase:* TLC was performed on 20 × 10 cm TLC F$_{254}$ silica gel plates.

*Mobile phase:* Chloroform:methanol:ammonia 25% (45:4.5:0.5 v/v/v).

Ten microliters of the studied solutions and reference substance were spotted in a form of 1-cm bands on TLC plates using Linomat 5 applicator; CAMAG (Muttenz,

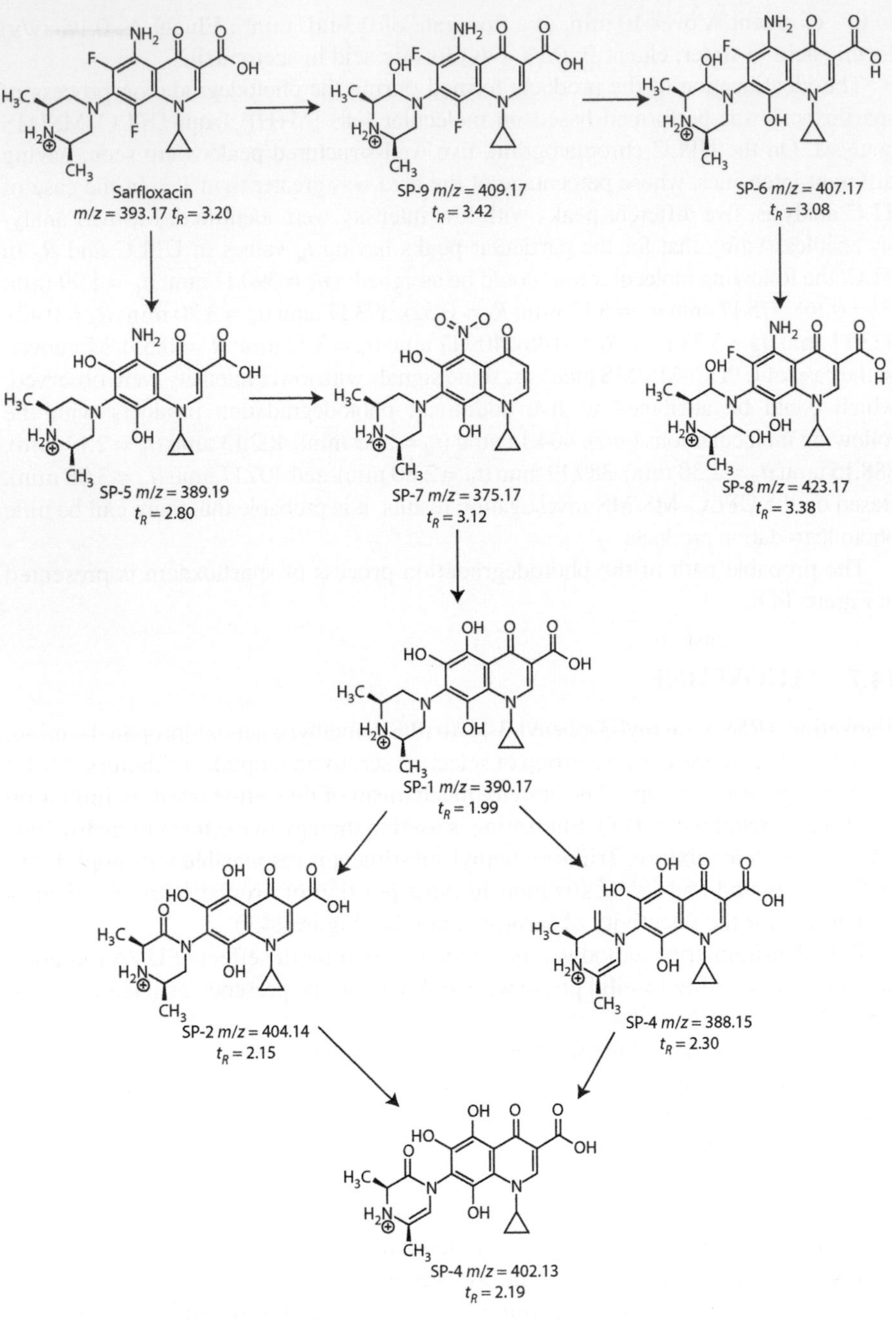

**FIGURE 14.8**   The path of the photodegradation process of sparfloxacin.

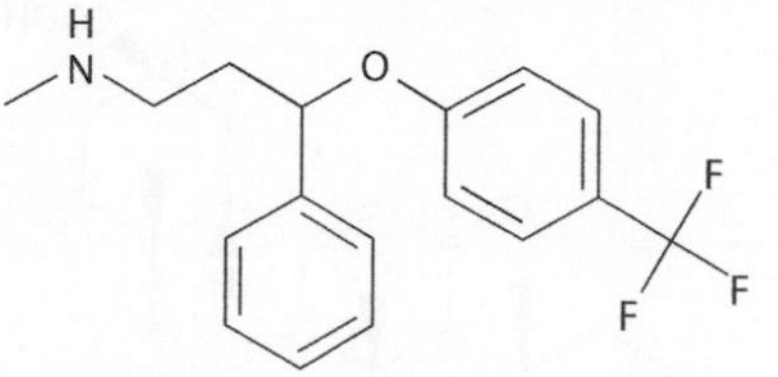

**FIGURE 14.9** Structure of fluoxetine.

Switzerland). The chromatograms were developed in the chromatographic chamber ($23 \times 12 \times 8$ cm in size) to a distance of 9.5 cm.

*Detection:* Densitometric registration was performed (TLC–Scanner-3 densitometer with WinCats Version 1.3.4 software, CAMAG, Muttenz, Switzerland), selecting the wavelength of $\lambda = 260$ nm corresponding to the maximum of fluoxetine absorption.

The method was validated and high sensitivity was shown ($LOD = 0.96$ μg per band, $LOQ = 2.91$ μg per band). Linearity range was 0.0505 mg mL$^{-1}$ to 2.0200 mg mL$^{-1}$.

In the presence of Al(III), Fe(II), and Fe(III) ions, one degradation product of $R_F \sim 0.24$ (P-A) is formed, while in the presence of Cu(II) ions, except the P-A product, an additional product of $R_F \sim 0.55$ is observed (P-B).

The kinetic studies demonstrated that fluoxetine photodegradation is the fastest in the presence of Cu(II) ions, decreases in the presence of Fe(III) and Fe(II) ions, and is the lowest in the presence of Al(III) ions. Under conditions established without the presence of metal ions, fluoxetine maintains photostability.

The changes in fluoxetine concentration during irradiation in time are consistent with kinetics for the first-order reaction.

*ESI–LC/MS analysis:* Triple quadrupole mass analyzer API 2000 was used. The chromatographic separation was performed using Xbridge C18 MS column, a mobile phase composed of water, acetonitrile, and 0.01% formic acid in gradient conditions. The flow rate was 600 μL min$^{-1}$. Twenty microliters of the studied solutions were injected on the column.

The analysis of mass spectra and literature data allows assigning the structure of 3-phenyl-3-hydroxypropylamine ($m/z = 152$) to degradation product A, and the structure of 4-trifluoromethylphenol ($m/z = 164$) to degradation product B. The signal on a mass spectra of $m/z = 310$ was identified as fluoxetine, and an additional signal of $m/z = 351$ as an adduct of fluoxetine and acetonitrile present in the mobile phase of chromatographic separation.

## 14.8 GLYCYRRHETIC ACID

Glycyrrhetic acid, (2S,4aS,6aS,6bR,8aR,10S,12aS,12bR,14bR)-10-hydroxy-2,4a,6a, 6b,9,9,12a-heptamethyl-13-oxo-1,2,3,4,4a,5,6,6a,6b,7,8,8a,9,10,11,12,12a,12b,-13,14b-icosahydropicene-2-carboxylic acid, is a pentacyclic triterpenoid derivative of the β-amyrin type obtained from the hydrolysis of glycyrrhizic acid, which was obtained from the herb licorice. It is used in flavoring and it masks the bitter taste of drugs such as aloe and quinine. It is effective in the treatment of peptic ulcer and has expectorant (antitussive) properties. It has some additional pharmacological

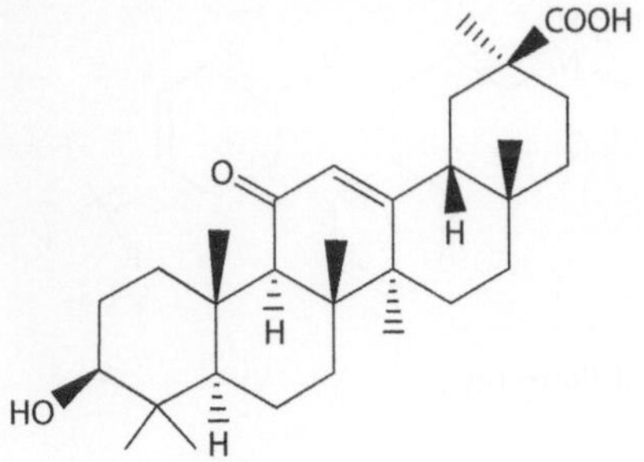

**FIGURE 14.10**    Structure of glycyrrhetic acid.

properties including antiviral, antifungal, antiprotozoal, and antibacterial activities. The TLC-densitometric method was developed for the determination of glycyrrhetic acid in the presence of its photodegradation products [13] (Figure 14.10).

*Sample preparation:* Stock solution containing 100 mg of glycyrrhetic acid in 100 mL of methanol was prepared. The stock solution of glycyrrhetic acid was irradiated by exposing to direct sunlight for 3 days from 8–18 h at 30°C.

*Stationary phase:* TLC silica gel 60 $F_{254}$ plates.

*Mobile phase:* Chloroform:methanol:formic acid (9:1:0.1 v/v/v).

1 µL (1000 ng·spot$^{-1}$) of resultant solutions after irradiation and 2 µL (1000 ng·spot$^{-1}$) of solution of glycyrrhetic acid were applied on a TLC sheet. The chromatogram was developed to a distance of 80 mm. The chromatographic chamber saturation time for mobile phase was 10 min.

*Detection:* Densitometry was carried out with CAMAG Reprostar III and scanning was performed on CAMAG TLC Scanner III at 254 nm.

The obtained values of retardation factors were as follows: $R_F \approx 0.42$ for glycyrrhetic acid and for peaks of degradation products: 0.35, 0.38, and 0.49. The calibration curve was established in the range of 200–1200 µg·spot$^{-1}$, the limit of detection and quantitation were, respectively, 1.56 and 4.74 ng·spot$^{-1}$.

*Preparation of samples for ESI–QqTOF–MS/MS analysis:* Photodegraded products were dissolved in methanol and working dilution was prepared in 50:50 acetonitrile/water, containing 0.1% tetrafluoro-acetic acid.

*ESI–QqTOF–MS/MS analysis:* Analysis was performed by ESI and collision-induced dissociation positive ion mode, on QqTOF–MS/MS instrument coupled with 1100 HPLC system (Agilent).

ESI–QqTOF–MS/MS spectrum of photodegradation products of glycyrrhetic acid showed peaks [M+H]$^+$ at $m/z = 485.3263$, $487.3450$, and $457.3636$ amu, corresponding to the molecular formula: $C_{30}H_{45}O_5$, $C_{30}H_{47}O_5$, and $C_{30}H_{49}O_3$.

## 14.9   ITRACONAZOLE

Itraconazole, (2*R*,4*S*)-*rel*-1-(butan-2-yl)-4-{4-[4-(4-{[(2*R*,4*S*)-2-(2,4-dichlorophenyl)-2-(1*H*-1,2,4-triazol-1-ylmethyl)-1,3-dioxolan-4-yl]methoxy}phenyl)piperazin-1-yl] phenyl}-4,5-dihydro-1*H*-1,2,4-triazol-5-one, is a synthetic tiazole antifungal. The

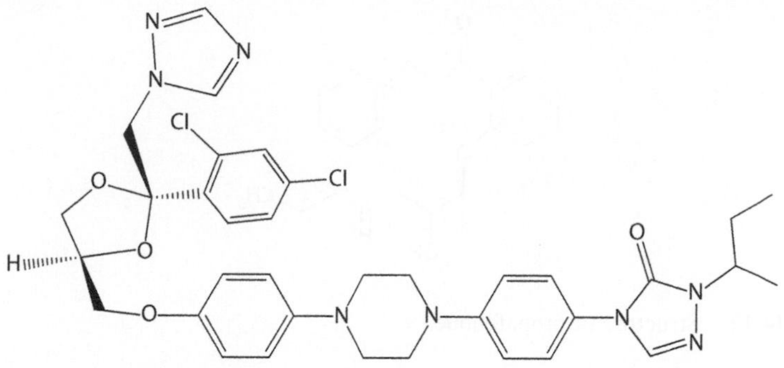

**FIGURE 14.11** Structure of itraconazole.

HPTLC-densitometeric method was developed for the determination of itraconazole in the presence of its photodegradation products [14] (Figure 14.11).

*Sample preparation:* To 5 mL of methanolic stock solution of itraconazole (100 µg mL$^{-1}$), 5 mL of methanol was added. The solution was exposed to direct sunlight for 3 days and UV irradiation at 254 nm for 8 h in a UV chamber.

*Stationary phase:* HPTLC silica gel 60 F$_{254}$ plates.

*Mobile phase:* Toluene:ethyl acetate:ammonia (1:5:0.1 v/v/v).

Aliquots of 2 µL of solution were applied to the chromatographic plates. The plates were developed by ascending migration over 8 cm. The chromatographic chamber was saturated with the mobile phase for 30 min.

*Detection:* Chromatograms were scanned at 254 nm (CAMAG TLC Scanner III).

The chromatogram of the sample exposed to photochemical degradation showed only one peak of itraconazole at $R_F \approx 0.60$. The calibration curve was established in the range of 50–2000 ng spot$^{-1}$, the limit of detection and quantitation were, respectively, 14.29 and 43.14 ng spot$^{-1}$.

Mass spectrum of the sample of itraconazole after irradiation showed the molecular ion peak ($m/z = 705.22$ amu) corresponding to the molecular weight of itraconazole.

## 14.10 PROPAFENONE HYDROCHLORIDE

Propafenone, 1-{2-[2-hydroxy-3-(propylamino)propoxy]phenyl}-3-phenylpropan-1-one, is a commonly used sodium and potassium channel blocker for the treatment of ventricular tachycardia and atrial fibrillation [15]. Propafenone hydrochloride is a class IC antiarrhytmic agent that shows structural similarity and activity related to β-adrenolytic agents. The drug is efficacious in suppressing supraventricular and ventricular rhythm disorders [15] (Figure 14.12).

The TLC method was developed for the determination of the photodegradated propafenone hydrochloride [15].

*Sample preparation:* The drug solution was prepared by adding 2.5 mL of the redistilled water to 10 mL of the methanolic solution of propafenone (1 mg mL$^{-1}$). The drug samples placed in a quartz cell were exposed to light at $\lambda = 254$ nm.

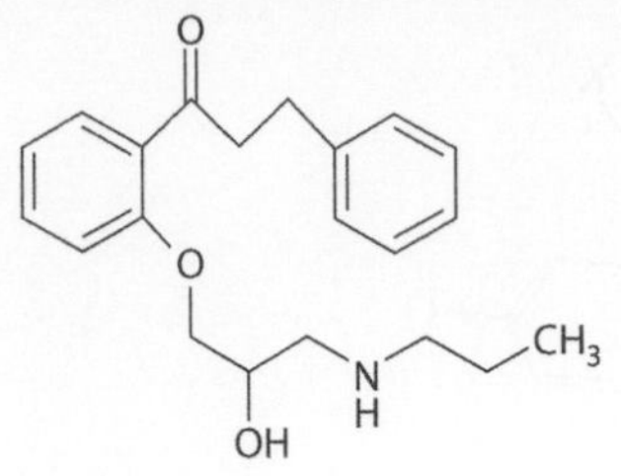

**FIGURE 14.12**   Structure of propafenone.

*Irradiation conditions:* The photolytic experiments were carried out in a UV chamber. Irradiation intensity was approximately 7.145 W/m$^2$.

*Stationary phase:* TLC was performed on $10 \times 20$ cm glass-backed HPTLC silica gel 60 with fluorescent indicator plates.

*Mobile phase:* Chloroform:methanol:acetic acid 99.5% (7.9:2.0:0.1, v/v/v).

The samples were applied in the form of spots using Desaga AS30 applicator (Heidelberg, Germany) equipped with a 10-mL Hamilton syringe (Bonaduz, Switzerland). The plates were developed at room temperature (22°C ± 2) to a distance of 90 mm in an unsaturated horizontal DS-type L chambers and dried in the air.

*Detection:* Densitometric scanning was performed on a Desaga CD60 in the reflectance/absorbance mode and the wavelength $\lambda = 316$ nm was found to be optimal for detection.

Good separation of propafenone hydrochloride from the degradation products was obtained and the received values of retardation factors were as follows: for propafenone hydrochloride $R_F \approx 0.64$, and for the degradation products 0.43, 0.82, and 0.88. The elaborated method was validated using ICH guidelines. The linear calibration function was obtained with respect to the peak area in the concentration range of 0.1–3.2 μg spot$^{-1}$, respectively. The limits of detection and quantification were, respectively, 0.02 and 0.08 μg per band.

The degradation of propafenone hydrochloride, reaching 38.5%, was observed because of exposure to UV irradiation.

*Preparation of samples for GC–MS analysis:* The solutions obtained in the forced degradation experiments were evaporated to dryness under a nitrogen stream. Then, the residues were reconstituted in hexane, and 2 μL of each sample were injected into GC–MS system.

*GC–MS analysis:* GC–MS analysis was performed using 7890A GC system coupled with 7000 triple quad mass spectrometer operated in an electron impact ionization mode. Separation was carried out using HP-5MS UI [(5% phenyl)-methylpolisiloxane, 30 m × 0.25 mm id., 0.25 μm film thickness] with helium of high purity as carrier gas (constant flow 1.5 mL min$^{-1}$). The system was operated by Agilent MassHunter B.05 software.

The identified photolytic degradation products of propafenone hydrochloride are benzoic acid/methyl ester ($m/z = 136.0$ amu), 2H-1-benzopyran/3,4-dihydro-2-phenyl ($m/z = 210.1$ amu), and 1-(2-hydroxyphenyl)-3-phenyl-1-propanone ($m/z = 226.1$ amu).

## 14.11 TIANEPTINE

Tianeptine, (*RS*)-7-(3-chloro-6-methyl-6,11-dihydrodibenzo[*c,f*][1,2]thiazepin-11-yl-amino)heptanoic acid *S,S*-dioxide, is an antidepressant effective against anxiety accompanying mood disorders. The drug is used primarily in the treatment of major depressive disorder, although it may also be used to treat asthma or irritable bowel syndrome. The TLC method was used to separate the photodegradation products of tianeptine [16] (Figure 14.13).

*Sample preparation:* A sample film of tianeptine sodium powder of approximately 0.1 mm thickness in a flat glass dish was exposed to UV light (254 nm) for a maximum of 24 h.

*Irradiation conditions:* Irradiation was conducted in a laminar flow cabinet, designed as germicidal UV light source. The distance between lamp and sample was 1 cm.

*Stationary phase:* TLC silica gel 60 $F_{254}$ plates.

*Mobile phase:* Ethyl acetate:*n*-hexane:glacial acetic acid:methanol (10:14:0.2:1 v/v/v/v).

Portions of the diluted and concentrated UV-degraded methanolic extract of tianeptine were evaporated to dryness, reconstituted in a minimal methanol, and spotted onto TLC plates. The chromatograms were developed to a distance of 15 cm. The spots were observed under UV light at $\lambda = 254$ and 366 nm and separated bands were scratched and extracted in methanol.

*Preparation of sample for GC–MS:* 1 mL methanolic solution of tianeptine (50 ng µL) was dried under nitrogen gas and reconstituted in dichloromethane. 50 µL of *N*-methyl-*N*-trimethylsilyltrifluoroacetamide and 50 µL of $CH_2Cl_2$ were added. The sample mixture was heated at 60°C for 5 min and cooled.

*GC–MS analysis:* 1 µL of solution was injected onto a GC–MS system. The software controller was TurboMass 4.5.0.007. An Elite 5MS GC capillary column (30 × 0.25 mm × 0.5 µm) was used. The carrier gas was helium at a flow rate of 2 mL min$^{-1}$. The column temperature program was as follows: 50°C for 5 min, increased to 220°C. MS scan was from 50 to 650 *m/z*.

Taneptine was detected only after silyliaton with *N*-methyl-*N*-trimethylsilyltri-fluoroacetamide in $CH_2Cl_2$. The most prominent peaks were recorded at *m/z* = 217 amu, which was assigned to the silylated amino acid chain [$NH_2$–$(CH_2)_6$–CO–O–Si(Me)$_3$], and *m/z* = 117 amu, which was assigned to the CO–O–Si(Me)$_3$ fragment.

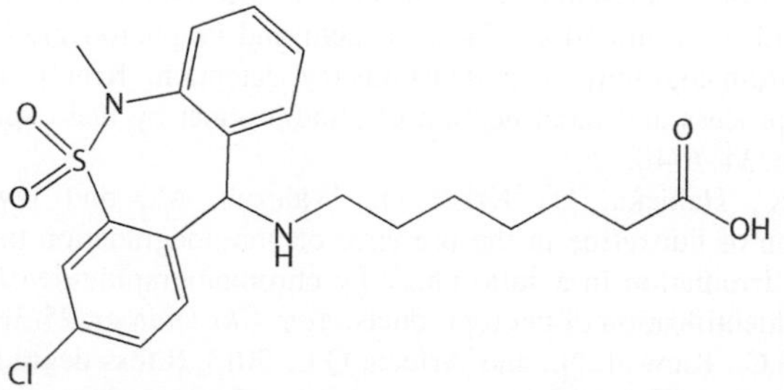

**FIGURE 14.13**  Structure of tianeptine.

## ACKNOWLEDGMENTS

The authors would like to dedicate this chapter to the memory of Professor Jan Krzek, our adviser, mentor, and head of Department of Inorganic and Analytical Chemistry.

## REFERENCES

1. Kleinman, M.H., Smith, M.D., Kurali, E., Kleinpeter, S., Jiang, K., Zhang, Y., Kennedy-Gabb, S.A., Lynch, A.M., and Geddes, Ch.D. 2010. An evaluation of chemical photoreactivity and the relationship to phototoxicity, *Regul. Toxicol. Pharmacol.*, 58: 224–232.
2. Kleinman, M.H. 2013. Using photoreactivity studies to provide insight into the photosafety of pharmaceutical therapies, *Trends Anal. Chem.*, 49: 100–107.
3. ICH Q1A(R2) Guideline, Stability testing of new drug substances and products, Comments for its application, February 6, 2003.
4. Blessy, M., Patel, R.D., Prajapati, P.N., and Agrawal, Y.K. 2014. Development of forced degradation and stability indicating studies of drugs—A review, *J. Pharm. Anal.*, 4(3): 159–165.
5. Khedr, A. and Sheha, M. 2008. Stress degradation studies on betahistine and development of a validated stability-indicating assay method, *J. Chromatogr. B*, 869: 111–117.
6. Miolo, G., Gallocchio, F., Levorato, L., and Dalzoppo, D. Beyersbergen van Henegouwen, G.M.J., Caffieri, S. 2009. UVB photolysis of betamethasone and its esters: Characterization of photoproducts in solution, in pig skin and in drug formulations, *J. Photochem. Photobiol. B*, 96: 75–81.
7. Vogna, D., Marotta, R., Andreozzi, R., Napolitano, A., and D'Ischia, M. 2004. Kinetic and chemical assessment of the UV/$H_2O_2$ treatment of antiepileptic drug carbamazepine, *Chemosphere*, 54: 49–505.
8. Breier, A.R., Nudelman, N.S., Steppe, M., and Schapoval, E.E.S. 2008. Isolation and structure elucidation of photodegradation products of fexofenadine, *J. Pharm. Biomed. Anal.*, 46: 250–257.
9. Hubicka, U., Żuromska-Witek, B., Żmudzki, P., Matwiej, B., and Krzek, J. 2013. Thin-layer chromatography with densitometry for the determination of difloxacin and its photodegradation products. Kinetic evaluation of the degradation process and identification of photoproducts by mass spectrometry, *J. Liq. Chromatogr. Relat. Technol.*, 36: 2431–2445.
10. Hubicka, U., Krzek, J., Żuromska, B., Walczak, M., Żylewski, M., and Pawłowski, D. 2012. Determination of photostability and photodegradation products of moxifloxacin in the presence of metal ions in solutions and solid phase. Kinetics and identification of photoproducts, *Photochem. Photobiol. Sci.*, 11: 351–357.
11. Hubicka, U., Żuromska-Witek, B., Żmudzki, P., Maślanka, A., Kwapińska, N., and Krzek, J. 2013. Determination of sparfloxacin and its photodegradation products by thin-layer chromatography with densitometry detection. Kinetic evaluation of the degradation process and identification of photoproduct by mass spectrometry, *Anal. Methods*, 5: 6734–6740.
12. Maślanka, A., Hubicka, U., Krzek, J., Walczak, M., and Izworski, G. 2013. Determination of fluoxetine in the presence of photodegradation products appearing during UVA irradiation in a solid phase by chromatographic-densitometric method, kinetics and identification of photoproducts, *Acta Chromatogr.* 25(3): 465–481.
13. Musharraf, S.G., Kanwal, N., and Arfeen, Q.U. 2013. Stress degradation studies and stability-indicating TLC-densitometric method of glycyrrhetic acid, *Chem. Cent. J.*, 7: 9.

14. Mirza, M.A., Talegaonkar, S., and Iqbal, Z. 2012. Quantitative analysis of itraconazole in bulk, marketed, and nano formulation by validated, stability indicating high performance thin layer chromatography, *J. Liq. Chromatogr. Relat. Technol.*, 35: 1459–1480.
15. Pietraś, R., Kowalczuk, D., Rutkowska, E., Komsta, Ł., and Gumieniczek, A. 2014. Validated stability-indicating HPTLC method for the determination of propafenone hydrochloride in tablets and the GC–MS identification of its degradation products, *J. Liq. Chromatogr. Relat. Technol.*, 37: 2942–2955.
16. Khedr, A. 2007. High-performance liquid chromatographic stability indicating assay method of tianeptine sodium with simultaneous fluorescence and UV detection, *J. Chromatogr. Sci.*, 45: 305–310.

# 15 Combination of Thin-Layer Chromatography with Laser Desorption Ionization and Electrospray Ionization–Mass Spectrometric Techniques for Screening of Organic Compounds

*Suresh Kumar Kailasa, Jigneshkumar V. Rohit, and Hui-Fen Wu*

## CONTENTS

## 15.1    INTRODUCTION

Among various chromatographic techniques, thin-layer chromatography (TLC) is an important planar chromatographic technique, and has proved to be a simple, rapid, and inexpensive chromatographic technique for the separation and visual semiquantitative assessment of a wide variety of chemical species. Moreover, it has come to rival liquid chromatography (LC) and gas chromatography (GC) in its ability to resolve complex mixtures and to provide quantitative results with minimal volume of samples and solvents [1]. The consistency of terminology should be reviewed owing to new developments regarding mass spectrometry (MS) as LC–MS = HPLC–MS + TLC/HPTLC–MS. Generally, LC comprises all chromatographic techniques that employ a liquid mobile phase. Therefore, planar chromatography is a subcategory of LC. LC–MS also includes coupling of high-performance thin-layer chromatography (HPTLC) with MS.

Recently, much efforts have been invested in the development of various versions of TLC (HPTLC, ultrathin-layer chromatography [UTLC], two-dimensional [2D] and three-dimensional [3D]) coupled with various detectors, including UV, fluorescence, infrared, and MS for the separation and identification of a wide variety of molecules in complex samples. In this connection, several reviews [2–8], book chapters, and edited books [9–12] have proposed new terminology related to LC–MS. As mentioned previously, a comprehensive review of TLC applications to specific compound classes is not possible in this chapter because of space restrictions. However, information on TLC/HPTLC/UTLC theory and their combination with several analytical techniques and applications are available in the above-mentioned reviews and books [2–12]. Because of the large number of published papers in this area, we chose to focus on fundamental and mechanistic aspects in conjunction with innovative applications of TLC/HPTLC/UTLC combining with laser desorption ionization (LDI), electrospray ionization (ESI), and ambient ionization/MS techniques rather than on an exhaustive coverage of all applications described in the current literature. In this chapter, we have highlighted some representative works in the area of TLC combined with LDI and ESI–MS techniques for the separation and identification of various molecules (lipids, gangliosides, dyes, drugs, and organic reaction products). Therefore, only a small part of the published papers were selected in this chapter, mainly based on relevance, innovation, and practical significance of TLC with LDI/ and ESI/MS for ultrasensitive assays.

Based on the flow of solvent, TLC can be divided into the capillary-flow (i.e., classical) and forced flow (overpressure layer chromatography [OPLC]) techniques according to the flow type of the mobile phase [13]. Thus, the separation efficiency of capillary-flow TLC is limited to the velocity at which the capillary forces drive the mobile phase through the stationary phase [14]. It was observed that the variable and nonoptimal mobile-phase velocity results in limited separation efficiency. In forced-flow technique, the velocity of the mobile phase is adjusted (i.e., increased) to give a constant and optimal velocity. This is done by applying external force, such as pressure, centrifugal force, or an electric field [15,16]. The flow velocity of the mobile phase is controlled in OPLC and new developments in TLC include high-pressure versions similar to HPLC, temperature-programmed OPLC, online one-dimensional OPLC, and two-dimensional OPLC.

Preparative-layer chromatography (PLC) can be used for the fractionation and/or isolation of compounds in amounts up to 1000 mg. According to the elution mode, it can be classified into classical PLC (i.e., conventional capillary-flow) and forced-flow PLC (e.g., OPLC and RPC). The main differences between analytical TLC/ HPTLC plates and preparative PLC plates are the layer thickness, mean particle size, and particle size distribution. In TLC and HPTLC, layer thickness is typically 0.2 or 0.25 mm. Mean particle size is about 12 μm in TLC and 5 μm in HPTLC, and the particle size distribution is up to 20 μm for TLC and about 10 μm for HPTLC. Consequently, HPTLC offers better resolution and lower limit of detections (LODs) than conventional TLC [17].

## 15.2 TWO-, THREE-, AND FOUR-DIMENSIONAL THIN-LAYER CHROMATOGRAPHY AND ULTRATHIN-LAYER CHROMATOGRAPHY SYSTEMS

Even though TLC has proved to be a simple tool for separation with low volumes of samples, unfortunately it has lower separation efficiency than, for example, HPLC. However, the separation efficiency of TLC can be improved by using 2D and 3D elution. In a 2D TLC system, the first-dimension elution (1D) is performed normally and, after drying, the plate is turned 90° and eluted again in the second dimension. Separation efficiency can be increased by applying different solvent compositions in the two dimensions. Three-dimensional TLC is a variation of planar chromatography, in which components of the mixture under investigation migrate under the action of the mobile phase flow in one direction, then in another direction at an angle to the first direction, and then in a third direction at an angle to the second direction; in this case, all elution processes are carried out using different selective eluents with drying of the plate between the elution processes [18]. It can be noticed that the smaller plates should be used in 2D TLC because the use of smaller plates decreases the time of analysis so that the method becomes more rapid. Similarly, in 3D TLC different sizes (5 × 5 cm, 7 × 7 cm, and standard 10 × 10 cm) of plates were used. It can be noticed that the angles of 90° are commonly used in both techniques.

Four-dimensional TLC is a new effective version of multidimensional planar chromatography [19]. In this method, the first separation of the mixture is carried out on a plate, and then, three groups of compounds (three fractions) with similar sorption characteristics are isolated. After elution of three group compounds, each isolated fraction is developed again along the direction perpendicular to the first development using the liquid mobile phase most suitable for compounds of this group (fraction). Methods for simultaneous separation of three samples on one plate using three different mobile phases do not exist and will hardly be developed. Therefore, for convenient implementation of this method, after the first separation, the plate with an aluminum foil substrate is cut into relatively narrow rectangular "daughter" plates in such a way that each one contains a fraction of compounds isolated after the first chromatographic separation [20].

The UTLC was developed by Hauck's group in 2001 to further improve sensitivity and reduce analysis time and amount of consumables required for TLC [21]. It significantly improved the analysis time and sensitivity over traditional TLC devices. UTLC devices have been reported to have lower LOD and faster analysis times but lower resolution when compared to HPTLC [22]. UTLC stationary phases are typically comprised of thinner monolithic silica gels with finer pore sizes than TLC or HPTLC media. As a result, UTLC media permit faster separations over shorter distances with better LOD.

## 15.3 APPLICATIONS OF THIN-LAYER CHROMATOGRAPHY COMBINED WITH MATRIX-ASSISTED LASER DESORPTION IONIZATION–MASS SPECTROMETRY

In recent years, TLC was successfully combined with different ionization techniques, matrix-assisted laser desorption/ionization (MALDI), ESI, atmospheric pressure chemical ionization (APCI), desorption electrospray ionization (DESI), electrospray-assisted laser desorption ionization (ELDI), and LDI for identification and quantification of organic and biomolecules. In this section, the interfacing of TLC techniques with MALDI–ESI/MS, DESI–MS, ELSI–MS, and LDI–MS will be described, performance will be discussed, and selected applications in the separation and identification of lipids, gangliosides, dyes, drugs, and medicinal compounds will be presented.

### 15.3.1 ANALYSIS OF LIPIDS

Lipids are a diverse and ubiquitous group of compounds that have many key biological functions in cell membranes and in signaling pathways [23]. A comprehensive analysis of lipid molecules, "lipidomics," in the context of genomics and proteomics is crucial to understanding cellular physiology and pathology; consequently, lipid biology has become a major research target of the postgenomic revolution and systems biology. Due to their diversity, separation and identification of lipids is a challenging task in analytical chemistry. Recently, the research field of lipidomics has been driven by rapid advances in a number of analytical technologies, in particular MS, nuclear magnetic resonance (NMR), and other spectroscopic methods [24,25]. Among these, TLC combined with MS techniques can provide a huge amount of information on lipidomics.

TLC is directly coupled with MALDI–MS for separation and identification of phospholipids from egg yolk [26]. Authors identified six phospholipids such as phosphatidylcholine (PC, 73%), lysophosphatidylcholine (LPC, 5.8%), sphingomyelin (SM, 2.5%), phosphatidylethanolamine (PE, 15.0%), lysophosphatidylethanolamine (LPE, 2.1%), and phosphatidylinositol (PI, 0.6%) in hen egg yolk by MALDI–MS using 2,5-dihydroxy benzoic acid (DHB). It was observed that PC (16:0/18:1) is the most abundant species among all the phospholipids and it gives two peaks at $m/z$ 760.6 and 782.6, which can be assigned to the $H^+$ and the $Na^+$ adducts, respectively. Stubiger and coworkers described an improved analytical strategy for the analysis of complex lipid mixtures using HPTLC coupled with MALDI–MS using trihydroxy acetophenone (THAP) as a matrix [27]. This method was effectively applied to separate and to detect various neutral (e.g., triacylglycerols) and polar (e.g., glycerophospholipids and sphingolipids) lipid classes derived from crude lipid extracts of, for example, human plasma as well as soybean lecithin. This technique provides a simple platform for the identification of neutral and polar lipids and their structures were confirmed by MALDI post-source decay (PSD). Recording of diagnostic losses and specific product ions was exploited for the determination of the headgroup composition (lipid class specific) as well as the identification of the constituent fatty acid (FA) residues of individual PL species [28]. Wegener's team developed a TLC–MALDI–MS method for the confirmation of whether spermatheca- and *in vitro*-stored honey bee sperm are indeed resistant to lipid peroxidation, and whether the nature of sperm lipids could explain this resistance [29]. They confirmed that drone sperm lipids are dominated by two glycerophosphocholine (GPC) species, although there were small amounts of SM and glycerophosphoethanolamines (GPE). It was also confirmed the alkyl/acyl and alkenyl/acyl compounds of GPC, and alkyl/acyl as well as diacyl compounds of GPE were detected containing oleyl, oleoyl, palmityl, and palmitoyl as the most abundant residues. It can be observed that several mass peaks were generated at their $m/z$ values and assigned as LPC, PI, PC, PE, phosphatidylglycerol (PG), phosphatidylserine (PS), and SM. Authors concluded that bee sperm lipids are mainly composed of 1-*O*-oleyl-2-oleoyl-*sn*-glycero-3-phosphocholine (GPC 18:1alkyl/18:1acyl) with a smaller contribution of GPC 18:0alkenyl/18:1acyl as the most prominent PL. It was also observed that all PL contain only moderately unsaturated (one double bond) residues, which are, therefore, only a little sensitive to oxidation.

Although a couple of different lipid extracts are effectively extracted using various extraction procedures, the extract from the avocado is unique because it yields nearly exclusively triacylglycerols (TAG), whereas the PLs content is extremely low. Eibisch and coworkers extracted lipid contents from hen egg yolk and purified PC and PE fractions [30]. Using this method, 1-palmitoyl-2-oleoyl-*sn*-phosphatidylcholine (POPC) and 1-palmitoyl-2-oleoyl-*sn*-phosphatidylethanolamine (POPE) were effectively separated and identified with good sensitivity. It was observed that the POPC ($m/z = 760.6$ and 782.6) is the most abundant species, which agrees favorably with the spectrum of isolated PC fraction. The reason for the much higher intensity of the Na$^+$ adduct ($m/z = 782.6$) in comparison to the H$^+$ adduct ($m/z = 760.6$) subsequent to the TLC separation is the use of physiological saline (NaCl—154 mM) to reelute the lipids from the silica gel. It was observed that PE moiety is easily appeared on the TLC plate but is exclusively detectable subsequent to separation from the PC that was clearly identified by MALDI mass spectra of the total extract. Therisod and coworkers developed a rapid method for the microscale extraction of lipopolysaccharides (endotoxins, LPSs) from rough-type gram-negative bacteria using TLC–MALDI–MS [31]. Phenol-killed cells from *B. pertussis* 1414 and *B. parapertussis* ATCC 15311 were separated and identified by TLC–MALDI–MS. The mass spectra of LPSs were greatly improved using malonic, oxalic, tartaric, and citric acid solutions (0.1 M) of the matrix in a 1:1 ratio with the LPS acid solutions. It can be noticed that three zones of signals corresponded to LPS molecular ion, core fragment ions, and lipid A fragment ions. In the lower mass range, the two major peaks at $m/z$ 1333 and 1559 corresponded to the tetra- and penta-acylated ion species of lipid A.

The middle range corresponded to the heterogeneous core moiety. The peak at $m/z$ 2293 corresponded to the anhydrododecasaccharide ion followed by its phosphoryl-, pyrophosphoryl-, and pyrophosphoryl-ethanolamine (PPEA) forms appearing at $m/z$ 2373, 2453, and 2496, respectively. The peaks at $m/z$ 3450 and 3257 correspond to $m/z$ 3626 minus the terminal galactosaminuronic acid (GalNA, 175 amu) and the sum GalNA plus the terminal Heptose (Hep, 192 amu).

Glycosphingolipids (GSLs) are a wide class of lipids sharing the same basic structure represented by ceramide. Gangliosides are a group of complex GSLs, which characteristically contain sialic acid as a component of their carbohydrate chain [32]. They appear to be ubiquitous in vertebrate tissues and have been found in some invertebrates, too [33]. Musken et al. described a method for the direct structural characterization of microbial GSL receptors using TLC overlay assay combined with IR–MALDI–oTOF–MS [34]. This technique was applied to separate the mixtures of GSLs, overlay of the chromatogram with GSLs-specific bacteria, detection of bound microbes with primary antibodies against bacterial surface proteins and appropriate alkaline phosphatase-labeled secondary antibodies, and *in situ* MS analysis of bacteria-specific GSLs receptors in the human urinary tract.

Guittard and coworkers illustrated the use of MALDI–MS for analysis of native GSLs after development on thin-layer chromatographic plates and after heat transfer of the GSLs from the plates to several types of polymer membranes [35]. The best results were obtained using a polyvinylidene difluoride (PVDF) as a membrane, with irradiation from a nitrogen laser. Samples containing both neutral and acidic components were characterized in a 1:1 combination of DHB and 2-amino-5-nitropyridine (ANP). GSLs show well the ability to bind antibodies in an overlay assay on the TLC plate, transfer to membranes, and then be analyzed by MALDI-TOF–MS without interference from the antibody or the salts and buffers used during the binding and visualization steps. Distler's group developed a bioanalytical method for structural characterization of GSLs [36]. The authors directly coupled TLC with IR–MALDI–oTOF–MS for structural confirmation of GSLs (Lc2Cer, globo series—Gb3Cer and Gb4Cer, ganglio series—Gg3Cer and Gg4Cer, and neolacto series—nLc4Cer, nLc6Cer, and nLc8Cer). Figure 15.1 shows the scheme of matching the TLC overlay assay with IR-MALDI–MS. TLC immunostain of neutral GSLs with Galâ4GlcNAc-specific polyclonal chicken IgY (pAb) and monoclonal mouse IgM antibody (mAb). It can be observed that the pAb positive nLc4Cer of band 4 is detected as monosodiated ion at $m/z$ 1249.72 and with lower abundance as disodiated ion at $m/z$ 1271.70 confirming the structure as nLc4Cer (d18:1, C16:0) (Figure 15.1c). The same results were obtained for mAb immunostained nLc4Cer of band 4 (Figure 15.1d). The mass spectra of pAb and mAb immunostained nLc4Cer of band 3, identified as nLc4Cer (d18:1, C24:1/C24:0) and the pAb-positive nLc6Cer of band 6 (Figure 15.1e) is detected as monosodiated ion at $m/z$ 1614.85 and with lower abundance as disodiated ion at $m/z$ 1636.83 confirming the structure as nLc6Cer (d18:1, C16:0). The authors observed similar results for mAb immunostained nLc6Cer of band 6 (Figure 15.1f). This method proves to be an efficient tool for high selective and sensitive identification of antibodies, bacterial toxins, and a plant lectin at <1 ng, and avoids GSL downstream purification procedures.

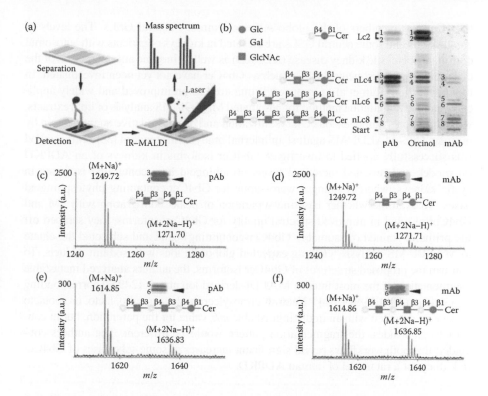

**FIGURE 15.1** Direct TLC–IR–MALDI–MS of immunodetected GSLs. (a) Scheme of matching the TLC overlay assay with IR–MALDI–MS. (b) TLC immunostain of neutral GSLs with Galâ4GlcNAc-specific polyclonal chicken IgY (pAb) and monoclonal mouse IgM antibody (mAb). Total amounts of 22.5 and 0.3 µg of neutral GSLs from human granulocytes were separated and detected by orcinol and TLC immunostain, respectively. For direct TLC–IR–MALDI–MS, amounts of 3.0 µg of total neutral GSLs were applied and mass spectra were acquired from 255 ng of pAb (c) and mAb (d) immunostained nLc4Cer (d18:1, C16:0) and from 45 ng of pAb (e) and mAb (f) immunostained nLc6Cer (d18:1, C16:0), all marked with arrowheads. (Reprinted from Distler, U. et al. 2008. *Anal. Chem.*, 80, 1835–1846. With permission.)

Kouzel's group developed a strategy to structurally characterize neutral GSLs in total lipid extracts prepared from *in vitro* propagated human monocytic THP-1 cells, which were used as a model cell line [37]. The entire structural analysis was completed by four steps: (1) extraction of total lipids from cellular material, (2) enzymatical disintegration of phospholipids by treatment of the crude lipid extract with phospholipase C (PLC), (3) subsequent multiple TLC overlay detection of individual GSLs with a mixture of various anti-GSL antibodies, and (4) structural analysis of immunostained GSLs directly on the TLC plate using IR–MALDI–oTOF–MS in combination with collision-induced dissociation (CID). This technique was successfully used to discriminate changes in the mutual ratios of lipoform doublets (C24:1/C24:0 carrying Lc2Cer, Gb3Cer, and Gb4Cer species) in kidneys of patients. Globotetraosylceramides

(Gb4Cer) are members of the globo series of complex neutral GSLs. The levels of gangliosides and some neutral GSLs are elevated in kidneys of patients with autosomal dominant polycystic kidney disease (ADPKD) as well as in some animal models of the disease, but complex neutral GSLs such as Gb4Cer have not yet been investigated. In this connection, Ruh et al. introduced Prima drop as an improved and widely applicable sample preparation method for automated MALDI–MS analysis of lipid extracts, which promotes homogeneous cocrystallization and enables relative quantification by indirect TLC–MALDI–MS against an internal bradykinin standard [38]. This method was successfully applied to investigate Gb4Cer isoforms in kidneys of an ADPKD rat model, and revealed increased levels of sphingoid base-containing isoforms in cystic kidneys, whereas changes were subtle for Gb4Cer-containing phytosphingoid bases. To examine whether baseline separation of peaks comigrating with SM and Gb4Cer resulted in improved spectral quality for Gb4Cer isoforms, they scraped off the primulin-stained (presumably Gb4Cer-containing) band and subjected the eluate to MALDI–MS analysis, yielding expected globoside ions with sodium adducts. To confirm the proposed structures of Gb4Cer isoforms, the authors analyzed metastable fragmentation of the most intense MALDI-derived ion at $m/z$ 1249.80 corresponding to [Gb4Cer (d18:1,16:0) + Na]$^+$. Neutral tetraosylceramides (ganglio, lacto, or neolacto series) are detected with an undistinguishable $m/z$ value for the parent ion, but in contrast to globosides, the fragmentation pattern would be different. The authors concluded that both workflows reveal significant increases of some subclasses of Gb4Cer in kidneys of a rat model of human ADPKD.

### 15.3.2 ANALYSIS OF GANGLIOSIDES

In view of gangliosides' importance and roles, TLC techniques coupled with MALDI–MS approaches were successfully applied to separate and detect GSLs in various samples. For example, Ivleva's team described the use of TLC coupled to an external ion source MALDI-Fourier transform (FT) MS for separation and identification of ganglioside mixtures without compromising mass accuracy and resolution of the spectra [39]. It was observed that the FT–MS has a vibrationally cooled MALDI ion source, fragile glycolipids are desorbed from TLC plates without fragmentation, even to the point that desorption of intact molecules from "hot" matrixes such as α-cyano-4-hydroxycinnamic acid (CHCA) are as a matrix. The authors investigated a set of 20 organic molecules as matrices for gangliosides and for phosphopeptide samples desorbed from TLC plates, as well as from a standard stainless steel target. They also studied the analyte mass spectral fragmentation patterns as a function of a laser power, enabling description of each matrix in "hot/cold" terms. Among the matrixes, DHB, 6-aza-2-thiothymine (ATT), and anthranilic acid had substantially reduced sialic acid loss. Similarly, the use of "hot" matrixes, such as CHCA, sinapinic acid (SA), or harmane, required maximum laser attenuation (minimum fluence) in order to obtain at least partially sialylated ganglioside peaks. Using this technique, whole-brain gangliosides are separated and the TLC plates are attached directly to the MALDI target, where the gangliosides are desorbed, ionized, and detected in the FTMS with >70,000 resolving power. The same group compared stabilization and detection of desorbed gangliosides on a commercial orthogonal time-of-flight (oTOF) instrument and on a home-built FT–MS [40]. It was proved that the coupling of the TLC method with the proTOF 2000 instrument yielded a simple and fast analysis for gangliosides. The authors optimized the conditions for desorbing the gangliosides off of the TLC plates, including the type and amount of matrix required for the best spectral performance. It was observed that SA was the best matrix for this purpose because it provides the most homogeneous cocrystallization within the bulk silica gel layer on the TLC plate and cocrystallizes with the gangliosides most efficiently. Furthermore, the authors used two lasers (infrared laser [Er:YAG, 2.94 μM] and UV laser). They showed that the sensitivity was increased, compared with UV–MALDI, for desorption of glycolipid ions from a TLC plate. Dreisewerd's group developed a novel method for direct coupling of HPTLC with MALDI–MS using Er:YAG infrared laser for soft desorption/ionization of biomolecules [41]. In this method, the authors used glycerol as a liquid matrix, which provides a homogeneous wetting of the silica gel and a simple and fast MALDI preparation protocol. Figure 15.2 shows the orcinol-stained HPTLC-separated GM3 double band. The direction of the chromatographic mobility is from bottom to top. It can be observed that the "lower band" contains the GM3 species with short-chain fatty acids (mainly C16:0), whereas the "upper band" contains the GM3 species with long-chain fatty acids (mainly C22:0, C24:1, and C24:0). A direct HPTLC-MALDI mass spectrum was shown in Figure 15.2a, which shows an unstained lower GM3 band. As minor components, deprotonated GM3 species with C14:0, C17:0, and C18:0 fatty acid residues were detected at $m/z$ values of 1123.69, 1165.74, and 1179.75, respectively. GM3 species with C22:0, C24:1, and C24:0 fatty acids, abundant in the total GM3 fraction, are completely absent in the direct infrared (IR) MALDI analysis of this band, which confirms that TLC combined IR–MALDI–MS plays a key role for separation and identification of GM3 species.

### 15.3.3 Analysis of Drugs

Complications of drug analysis were successfully resolved by the combination of TLC with MALDI–MS. TLC combined with MALDI–MS was used for analysis of psychotropic drugs (3,4-methylenedioxy methamphetamine, 4-hydroxy-3-methoxy methamphetamine, 3,4-methylenedioxy amphetamine, methamphetamine, p-hydroxy methamphetamine, amphetamine, ketamine, caffeine, chlorpromazine, triazolam, and morphine) in biological samples [42]. This technique was able to analyze 3,4-methylenedioxy methamphetamine (MDMA) and its metabolites in urine samples without sample dilution, and the detection limit of the MDMA spot was 0.05 ng/ spot. Crecelius and coworkers described the use of TLC with MALDI–MS/MS for the structural analysis of small drug molecules [43]. This method was successfully applied to analyze two representatives of nonsteroidal antiinflammatory drugs (tenoxicam and piroxicam), and pharmaceutically active compound UK-137,457 and one of its related substances UK-124,912. The feasibility of UTLC-atmospheric pressure (AP)-MALDI-MS was described for the analysis of small molecules (triazole, midazolam, verapamil, and metaprolol) [44]. The authors compared the selectivity and sensitivity between UTLC- and HPTLC–AP–MALDI–MS. It was observed that UTLC plates provided 10–100 times better sensitivity in MALDI analysis than the conventional

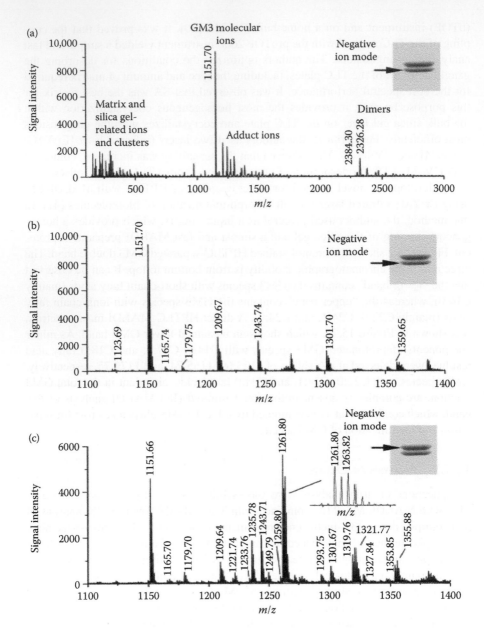

**FIGURE 15.2** Direct HPTLC–IR–MALDI mass spectra recorded in the negative ion mode. (a) Mass spectrum acquired from the lower GM3 HPTLC band. (b) Enlarged section showing the *m/z* region between 1100 and 1400. (c) Enlarged section of a mass spectrum acquired from the upper GM3 HPTLC band showing the *m/z* region between 1100 and 1400. (Reprinted from Dreisewerd, K. et al. 2005. *Anal. Chem.*, 77, 4098–4107. With permission.)

HPTLC. Moreover, UTLC provides faster separations and lower solvent consumption and allows detecting analytes at the picomole range. In addition, Solo's group studied the feasibility of UTLC–AP–MALDI–MS for bioassays using benzodiazepines as model substances in human urine [45]. The separation efficiency of benzodiazepines was studied using 1D UTLC and 2D UTLC. Between two TLC methods, 2D UTLC was shown to be an efficient technique for the separation of benzodiazepines. This method provides LOD within the picomole range for benzodiazepine metabolites in an authentic urine sample.

## 15.3.4 Analysis of Other Organic Compounds and Reaction Products

In recent years, several groups have proved that TLC–MALDI enables the convenient separation and characterization of oligosaccharides [46,47] and carbohydrates [48] in milk and *Quercus robur* extract with reduced sample pretreatments. In these methods, glycerol, 2,5-DHB, and 9-aminoacridine (9-AA) were used as matrices and provided homogeneous crystals on TLC plate to create efficient material ablation and particular soft desorption/ionization conditions, which allows separating and detecting carbohydrates with high sensitivity. The native milk oligosaccharides were successfully analyzed even at 10 pmol [46]. The online hyphenation of TLC with matrix-free material-enhanced LDI–MS was developed by immobilizing bradykinin a peptide on silica gel coupled to 4-(3-triethoxysilylpropylureido)azobenzene and applied for the analysis of carbohydrates (glucose, sucrose, raffinose) in plant extract of *Quercus robur* [48]. Even through TLC–MALDI–MS techniques have proved to be efficient analytical tools for separation and quantification of a wide variety of molecules, analysis of low-molecular weight analytes might be difficult due to the background ions from the matrix often causing serious interferences. To accomplish on-spot mass analysis of low-molecular weight organic compounds, TLC techniques were successfully coupled with MALD–MS [49,50]. Three arborescidine alkaloids (anesthesics, levobupivacaine, and mepivacaine) and the antibiotic tetracycline were readily characterized by TLC followed by direct on spot MALDI–MS with "matrix-free" mass spectra using a UV-absorbing ionic liquid matrix (triethylamine/CHCA) [49]. Chen et al. developed nanomaterial-assisted TLC–MALDI–MS for direct monitoring of chemical transformations in nucleophilic substitution reaction products [50]. The authors constructed a hybrid system using DHB-iron oxide magnetic nanoparticles (MNPs)-assisted TLC–MALDI–MS for efficient separation of TLC with matrix-MNPs to identify unknown compounds from ongoing chemical reactions on TLC by MALDI–MS. The key advantage of this approach is that it involves direct "on-plate" separation of multiple organic reaction products by TLC, essentially allowing the reaction products to be directly "read out" by MALDI–MS. St. Hilaire and coworkers developed TLC–MALDI–MS for the separation and identification of various molecules including crude mixtures of peptides and glycopeptides, and complex carbohydrate reactions [51]. Further, this technique was applied to monitor base-catalyzed condensation between benzaldehyde and cyclohexanone. These results indicated that TLC is a simple, inexpensive, and convenient analytical method that can easily interface with MALDI–MS for separation and identification of a wide variety of molecules in complex samples with high sensitivity. Since desorption techniques hit only an aliquot of the zone size on its very surface, sputtering and conduction into the MS must be constructed very effectively to guarantee the respective sensitivity and reliability. Table 15.1 summarizes the references on TLC combined with MALDI–MS for lipids, GSLs, dyes, drugs, and other organic compounds.

## 15.4 ENHANCEMENT OF CHROMATOGRAPHIC BANDS DESORPTION

The detection and quantitation of biomolecules, drugs, and organic molecules has been greatly improved in recent years by the combination of TLC with advanced MS techniques, in particular MALDI, ESI, DESI, APCI, and other ionization techniques, which allows efficient separation and a user to enter an $m/z$ value of interest and view a list of matching structure candidates, along with a list of calculated "high-probability" product ions where appropriate. In recent years, considerable effort has been made to develop new ionization techniques to deconvolute and identify target analytes from complex samples in conjunction with TLC techniques. For example, Shiea's group developed two interfaces to connect small size TLC with ESI for the continuous analysis of organic mixtures (clindamycin and sildenafil) [52]. They interfaced two bound optical fibers inserted into the C18-bonded particles at the exit of a small TLC channel and a small commercial TLC strip with a sharpened tip. The high voltage required for ESI was introduced into the makeup solution or mobile phase through a Pt wire, and electrospray was generated at the tip of the bonded optical fibers and at the sharp end of the TLC strip. The same group developed a laser-induced acoustic desorption and electrospray ionization mass spectrometry (LIAD/ESI/MS) combined with TLC for the rapid characterization of chemical compounds [53]. The authors performed LIAD analysis by irradiating the rear side of an aluminum-based TLC plate with a pulsed IR laser. They attached a glass slide to the rear of the TLC plate and the gap between the glass slide and the TLC plate was filled with a glycerol solution, which allows efficient generation and transfer of acoustic and shock waves to ablate the analyte-containing TLC gels. The ablated analyte molecules were ionized in an ESI plume and then detected by an ion trap mass analyzer. Similarly, Van Berkel and coworkers described the use of TLC combined with ESI–MS for the quantification of dyes [54] and caffeine [55]. They combined surface sampling probe and electrospray emitter for the direct readout of TLC plates by ESI–MS. The TLC–ESI–MS was successfully applied to detect caffeine in Diet Cherry Coke and diet sports drinks with high accuracy and precision.

The greater spatial resolution achieved in HPTLC and continuing improvements in the variety of stationary phases available complement the basic simplicity and versatility of planar chromatography. In this connection, Chai et al. have successfully combined OPLC with ESI–MS for the quantification of glycolipids [56]. In OPLC, the TLC plate is covered with an inert membrane sheet under external pressure, and the mobile phase is pumped through the sealed layer of stationary phase (silica gel). The plate equates to a planar column and results in a substantially shorter analysis time, higher efficiency, and lower consumption of solvent as compared with conventional TLC. This method was successfully applied to detect glycosphingolipid at 5 pmol by TLC/ESI–MS and at 20 pmol by TLC/ESI–MS/MS.

**TABLE 15.1**

**TLC Combined with MALDI–MS Techniques for Identification of Lipids, Gangliosides, Drugs, and Other Organic Compounds**

| Type of TLC | Stationary Phase | Mobile Phase | Matrix | MS Technique | Analytes | Reference |
|---|---|---|---|---|---|---|
| HPTLC | HPTLC silica gel 60 plates | $CHCl_2$/EtOH/$H_2O$/$Et_3N$ (35:35:7:35, v/v/v/v) | DHB | MALDI–MS | Phospholipids | [26] |
| HPTLC | Silica gel 60 HPTLC aluminum plates | Solvent system 1: (methyl acetate/1-propanol/$CHCl_3$/MeOH/0.25% KCl, 25:25:25:10:9, v/v/v/v/v) Solvent system 2: (toluene/diethylether/EtOH/AcOH, 60:40:1:0.05, v/v/v/v) | THAP | MALDI–MS | Various neutral triacylglycerols and polar glycerophospholipids and sphingolipids | [27] |
| HPTLC | HPTLC silica gel 60 plates | $CHCl_2$/EtOH/$H_2O$/$Et_3N$ (30:35:7:35, v/v/v/v) | DHB | MALDI–MS | GPC species, SM and GPE | [29] |
| TLC | Aluminum backed silica gel plates | Isobutyric acid/$NH_4OH$ (5:3, v/v) and MeOH/$H_2O$ (1:1, v/v) | DHB | MALDI–MS | Lipopoly-saccharides | [31] |
| HPTLC | Silica gel 60 precoated glass plates | $CHCl_2$/MeOH/$H_2O$ (120:70:17, v/v/v) | Glycerol | IR/MALDI–MS | Glycosphingo-lipids | [34] |
| TLC | Silica gel TLC plate | Method-I: $CHCl_3$/MeOH/$H_2O$/0.2% $CaCl_2$ (w/v) (55:45:10, v/v/v) Method-II: isopropyl alcohol/MeOH/$H_2O$/0.2% $CaCl_2$ (w/v) (40:7:20, v/v/v) | DHB and ANP | MALDI–MS | Glycosphingo-lipids | [35] |
| HPTLC | Glass-backed silica gel 60 precoated HPTLC plates | Solvent 1: $CHCl_3$/MeOH/$H_2O$ (120/70/17, v/v/v) and solvent 2: $CHCl_3$/MeOH/$H_2O$ (120/85/20, v/v/v), both supplemented with $CaCl_2$ (2 mM) | Glycerol | MALDI–MS | Glycosphingo-lipids | [36] |
| HPTLC | Silica gel of TLC plates was fixed with poly isobutyl methacrylate | $CHCl_3$/MeOH/$H_2O$ (120/85/20, v/v/v) supplemented with $CaCl_2$ (2 mM) | Glycerol | IR–MALDI–MS | Glycosphingo-lipids | [37] |

*(Continued)*

**TABLE 15.1 (Continued)**
**TLC Combined with MALDI–MS Techniques for Identification of Lipids, Gangliosides, Drugs, and Other Organic Compounds**

| Type of TLC | Stationary Phase | Mobile Phase | Matrix | MS Technique | Analytes | Reference |
|---|---|---|---|---|---|---|
| HPTLC | Silica HPTLC plates | CHCl$_3$/MeOH/0.2% CaCl$_2$ (50/35/8, v/v/v) | DHB, ATT, and THAP | MALDI-MS | Glycosphingo-lipids | [38] |
| TLC | Silica–aluminum TLC plates | CHCl$_3$/MeOH/0.2% CaCl$_2$ (55:45:10, v/v/v) or CHCl$_3$/2-propanol/50 mM KCl (2:13.4:4.6, v/v/v) | Matrix mixtures | MALDI/FT-MS | Ganglioside mixtures | [39] |
| TLC | Silica gel on aluminum TLC plates | SA in MeOH/ACN/H$_2$O (2:2:1, v/v/v) | SA | MALDI-FT-MS | Gangliosides | [40] |
| HPTLC | Silica gel 60 precoated HPTLC plates | CHCl$_3$/MeOH/H$_2$O (120:85:20, v/v/v) | Glycerol | IR–MALDI-MS | Gangliosides | [41] |
| TLC | TLC plate | Acetone/28% NH$_3$ (99:1, v/v) | CHCA | MALDI-MS | Psychotropic drugs | [42] |
| TLC | 0.2-mm layers of silica gel 60 F254 | CHCl$_3$/MeOH (9:1, v/v), CHCl$_3$/MeOH/AcOH (60:5:1, v/v/v) | CHCA | MALDI/MS | Tenoxicam and piroxicam | [43] |
| UTLC and HPTLC | Silica gel 60 F254 HPTLC plates and monolithic UTLC plates | Ethyl acetate/hexane (1:2, v/v) containing 2% acetic acid | CHCA | AP-MALDI-MS | Triazole, midazolam, verapamil, and metaprolol | [44] |
| 2D UTLC | Monolithic UTLC plates | CH$_2$Cl$_2$/acetone (93:7, v/v) and toluene/acetone/EtOH/25% NH$_3$ (70:20:3:1, v/v/v) | CHCA | AP-MALDI-MS | Benzodiazepines | [45] |
| HPTLC | Glass backed silica gel 60 precoated HPTLC plates | n-Butanol/AcOH/H$_2$O (110:45:45, v/v/v) | Glycerol | MALDI-MS | Milk oligosaccharides | [46] |
| TLC | Silica gel 60 plates | n-butanol/HCOOH/H$_2$O (3:4:1, v/v/v) | DHB or 9-AA | MALDI-MS | Complex oligosaccharides | [47] |

(Continued)

**TABLE 15.1 (Continued)**
**TLC Combined with MALDI–MS Techniques for Identification of Lipids, Gangliosides, Drugs, and Other Organic Compounds**

| Type of TLC | Stationary Phase | Mobile Phase | Matrix | MS Technique | Analytes | Reference |
|---|---|---|---|---|---|---|
| TLC | Modified silica gel | n-Butanol/acetone/AcOH/H$_2$O (35:35:10:20, v/v/v/v) | Matrix-free | MALDI-MS | Carbohydrates | [48] |
| TLC | Commercial TLC aluminum sheets | CHCl$_3$/MeOH (9:1, v/v) | Et$_3$N/CHCA | MALDI-MS | Alkaloids | [49] |
| TLC | TLC plates with an aluminum substrate | MeOH/CH$_2$Cl$_2$ (1:9, v/v) | DHB and CHCA | MALDI-MS | Chemical reaction products | [50] |
| TLC | Silica gel 60 F254 aluminum or glass-backed TLC plates | Ethyl acetate/MeOH/AcOH/H$_2$O (4:3:3:1, v/v/v/v) | DHB | MALDI-MS | Peptides and glycopeptides, and complex carbohydrate reactions | [51] |

A novel, sensitive, convenient, rapid, and cost-effective HPTLC was successfully coupled with ESI–MS for the qualitative and quantitative analysis of small saturated hyaluronan oligosaccharides consisting of 2–4 hyalobiuronic acid moieties [57]. The authors used amino-modified silica as a stationary phase, which allows a simple reagent-free *in situ* derivatization by heating, resulting in a very low limit of detection (7–19 pmol per band, depending on the analyzed saturated oligosaccharide). Chen and Schwack illustrated the use of HPTLC–ESI–MS for the rapid screening of 12 sulfonamides (sulfadoxin, sulfadiazine, sulfamethazine, sulfanilamide, sulfamethiozole, sulfachloropyridazine, sulfathiazole, sulfapyridine, sulfamerazine, sulfisoxazole, sulfaquinoxaline, and sulfacetamide) in foods of animal origin [58]. The authors studied the separation efficiency of target analytes using derivatized and nonderivatized plates, indicating that derivatized plates are to be favored for confirmation purposes of suspicious findings. A straightforward procedure was developed for direct mass spectrometric analysis of spots from TLC plates using the aluminum plate backing as a spray tip [59]. In this method, the spots were cut out shaped as a tip with a 60° angle, mounted in front of the MS orifice, and, after addition of spray solvent, spectra were obtained immediately, which leads to avoiding an external ion source. The authors described the practical benefits of this technique for detection of by-products of organic reactions and of degradation products, and for accurate confirmation of UV filters in sunscreens. Recently, Naumoska and Vovk performed three TLC separations on Merck 20 cm × 10 cm glass-backed HPTLC silica gel 60 (Art. No. 1.05641) and HPTLC $C_{18}$ RP (Art. No. 1.05914) plates predeveloped with chloroform–methanol (1:1, *v/v*) and acetone and coupled with ESI–MS for screening of some common plant triterpenoids and phytosterols in cuticular wax extracts of different vegetables (zucchini, eggplant, tomato, red pepper, mangold, spinach, lettuce, white-colored radicchio di Castelfranco, raddichio Leonardo, white cabbage, red cabbage, and savoy cabbage) [60]. Using this method, eight triterpenoids (lupeol, α-amyrin, β-amyrin, cycloartenol, cycloartenol acetate, lupeol acetate, lupenone, and friedelin) and two phytosterols (β-sitosterol and stigmasterol) were effectively separated and identified by their differentiation according to the band colors.

Desorption ionization is a phrase that describes a diverse set of ionization methods for mass spectrometry in which the rapid addition of energy into a condensed phase sample results in the production of gas-phase ions. Cooks and coworkers introduced a new atmospheric pressure desorption ionization method that is, DESI for the analysis of analytes on surfaces [61]. The technique has the ability to directly analyze compounds on a number of different surface types using DESI–MS, including leather and nitrile gloves, a tomato skin, a medicine tablet, and even a blood drop on a finger, for a variety of analytes, from small pharmaceutical molecules to large biopolymers. Due to its feasibility, Van Berkel's group combined TLC with DESI–MS for direct analysis of various compounds [62–64]. They successfully coupled TLC with MS using DESI for a variety of hydrophobic and wettable TLC stationary phases. The basic experimental setup and the optimization of TLC/DESI–MS conditions are discussed by studying solvent flow rate, solvent composition, nebulizing gas flow rate, DESI emitter-to-surface distance, and the effect of surface scan rate on signal levels and chromatographic readout resolution for identification of various compounds (rodhamaines, dyes, and drugs). Similarly, modest modifications to the atmospheric sampling capillary of a commercial ESI–MS and upgrades to an in-house-developed surface positioning control software package (Hands Free TLC–MS) were used to enable the automated sampling and imaging of analytes on and within large area surface substrates using DESI–MS [63]. Using this technique, sampling and imaging of rhodamine dyes were separated on TLC plates and shown for user-defined spot sampling from separated bands on a TLC plate (one or multiple spots), scanning of a complete development lane (one or multiple lanes), or imaging of analyte bands in a development lane (i.e., multiple lane scans with close spacing). Further, the atmospheric sampling capillary of a commercial ion trap mass spectrometer was extended to permit sampling and ionization of analytes in bands separated on intact TLC plates (10 cm × 10 cm) [64]. This technique was successfully applied to separate and to detect goldenseal (*Hydrastis canadensis*) and related alkaloids, and the detection levels were found to be 5 ng each or 14–28 pmol in mass spectral full-scan mode and 2.5–100 pmol in from the calibration curves.

DESI is as a sample introduction method for MS and ideally suited to combination with TLC for the analysis of drugs [65,66], porcine brain lipids [67], and peptides [68]. Nonbonded reversed-phase (RP) TLC plates coupled with DESI ion mobility mass spectrometry (IM–MS) was developed for the direct analysis of pharmaceutical formulations and active ingredients. This method shows high potentiality for the analysis of analgesic (paracetamol), decongestant (ephedrine), opiate (codeine), and stimulant (caffeine) in their active pharmaceutical ingredients. TLC–DESI–MS was used for the analysis of intact *S. divinorum* leaves for salvinorin A (SA) and of acetone extracts [66]. This technique detected several ions of SA that are useful for both the direct analysis of intact plant materials for screening illicit substances and for the examination of natural products. The direct analysis of porcine brain lipids was performed on HPTLC–DESI–MS [67]. Using this technique, eight class-specific spots were imaged in the negative ion mode and shown to contain more than 50 lipids. Han's team prepared superhydrophobic monolithic porous polymer layers with a photopatterned hydrophilic channel on TLC for the separation of peptide mixtures (human angiotensin II, bradykinin acetate salt, leucine-enkephalin acetate salt hydrate, and val-tyr-val), and visualized by UV light and then directly monitored by DESI–MS [68]. These results illustrated that the unidirectional surface scanning with the DESI source was found suitable to determine both their location of each separated analyte and their *m/z* values.

Interfacing TLC with ambient mass spectrometry (AMS) has been an important area of analytical chemistry because of its capability to rapidly separate and characterize the chemical compounds, which allows detecting analytes by reducing or eliminating the use of materials and by avoiding the generation of hazardous waste. Shiea and coworkers integrated ELDI that combines laser desorption and ESI–MS with TLC plate coated with either reversed-phase C18 particles or normal-phase silica gel for separation and identification of dyes, amines, and drugs [69]. In this technique, the authors placed a TLC plate on an acrylic sample holder set in front of the sampling skimmer of an ion trap mass analyzer and then the analytes at the center of the TLC plate were analyzed by pushing the sample holder into the path of a laser beam with a syringe pump. The target analytes in the sample spot were desorbed by continuously irradiating the surface of the TLC plate with a pulsed nitrogen laser and then the desorbed sample molecules entered an ESI plume where they were ionized through the reactions with the charged species. The same group developed a novel high-throughput TLC–AMS system for the analysis of dyes and drugs using building blocks to deal, deliver, and collect the TLC plate through an ELDI source [70]. This technique shows several advantages such as readily available, cheap, reusable, and extremely easy to modify without consuming any material or reagent, the use of building blocks to develop the TLC–AMS interface, which is undoubtedly a green methodology. In order to examine the usability of the new TLC–ELDI–MS system, this technique was successfully applied to detect acetaminophen, ethenzamide, and chlorpheniramine in three over-the-counter drugs (Chyrtongdan, Noharege, and Panadol). TLC remains a popular chromatographic technique for the screening of drugs in a biological sample. Tames' group described the application of fast atom bombardment (FAB) tandem MS for the analysis and identification of morphine in a urine sample following TLC [71]. The authors completed the whole TLC–FAB–MS/MS for confirmation of morphine in urine samples within 5–10 min. Unique applications were enabled by HPTLC combined with LDI MS to differentiate blue ballpoint inks [72]. The authors analyzed ink entries on paper from 31 blue ballpoint pens. Their dye ink formulations were compared and the pens were classified into 26 classes by LDI–MS against 18 for HPTLC.

Great progress has been recently made on spot detection and analyte characterization by performing TLC via ambient desorption/ionization MS/MS, that is, via easy ambient sonic spray ionization mass spectrometry (EASI–MS) [73]. This technique was successfully applied to monitor a chemical reaction of synthetic importance and analytes were separated and ionized at ambient condition without the use of voltages, electrical discharges, UV or laser beams, and high temperature. Recently, Zhang's group developed a novel plasma-assisted multiwavelength (1064, 532, and 355 nm) laser desorption ionization mass spectrometry (PAMLDI–MS) system and applied it in the analysis of low-molecular weight compounds by combining with TLC [74]. The TLC/PAMLDI–MS system successfully integrated TLC, the multiwavelength laser ablation, and the excited state plasma from direct analysis in real time and was proved to be effective in the facile separation and selective identification of dyes (rhodamine B, Sudan III, and fluorescein) and drugs (quinine, chloramphenicol, and gliclazide). The three-wavelength laser system provides great advantages in detecting different species with minimal sample preparations and reduced analysis time. As seen in Table 15.2, TLC combined with ESI, DESI, ELDI, and other MS techniques has been used for the separation and identification of lipids, dyes, and drugs in complex samples.

## 15.5  CONCLUSIONS

A multitude of TLC–MS-based techniques aimed at separation, purification, and identification of biomolecules and organic molecules in mixtures is conventional tools and represents mostly the first step in the analysis. Two-dimensional TLC and multidimensional TLC increase the resolution capability of TLC by affording separations with reduced time and solvents. The TLC and HPTLC coupled with MS belong to the principal analytical techniques that can be used for correct identification of

**TABLE 15.2**

**An Overview of Research Involving TLC Combined with ESI, DESI, ELSI, and Other Ionization MS Techniques for the Separation and Identification of Lipids, Carbohydrates, Drugs, and Natural Products**

| Type of TLC | Mobile Phase | Volume of Sample | Volume of Solvent | MS Technique | Analyte | Reference |
|---|---|---|---|---|---|---|
| TLC | MeOH/CHCl$_3$ (85:15, v/v) | 0.2 μL | 200 μL | ESI–MS | Clindamycin and sildenafil | [52] |
| TLC | CHCl$_3$/MeOH (9:1, v/v) | 1 μL | – | LIAD/ESI–MS | Drugs | [53] |
| TLC | MeOH/THF (60:40, v/v) and MeOH/H$_2$O (70:30, v/v) | – | – | ESI–MS | Dyes | [54] |
| TLC | MeOH/H$_2$O (60/40, v/v) | – | 15 μL | ESI–MS | Caffeine | [55] |
| TLC and OPLC | CHCl$_3$/MeOH/H$_2$O (60:35:8, v/v) | – | 100–125 μL | ESI–MS | Glycolipids | [56] |
| HPTLC | ACN/H$_2$O/HCOOH (90:10:0.1, v/v/v) | 5–10 μL | – | ESI–MS | Oligosaccharides | [57] |
| HPTLC | ACN/20 mM NH$_4$HCO$_2$ (7:3, v/v), and MeOH/20 mM NH$_4$HCO$_2$ (7:3, v/v) | 200 μL | 0.2 mL | ESI–MS | Sulfonamides | [58] |
| TLC | Ethyl acetate/heptane (1:1, v/v) and ethyl acetate/heptane (10:1, v/v) | 10 μL | 1.5 mL | ESI–MS | Synthesis products and UV filters | [59] |
| TLC and HPTLC | n-Hexane/ethyl acetate (5:1, v/v) acetone/ACN (5:1, v/v) and ethyl acetate/ACN (3:2, v/v) | – | 6 mL | ESI–MS | Triterpenoids and phytosterols | [60] |
| TLC | MeOH/H$_2$O (80:20, v/v), H$_2$O/acetone (70:30, v/v) and ethyl acetate/AcOH (99:1, v/v) | – | – | DESI–MS | Rhodamines and drugs | [62] |
| TLC | MeOH/H$_2$O (75:25, v/v) | 1.0 μL | – | DESI–MS | Rhodamines | [63] |
| TLC | Ethyl acetate/MeOH/HCOOH/H$_2$O (50:10:6:3, v/v/v/v) | – | – | DESI–MS | Alkaloids | [64] |
| RP-TLC | HCOOH/H$_2$O (0.1:100, v/v) and HCOOH/ACN (0.1:100, v/v) | – | 25 μL | DESI–MS | Drugs | [65] |
| TLC | CHCl$_3$ or CHCl$_3$/MeOH | 5 μL | – | DESI | Salvinorin A | [66] |
| HPTLC | CHCl$_3$/Et$_3$N/MeOH/H$_2$O (35:35:35:7, v/v/v/v) and CHCl$_3$/MeOH/AcOH (65:35:8 v/v/v) | – | – | DESI | Porcine brain lipids | [67] |

*(Continued)*

**TABLE 15.2 (Continued)**

**An Overview of Research Involving TLC Combined with ESI, DESI, ELSI, and Other Ionization MS Techniques for the Separation and Identification of Lipids, Carbohydrates, Drugs, and Natural Products**

| Type of TLC | Mobile Phase | Volume of Sample | Volume of Solvent | MS Technique | Analyte | Reference |
|---|---|---|---|---|---|---|
| 2D-TLC | ACN/0.2 M C$_2$H$_3$O$_2$NH$_4$ (30:70, v/v) | – | – | DESI–MS | Peptides | [68] |
| TLC | 500 mM NH$_4$OH/acetone (70/30, v/v) | – | – | ELDI–MS | Dyes, amines, and drugs | [69] |
| TLC | Ethyl acetate/AcOH/CHCl$_3$ (98:1:1, v/v/v) | 5 μL | 10 μL | ELDI–MS | Dyes and drugs | [70] |
| HPTLC and TLC | Ethyl acetate/MeOH/NH$_4$OH (8:2:0.2, v/v) | 0.5 mL | 1–10 mL | FAB–MS | Morphine | [71] |
| HPTLC and TLC | 1-Butanol/2-propanol/H$_2$O/AcOH (10:5:5:0.5, v/v/v/v) and 1-butanol/ethanol/H$_2$O/AcOH (15:3:3.9:0.45, v/v/v/v) | 2.5 and 5 μL | – | LDI–MS | Ink entries | [72] |
| TLC | H$_2$O/NH$_4$OH (pH 8.0)/ethyl acetate | 10 mL | – | EASI–MS | Propranolol and amlodipine besylate | [73] |
| TLC | CH$_2$Cl$_2$/EtOH/NH$_3$ (66.1:33.1:0.8, v/v/v), hexane/EtOH/HCOOH (64.7:32.4:2.9, v/v/v) and hexane/EtOH (1:2, v/v) | – | – | PAMLDI–MS | Dyes and drugs | [74] |

a wide variety of molecules in various samples. Hyphenation of TLC/HPTLC with MS greatly contributes to the progress of planar chromatography. Direct coupling of TLC with various ionization (MALDI, ESI, DESI, ELDI, and EASI) MS techniques separated analytes on the plate followed by MS analysis is especially attractive, providing chromatographic and at least partial structural information simultaneously to many analytical tasks such as drug and oil analysis, reaction monitoring, phytochemistry and synthetic chemistry, forensic counterfeit screening, and quality control. Integration of TLC techniques with MS progressively more powerful and portable TLC-mass spectrometers will enable reaching the full *in situ* direct analysis potential promised by ambient MS. Further increase in the spatial resolution and mass accuracy of TLC combined with MALDI, ESI, and ambient MS experiments should continue to receive attention from the leading groups in the field.

## ACKNOWLEDGMENTS

The authors thank Hani Abdelhamid (Department of Materials and Environmental Chemistry, Stockholm University, Sweden) and Ganga Raju (Doctoral Degree in Marine Biotechnology, National Sun Yat-Sen University) for their assistance in literature collection. We thank the American Chemical Society for giving copyright permission to reuse figures in this chapter.

## REFERENCES

1. Striegel, M.F. and Hill J. 1996. *Thin-Layer Chromatography for Binding Media Analysis,* Scientific Tools for Conservation, Getty Conservation Institute, Los Angeles, CA, p. 2–6.
2. Sherma, J. 2008. Planar chromatography, *Anal. Chem.*, 80: 4253–4267.
3. Tuzimski, T. 2011. Application of different modes of thin-layer chromatography and mass spectrometry for the separation and detection of large and small biomolecules, *J. Chromatogr. A*, 1218: 8799–8812.
4. Fuchsa, B., Süss, R., Teubera, K., Eibischa, M., and Schiller, J. 2011. Lipid analysis by thin-layer chromatography-A review of the current state, *J. Chromatogr. A*, 1218: 2754–2774.
5. Wilson, I.D. 1999. The state of the art in thin-layer chromatography–mass spectrometry: A critical appraisal, *J. Chromatogr. A*, 856: 429–442.
6. Meisen, I., Mormann, M., and Müthing, J. 2011. Thin-layer chromatography, overlay technique and mass spectrometry: A versatile triad advancing glycosphingolipidomics, *Biochim. Biophys. Acta*, 1811: 875–896.
7. Huber, C.G. and Oberacher, H. 2001. Analysis of nucleic acids by on-line liquid chromatography–mass spectrometry, *Mass Spectrom. Rev.*, 20: 310–343.
8. Morlock, G. and Schwack, W. 2010. Coupling of planar chromatography to mass spectrometry, *Trends Anal. Chem.*, 29: 1157–1171.
9. Srivastava, M.M. 2011. An overview of HPTLC: A modern analytical technique with excellent potential for automation, optimization, hyphenation, and multidimensional applications. In: Srivastava, M. (Ed.), *High Performance Thin Layer Chromatography (HPTLC)*, Springer, Heidelberg, Germany, pp. 3–26, Chapter 1.
10. Bhushan, R. 2008. Amino acids, in thin-layer chromatography in phytochemistry. In: Waksmundzka-Hajnos, M., Sherma, J., and Kowalska T. (Eds.), *Thin-Layer Chromatography in Phytochemistry*, CRC Press/Taylor & Francis Group, Boca Raton, FL, p. 299, Chapter 13.

11. Bhushan, R. and Martens, J. 2003. Amino acids and their derivatives. In: Sherma J. and Fried B. (Eds.), *Handbook of Thin-Layer Chromatography*, 3rd ed., Marcel Dekker, New York, p. 373, Chapter 14.

12. Tuzimski, T. 2011. Basic principles of planar chromatography and its potential for hyphenated techniques. In: Srivastava, M.M. (Ed.), *High-Performance Thin-Layer Chromatography (HPTLC)*, Springer, Heidelberg, p. 247, Chapter 14.

13. Poole, C.F. 2003. Thin-layer chromatography: Challenges and opportunities, *J. Chromatogr. A*, 1000: 963–984.

14. Poole, C.F. 1989. Solvent migration through porous layers, *J. Planar Chromatogr.*, 2: 95–98.

15. Nurok, D. 2000. Analytical chemistry: Forced-flow techniques in planar chromatography, *Anal. Chem.*, 72: 634A–641A.

16. Sherma, J. 2003. Basic techniques, materials and apparatus, In: Sherma J. and Fried, B. (Eds.), *Handbook of Thin-Layer Chromatography*, Marcel Dekker, Inc., New York, Vol. 55, p. 3–41.

17. Sherma, J. and Fried, B. 2005. Thin layer chromatographic analysis of biological samples—A review, *J. Liq. Chromatogr. Relat. Technol.*, 28: 2297–2314.

18. Berezkin, V.G. and Kulakova, N.Y. 2009. Three dimensional thin layer chromatography, *Russ. J. Phys. Chem. A*, 83: 1961–1965.

19. Berezkin, V.G., Khrebtova, S.S., and Kulakova, N. Y. 2009. Four-dimensional thin-layer chromatography, *Dokl. Phys. Chem.*, 429: 229–232.

20. Berezkin, V., Khrebtova, S., and Kulakova, N. 2010. Four-dimensional TLC on plates with open and closed adsorbent layers, *Chromatographia*, 71: 907–911.

21. Hauck, H.E., Bund, O., Fischer, M., and Schulz, M. 2001. Ultra-thin layer chromatography (UTLC)—A new dimension in thin-layer chromatography, *J. Planar Chromatogr.*, 14: 234–236.

22. Clark, J.E. and Olesik, S.V. 2009. Technique for ultrathin layer chromatography using an electrospun, nanofibrous stationary phase, *Anal. Chem.*, 81: 412–4129.

23. Oresic, M., Hänninen, V.A., and Vidal-Puig, A. 2008. Lipidomics: A new window to biomedical frontiers, *Trends Biotechnol.*, 26: 647–652.

24. Fahy, E., Cotter, D., Sud, M., and Subramaniam, S. 2011. Lipid classification, structures and tools, *Biochim. Biophys. Acta*, 1811: 637–647.

25. Li, M., Yang, L., Bai, Y., and Liu, H. 2014. Analytical methods in lipidomics and their applications, *Anal. Chem.*, 86: 161–175.

26. Fuchs, B., Schiller, J., Süss, R., Schürenberg, M., and Suckau, D. 2007. A direct and simple method of coupling matrix-assisted laser desorption and ionization time-of-flight mass spectrometry (MALDI-TOF MS) to thin-layer chromatography (TLC) for the analysis of phospholipids from egg yolk, *Anal. Bioanal. Chem.*, 389: 827–834.

27. Stubiger, G., Pittenauer, E., Belgacem, O., Rehulka, P., Widhalm, K., and Allmaier, G. 2009. Analysis of human plasma lipids and soybean lecithin by means of high-performance thin-layer chromatography and matrix-assisted laser desorption/ionization mass spectrometry, *Rapid Commun. Mass Spectrom.*, 23: 2711–2723.

28. Schiller, J., Müller, K., Süss, R., Arnhold, J., Gey, C., Herrmann, A., Lessig J., Arnold, K., and Müller, P. 2003. Analysis of the lipid composition of bull spermatozoa by MALDI-TOF mass spectrometry–A cautionary note, *Chem. Phys. Lipids*, 126: 85–94.

29. Wegener, J., Zschörnig, K., Onischke, K., Fuchs, B., Schiller J., and Müller, K. 2013. Conservation of honey bee (*Apis mellifera*) sperm phospholipids during storage in the bee queen—A TLC/MALDI-TOF MS study, *Exp. Geront.*, 48: 213–222.

30. Eibisch, M., Fuchs, B., Schiller, J., Suß, R., and Teuber, K. 2011. Analysis of phospholipid mixtures from biological tissues by matrix-assisted laser desorption and ionization time-of-flight mass spectrometry (MALDI-TOF MS): A laboratory experiment, *J. Chem. Educ.*, 88: 503–507.

31. Therisod, H., Labas, V., and Caroff, M. 2001. Direct microextraction and analysis of rough-type lipopolysaccharides by combined thin-layer chromatography and MALDI mass spectrometry, *Anal. Chem.*, 73: 3804–3807.

32. Scandroglio, F., Loberto, N., Valsecchi, M., Chigorno, V., Prinetti, A., and Sonnino, S. 2009. Thin layer chromatography of gangliosides, *Glycoconj. J.*, 26: 961–973.

33. Huwiler, A., Kolter, T., Pfeilschifter, J., and Sandhoff, K. 2000. Physiology and pathophysiology of sphingolipid metabolism and signaling, *Biochim. Biophys. Acta*, 1485: 63–99.

34. Musken, A., Souady, J., Dreisewerd, K., Zhang, W., Distler, U., Peter-Katalinic, J., Miller-Podraza, H., Karch, H., and Muthing, J. 2010. Application of thin-layer chromatography/infrared matrix-assisted laser desorption/ionization orthogonal time-of-flight mass spectrometry to structural analysis of bacteria-binding glycosphingolipids selected by affinity detection, *Rapid Commun. Mass Spectrom.*, 24: 1032–1038.

35. Guittard, J., Hronowski, X.L., and Costello, C.E. 1999. Direct matrix-assisted laser desorption/ionization mass spectrometric analysis of glycosphingolipids on thin layer chromatographic plates and transfer membranes, *Rapid Commun. Mass Spectrom.*, 13: 1838–1849.

36. Distler, U., Hülsewig, M., Souady, J., Dreisewerd, K., Haier, J., Senninger, N., Friedrich, A.W. et al. 2008. Matching IR-MALDI-o-TOF Mass spectrometry with the TLC overlay binding assay and its clinical application for tracing tumor-associated glycosphingolipids in hepatocellular and pancreatic cancer, *Anal. Chem.* 80: 1835–1846.

37. Kouzel, I.U., Pirkl, A., Pohlentz, G., Soltwisch, J., Dreisewerd, K., Karch, H., and Müthing, J. 2014. Progress in detection and structural characterization of glycosphingolipids in crude lipid extracts by enzymatic phospholipid disintegration combined with thin-layer chromatography immune detection and IR-MALDI mass spectrometry, *Anal. Chem.*, 86: 1215–1222.

38. Ruh, H., Sandhoff, R., Meyer, B., Gretz, N., and Hopf, C. 2013. Quantitative characterization of tissue globotetraosylceramides in a rat model of polycystic kidney disease by primadrop sample preparation and indirect high-performance thin layer chromatography-matrix-assisted laser desorption/ionization-time-of flight-mass spectrometry with automated data acquisition, *Anal. Chem.*, 85: 6233–6240.

39. Ivleva, V.B., Elkin, Y.N., Budnik, B.A., Moyer, S.C., O'Connor, P.B., and Costello, C.E. 2004. Coupling thin-layer chromatography with vibrational cooling matrix-assisted laser desorption/ionization fourier transform mass spectrometry for the analysis of ganglioside mixtures, *Anal. Chem.*, 76: 6484–6491.

40. Ivleva, V.B., Sapp, L.M., O'Connor, P.B., and Costello, C.E. 2005. Ganglioside analysis by thin-layer chromatography matrix-assisted laser desorption/ionization orthogonal time-of-flight mass spectrometry, *J. Am. Soc. Mass Spectrom.*, 16: 1552–1560.

41. Dreisewerd, K., Müthing, J., Rohlfing, A., Meisen, I., Vukelić, Z., Peter-Katalinić, J., Hillenkamp, F., and Berkenkamp, S. 2005. Analysis of gangliosides directly from thin-layer chromatography plates by infrared matrix-assisted laser desorption/ionization orthogonal time-of-flight mass spectrometry with a glycerol matrix, *Anal. Chem.*, 77: 4098–4107.

42. Kuwayama, K., Tsujikawa, K., Miyaguchi, H., Kanamori, T., Iwata, Y.T., and Inoue, H. 2012. Rapid, simple, and highly sensitive analysis of drugs in biological samples using thin-layer chromatography coupled with matrix-assisted laser desorption/ionization mass spectrometry, *Anal. Bioanal. Chem.*, 402: 1257–1267.

43. Crecelius, A., Clench, M.R., Richards, D.S., Evason, D., and Parr, V. 2002. Thin-layer chromatography-postsource-decay matrix-assisted laser desorption/ionization time-of-flight mass spectrometry of small drug molecules, *J. Chromatogr. Sci.*, 40: 614–620.

44. Salo, P.K., Salomies, H., Harju, K., Ketola, R.A., Kotiaho, T., Yli-Kauhaluoma, J., and Kostiainen, R. 2005. Analysis of small molecules by ultra thin-layer chromatography-atmospheric pressure matrix-assisted laser desorption/ionization mass spectrometry, *J. Am. Soc. Mass Spectrom.*, 16: 906–915.

45. Salo, P.K., Vilmunen, S., Salomies, H., Ketola, R.A., and Kostiainen, R. 2007. Two-dimensional ultra-thin-layer chromatography and atmospheric pressure matrix-assisted laser desorption/ionization mass spectrometry in bioanalysis, *Anal. Chem.*, 79: 2101–2108.

46 Dreisewerd, K., Kölbl, S., Peter-Katalinić, J., Berkenkamp, S., and Pohlentz, G. 2006. Analysis of native milk oligosaccharides directly from thin-layer chromatography plates by matrix-assisted laser desorption/ionization orthogonal-time-of-flight mass spectrometry with a glycerol matrix, *J. Am. Soc. Mass Spectrom.*, 17: 139–150.

47. Nimptsch, K., Süss, R., Riemer, T., Nimptsch, A., Schnabelrauch, M., and Schiller, J. 2010. Differently complex oligosaccharides can be easily identified by matrix-assisted laser desorption and ionization time-of-flight mass spectrometry directly from a standard thin-layer chromatography plate, *J. Chromatogr. A*, 1217: 3711–3715.

48. Qureshi, M.N., Stecher, G., Huck, C., and Bonn, G.K. 2010. Online coupling of thin layer chromatography with matrix-assisted laser desorption/ionization time-of-flight mass spectrometry: Synthesis and application of a new material for the identification of carbohydrates by thin layer chromatography/matrix free material enhanced laser desorption/ionization mass spectrometry, *Rapid Commun. Mass Spectrom.*, 24: 2759–2764.

49. Santos, L.S., Haddad, R., Höehr, N.F., Pilli, R.A., and Eberlin, M.N. 2004. Fast screening of low molecular weight compounds by thin-layer chromatography and "on-spot" MALDI-TOF mass spectrometry, *Anal. Chem.*, 76: 2144–2147.

50. Chen, C.C., Yang, Y.L., Ou, C.L., Chou, C.H., Liaw, C.C., and Lin, P.C. 2013. Direct monitoring of chemical transformations by combining thin layer chromatography with nanoparticle-assisted laser desorption/ionization mass spectrometry. *Analyst*, 138: 1379–1385.

51. St Hilaire, P.M., Cipolla, L., Tedebark, U., and Meldal, M. 1998. Analysis of organic reactions by thin layer chromatography combined with matrix-assisted laser desorption/ionization time-of-flight mass spectrometry, *Rapid Commun. Mass Spectrom.*, 12: 1475–1484.

52. Hsu, F.L., Chen, C.H., Yuan, C.H., and Shiea, J. 2003. Interfaces to connect thin-layer chromatography with electrospray ionization mass spectrometry, *Anal. Chem.*, 75: 2493–2498.

53. Cheng, S.C., Huang, M.Z., and Shiea, J. 2009. Thin-layer chromatography/laser-induced acoustic desorption/electrospray ionization mass spectrometry, *Anal. Chem.*, 81: 9274–9281.

54. Van Berkel, G.J., Sanchez, A.D., and Quirke, J.M.E. 2002. Thin-layer chromatography and electrospray mass spectrometry coupled using a surface sampling probe, *Anal. Chem.*, 74: 6216–6223.

55. Ford, M.J., Deibel, M.A., Tomkins, B.A., and Van Berkel, G.J. 2005. Quantitative thin-layer chromatography/mass spectrometry analysis of caffeine using a surface sampling probe electrospray ionization tandem mass spectrometry system, *Anal. Chem.*, 77: 4385–4389.

56. Chai, W., Leteux, C., Lawson, A.M., and Stoll, M.S. 2003. On-line overpressure thin-layer chromatographic separation and electrospray mass spectrometric detection of glycolipids, *Anal. Chem.*, 75: 118–125.

57. Rothenhöfera, M., Scherüblb, R., Bernhardta, G., Heilmannb, J., and Buschauer, A. 2012. Qualitative and quantitative analysis of hyaluronan oligosaccharides with high performance thin layer chromatography using reagent-free derivatization on amino-modified silica and electrospray ionization-quadrupole time-of-flight mass spectrometry coupling on normal phase, *J. Chromatogr. A*, 1248: 169–177.

58. Chen, Y. and Schwack, W. 2014. Rapid and selective determination of multi-sulfonamides by high-performance thin layer chromatography coupled to fluorescent densitometry and electrospray ionization mass detection, *J. Chromatogr. A*, 1331: 108–116.

59. Himmelsbach, M., Waser, M., and Klampfl, C.W. 2014. Thin layer chromatography-spray mass spectrometry: A method for easy identification of synthesis products and UV filters from TLC aluminum foils, *Anal. Bioanal. Chem.*, 406: 3647–3656.

60. Naumoska, K. and Vovk, I. 2015. Analysis of triterpenoids and phytosterols in vegetables by thin-layer chromatography coupled to tandem mass spectrometry, *J. Chromatogr. A*, 1381: 229–238.

61. Takats, Z., Wiseman, J. M., Golagan, B., and Cooks, R.G. 2004. Mass spectrometry sampling under ambient conditions with desorption electrospray ionization, *Science*, 306: 471–473.

62. Van Berkel, G.J., Ford, M.J., and Deibel, M.A. 2005. Thin-layer chromatography and mass spectrometry coupled using desorption electrospray ionization, *Anal. Chem.*, 77: 1207–1215.

63. Van Berkel, G.J. and Kertesz, V. 2006. Automated sampling and imaging of analytes separated on thin-layer chromatography plates using desorption electrospray ionization mass spectrometry, *Anal. Chem.*, 78: 4938–4944.

64. Van Berkel, G.J., Tomkins, B.A., and Kertesz, V. 2007. Thin-layer chromatography/desorption electrospray ionization mass spectrometry: Investigation of goldenseal alkaloids, *Anal. Chem.*, 79: 2778–2789.

65. Harry, E.L., Reynolds, J.C., Bristow, A.W., Wilson, I.D., and Creaser, C.S. 2009. Direct analysis of pharmaceutical formulations from non-bonded reversed-phase thin-layer chromatography plates by desorption electrospray ionisation ion mobility mass spectrometry, *Rapid Commun. Mass Spectrom.*, 23: 2597–2604.

66. Kennedy, J.H. and Wiseman, J.M. 2010. Direct analysis of *Salvia divinorum* leaves for salvinorin A by thin layer chromatography and desorption electrospray ionization multistage tandem mass spectrometry, *Rapid Commun. Mass Spectrom.*, 24: 1305–1311.

67. Paglia, G., Ifa, D.R., Wu, C., Corso, G., and Cooks, R.G. 2010. Desorption electrospray ionization mass spectrometry analysis of lipids after two-dimensional high-performance thin-layer chromatography partial separation, *Anal. Chem.*, 82: 1744–1750.

68. Han, Y., Levkin, P., Abarientos, I., Liu, H., Svec, F., and Fréchet, J.M. 2010. Monolithic superhydrophobic polymer layer with photopatterned virtual channel for the separation of peptides using two-dimensional thin layer chromatography–desorption electrospray ionization mass spectrometry, *Anal. Chem.*, 82: 2520–2528.

69. Lin, S.Y., Huang, M.Z., Chang, H.C., and Shiea, J. 2007. Using electrospray-assisted laser desorption/ionization mass spectrometry to characterize organic compounds separated on thin-layer chromatography plates, *Anal. Chem.*, 79: 8789–8795.

70. Cheng, S.C., Huang, M.Z., Wu, L.C., Chou, C.C., Cheng, C.N., Jhang, S.S., and Shiea, J. 2012. Building blocks for the development of an interface for high-throughput thin layer chromatography/ambient mass spectrometric analysis: A green methodology, *Anal. Chem.*, 84: 5864–5868.

71. Tames, F., Watson, I.D., Morden, W., and Wilson, I.D. 1999. Detection and identification of morphine in urine extracts using thin-layer chromatography and tandem mass spectrometry, *J. Chromatogr. B*, 729: 341–346.

72. Weyermann, C., Marquis, R., Mazzella, W., and Spengler, B. 2007. Differentiation of blue ballpoint pen inks by laser desorption ionization mass spectrometry and high-performance thin-layer chromatography, *J. Forensic Sci.*, 52: 216–220.

73. Haddad, R., Milagre, H.M.S., Catharino, R.R., and Eberlin, M.N. 2008. Easy ambient sonic-spray ionization mass spectrometry combined with thin-layer chromatography, *Anal. Chem.*, 80: 2744–2750.

74. Zhang, J., Zhou, Z., Yang, J., Zhang, W., Bai, Y., and Liu, H. 2012. Thin layer chromatography/plasma assisted multiwavelength laser desorption ionization mass spectrometry for facile separation and selective identification of low molecular weight compounds, *Anal. Chem.*, 84: 1496–1503.

# 16 Application of TLC–MS to Analysis of Drugs of Abuse

*Bruno D. Sabino, Amadeu Cardoso Jr.,
and Wanderson Romão*

## CONTENTS

## 16.1 CANNABINOID ANALYSIS

In analysis of the primary cannabinoids (Δ9-tetrahydrocannabinol, cannabidiol, and cannabinol) in marijuana samples (*Cannabis sativa* L.), diverse eluent systems have been described in the literature for use in chromatographic runs, such as ethyl acetate:methanol:water:concentrated ammonium (12:5:0.5:1), toluene:chloroform (7:3), and *n*-hexane:diethyl ether (80:20) [1]. The detection of cannabinoids can be accomplished using diverse diazonium salts, such as Fast Blue B, or with Duquenois–Levine reagent (Table 16.1) [2]. The limit of detection (LOD) varies from 2 to 10 ng mL$^{-1}$ (Figure 16.1).

## 16.2 OPIATE ANALYSIS

Opiates include heroin (obtained from morphine), morphine, and codeine. In the analysis of heroin, opium, and morphine, 5 mg of the sample should be dissolved in 1 mL

## TABLE 16.1
## Reagents Used in the Identification of Natural Sources Compounds

| Reagent | Application | Reagent Description | Staining |
|---|---|---|---|
| Dragendorff | Alcaloids (cocaine and opiates) | Bismuth subnitrate<br>Concentrated acetic acid (glacial)<br>Potassium iodide | Varies according to the compound |
| Fast Blue B | Cannabinoids | Sodium hydroxide solution<br>Fast Blue B salt<br>Chloroform | Bright red |
| Duquenois | Cannabinoids | Acetaldehyde—vaniline<br>Concentrated chloridric acid<br>Chloroform | Bluish purple |
| Acidified platinum iodine | Alkaloids (cocaine and opiates) | Platinum chloride<br>Potassium iodide<br>Concentrated chloridric acid | Varies according to the compound |
| Marquis | Aromatics | Acetic acid solution—formaldehyde<br>Concentrated sulfuric acid | Varies according to the compound |
| Ehrilich | LSD | p-Dimethylaminobenzaldehyde<br>Concentrated orthophosphoric acid | Purple |
| Scott | Cocaine | Cobalt thiocyanate (II) solution<br>Concentrated chloridric acid<br>chloroform | In the presence of cocaine turns from pink to blue |

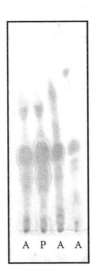

**FIGURE 16.1**  Analysis of a *C. sativa* extract by TLC (silica). Elution system comprising toluene:chloroform 7:3. Revealing: FBS. Carmine blots indicate the presence of cannabinoids. P = standard and A = sample.

of methanol and 1–5 μL aliquots should be spotted on the chromatographic plate. The following elution systems have been used for chromatographic runs: toluene:acetone:methanol:concentrated ammonium (45:45:7:3); ethyl acetate:methanol:concentrated ammonium (85:10:5); and methanol:concentrated ammonium (100:1.5). Alternatively, a combination of two different elution systems could be used to facilitate optimal separation. For example, ethyl acetate:isopropylalcohol:ammonium (80:15:3:8) or 1,2-dichloroethane:isopropyl alcohol:methanol:ammonium (20:20:20:7) have been utilized. The LOD of opiates when using platinum iodide varies from 100 to 500 ng mL$^{-1}$ depending on the compound that is being analyzed [3].

## 16.3  LYSERGIC ACID DIETHYLAMIDE ANALYSIS

In the qualitative analysis of seized samples that are suspected to have the semisynthetic substance lysergic acid diethylamide (LSD) (blotters or papers) via chromatographic techniques, simple extraction of this compound with methanol is sufficient, in general. The sample that is suspected to contain LSD should be mixed for 30 s with enough methanol in order to obtain a concentration of about 1 mg of LSD per mL of solution. After filtration, the extract can be spotted directly on the chromatographic plate. The following elution systems can be used in chromatographic runs: toluene:methanol (90:10); and chloroform:acetone (20:80) [1]. The detection of LSD can be carried out using Ehrilich's reagent (Table 16.1) [2].

## 16.4  COCAINE ANALYSIS

In the identification of products that are suspected to contain illicit compounds, the use of reference materials (controls) for the main compounds analyzed, as well as for the main adulterants that could be present, is recommended. As an example, seized cocaine samples could have the following adulterants: caffeine, lidocaine, benzocaine, ketamine, and procaine among others. The samples and controls used in chromatographic runs can be dissolved in methanol at a final concentration of 1 mg mL$^{-1}$. The chemical form of the controls (i.e., freebase or salt) that will be spotted on the plates is not important. Both forms are acceptable because the compounds always move as freebases on TLC plates [3].

The following elution systems can be used in chromatographic runs: chloroform:dioxane:ethylacetate:ammonium (29% solution) (25:60:10:5); methanol:ammonium (29% solution) (100:1.5); and cyclohexane:toluene:diethylamine (75:15:10). The plates must be dried prior to use. This could be done at room temperature or using hot air. With the application of hot air, caution must be exercised in case thermally sensitive compounds are present in the sample. In order to ensure the correct progress of color reactions, it is crucial that traces of ammonium or other bases be removed from the plate [1]. The detection of cocaine can be carried out using a UV lamp at 254 nm, acidified platinum iodine reagent, or Dragendorff's reagent (Table 16.1) [2].

Recently, our group developed a method for the analysis of cocaine mixed with adulterants (benzocaine, lidocaine, and caffeine) using two-dimensional TLC. In this technique, two different elution systems were utilized in sequence, in order to

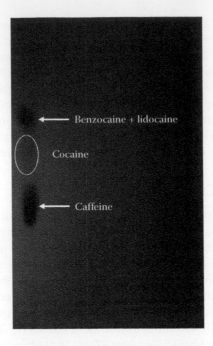

**FIGURE 16.2**  Analysis of cocaine by TLC (silica) with an elution system comprising acetone 100%. Revealing: UV lamp at 254 nm.

optimize the separation of the analytes. Initially, the chromatographic run was carried out using 100% acetone (system 1) (Figure 16.2). However, this chromatographic system did not allow for the adequate separation of benzocaine and lidocaine (Table 16.2). Thus, a two-dimensional run was conducted on the same plate, using elution system 2, which was composed of $CHCl_3$:methanol (9:1) (Figure 16.3).

The use of elution system 1 followed by elution system 2 led to the adequate separation of benzocaine and lidocaine and from all other analytes (Table 16.3). Thus, this two-dimensional system was adequate for the analysis of cocaine mixed with adulterants. Figure 16.4 shows a picture of the chromatoplate used in the two-dimensional system; the analytes were isolated using the following systems: modified Dragendorff (bismuth carbonate solution + concentrated HCl + potassium

**TABLE 16.2**

**Retention Factor ($R_f$) of Analytes Using the Elution System 1 (Acetone 100%)**

| Analyte | Retention Factor ($R_f$) |
| --- | --- |
| Cocaine | 0.59 |
| Lidocaine | 0.70 |
| Benzocaine | 0.70 |
| Caffeine | 0.40 |

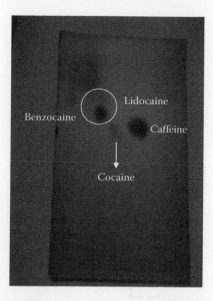

**FIGURE 16.3** TLC cocaine analysis (silica) with an elution system comprised by methanol 9:1. Revealing: UV lamp at 254 nm.

**TABLE 16.3**
**Retention Factor ($R_f$) of Analytes When Using the Elution System 1 (Acetone 100%) Followed by Elution System 2 (CHCl$_3$:MeOH 9:1)**

| Analyte | Retention Factor ($R_f$) |
| --- | --- |
| Cocaine | 0.61 |
| Lidocaine | 0.80 |
| Benzocaine | 0.70 |
| Caffeine | 0.65 |

iodide) for cocaine, lidocaine, and caffeine; and diazotization using β-naphthol for benzocaine.

## 16.5 AMBIENT IONIZATION MASS SPECTROMETRY APPLIED TO THIN-LAYER CHROMATOGRAPHY ANALYSIS

This chapter highlights various ionization techniques that can be conducted under atmospheric conditions for the analysis of drugs of abuse and controlled substances, with particular emphasis on TLC, a technique in which mixtures are separated on a thin layer of an adsorbent material. Recent advances in chromatography, such as planar chromatography coupled to MS, have allowed for significant progress in the field [4].

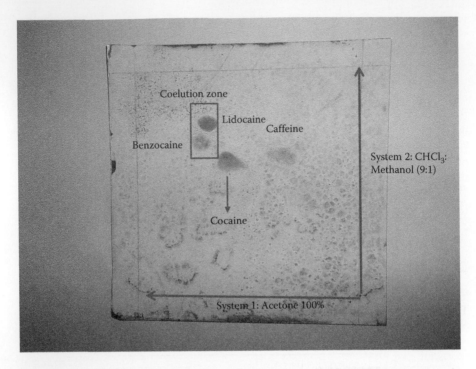

**FIGURE 16.4** Chromatoplate picture after elution with two-dimensional system and revelation with modified Dragendorff (bismuth carbonate solution + potassium iodide +concentrated HCl) for cocaine, lidocaine caffeine; followed by revelation with diazotization reaction by using β-naphthol for benzocaine.

The detection of several drugs of abuse and metabolites in biological matrices using desorption ionization (DESI) has been reported in the literature; for example, amphetamines, opiates, cannabinoids, and benzodiazepines were analyzed in urine [5]. In this study, very low concentrations (picograms) of the material were analyzed, thus demonstrating the high sensitivity of the technique. Moreover, DESI was revealed to be a very powerful tool for the analysis of analytes in complex biological matrices, in which the analytes were only present in trace amounts. According to the authors, the use of a higher proportion of polar solvents facilitated the acquisition of polar analytes such as benzodiazepines, while the use of less polar solvents allowed for the detection of less polar substances such as morphine and codeine, both of which are opiates. Notably, methamphetamine monitoring in raw urine using DESI–MS analysis was also reported. The mass spectra revealed numerous sodium and potassium adducts, owing to the high concentration of electrolytes present in this kind of matrix [6]. The analysis of anabolic steroid esters in hair also was reported using a simplified ultrasonic liquid extraction procedure [7].

Leuthold et al. analyzed illicit ecstasy tablets and powders using a homemade DESI system. The samples were submitted to pneumatically assisted electrospray without pretreatment. The authors showed that the nonhomogeneous surface led to distinct mass spectra, suggesting that DESI could be used for imaging. A notable feature of the mass spectra acquired by DESI–MS is the presence of ions, which result from the protonation or deprotonation of certain molecules [8].

DESI–MS is an alternative and powerful tool employed in the analysis of seized materials for the qualitative identification of the components and profile definition. Stojanovska et al. [9] analyzed seized cocaine samples and revealed that this technique could also be used to determine the geographic origin of the drug, that is, Bolivia, Peru, or Columbia. Truxilines extracted from *Erythroxylum coca* leaves during the refining process also can be used to identify the drug production region. In this study, adulterants including caffeine, procaine, levamisole, lignocaine, and paracetamol were also investigated. Using DESI–MS, seized samples were screened, the active ingredients were easily detected, and various adulterants were identified [9].

DESI mass ionization was coupled to TLC. In this study, rhodamine dyes were separated using reverse-phase hydrophobic C8 plates. In this technique, a spray containing charged droplets of a solvent is directed to a certain spot on the chromatographic plate. Then, the solvent impacts the TLC adsorbent and desorption and ionization of the components occurs on the plate. Selective reaction monitoring (SRM) mode was employed during the acquisition of the mass spectra. Moreover, medications containing acetaminophen, aspirin, and caffeine were also analyzed; they were separated on a normal-phase silica gel plate and data acquisition was subsequently carried out in positive-ion full-scan mode [10].

Another ionization technique that can be carried out under atmospheric conditions and is utilized for direct analysis in real time is DART–MS. Similar to DESI–MS, samples do not require pretreatment, and thus, the time required for DART–MS analysis decreases. The DART ion source has been used to analyze a number of substances such as drugs in seized materials and biological fluids, dyes and inks, food, and environmental compounds. All of these analytes can be ionized directly on surfaces such as glass, TLC plates, concrete, and paper [11].

Several applications of forensic science were reported. Methilenedioxymethamphetamine (MDMA) was detected by placing ecstasy pills in front of the DART ion source. Ropero Miller et al. characterized 25 cocaine samples acquired by local police. The use of DART–MS allowed for the detection of adulterants and other components, thus generating a complete profile of the samples [12,13].

The first use of TLC–DART–MS was described in the analysis of milk products [14]. Since then, innovations in ionization techniques under atmospheric conditions were made, which led to increased precision in the quantitative assessment of substances present on TLC plates. Currently, a new version of DART–MS is available in which the angle of the carrier gas flow can be adjusted and a motorized rail can be used to adjust the position of the ion source toward spots on the TLC plates [15]. TLC–DART–MS also has been used for the detection of organophosphorus in fatty foods [16].

There are reports in the literature regarding cocaine and methadone analysis in urine for antidoping programs. In the procedure described by Rodriguez-Lafuente, Mirnaghi, and Pawliszyn, solid-phase microextraction (SPME) was employed as a sample preparation technique for matrix cleanup prior to analysis using DART–MS; the use of SPME reduced the possibility of adducts due to salts present in urine [17]. Analysis of cocaine and its metabolites in seized samples and biological matrices is very well documented [18,19].

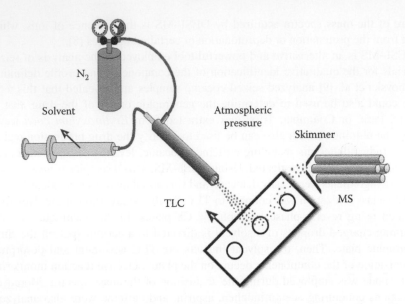

**FIGURE 16.5** Schematic of the TLC/EASI–MS system in operation to analysis of ecstasy tablets. (From Sabino, B.D. et al. 2010. *Braz. J. Anal. Chem.*, 1: 6–11. With permission.)

A set of designer drugs has been produced to circumvent legal restrictions and generate structural analogs with psychoactive effects similar to the parent drugs available in illicit markets. In addition, the lack of uniform methods for the detection of designer drugs presents a great challenge. Musah et al. utilized DART–MS for the direct identification of trace synthetic cannabinoids in a botanical matrix without prior extraction, which allowed for a simple and rapid analysis with high sensitivity [20].

Among the available ionization/desorption techniques, easy ambient sonic spray ionization (EASI) (originally termed desorption sonic spray ionization) is one of the most simple, gentle, and easily implemented methods. An EASI source can be constructed and installed in a few minutes using common MS parts (Figure 16.5 for analysis performed directly on TLC plate). It does not require high voltage, UV lights, laser beams, corona or glow discharges, or heating. Compressed $N_2$ is used to form a supersonic spray [21]. EASI was developed by Eberlin et al. [21] and has been successfully applied in the analysis of various analytes in matrices such as ecstasy, m-CPP, and ecstasy tablets [22,23], as well as LSD [24] and cocaine samples [25], banknotes [26], perfumes [27], surfactants [28], and biodiesel [29].

### 16.5.1 QUALITATIVE THIN-LAYER CHROMATOGRAPHY–EASY AMBIENT SONIC SPRAY IONIZATION ANALYSIS OF SEIZED ECSTASY TABLETS

Ecstasy is the common name for 3,4-methylenedioxymethamphetamine (MDMA). MDMA is a methamphetamine derivative and is also know on the streets as "candy,"

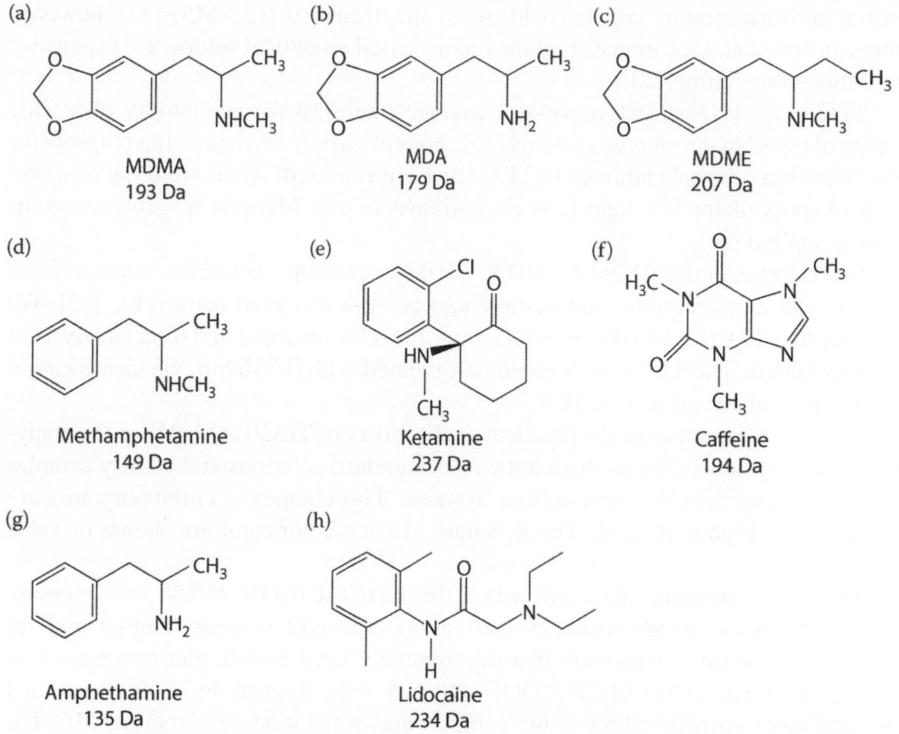

(a)

MDMA
193 Da

(b)

MDA
179 Da

(c)

MDME
207 Da

(d)

Methamphetamine
149 Da

(e)

Ketamine
237 Da

(f)

Caffeine
194 Da

(g)

Amphetamine
135 Da

(h)

Lidocaine
234 Da

**FIGURE 16.6** Structures of compounds normally found in ecstasy tablets. (From Sabino, B.D. et al. 2010. *Braz. J. Anal. Chem.*, 1: 6–11. With permission.)

"XTC," and "Adam" [22]. Its name is effectively used with a nonselective form and is applied to 3,4-methylenedioxyamphetamine (MDA), and to 3,4-methylenedioxy-ethylamphetamine (MDEA) that is also known on the streets as "Eve." These three compounds are quite similar in their chemical compositions and biological effects [23]. Their structures and *m/z* values are shown in Figure 16.6a–c.

Ecstasy tablets sometimes contain other amphetamine analogs such as methamphetamine (Figure 16.6d) and other psychoactive substances including ketamine (Figure 16.6e). Ecstasy pills come in different colors and with different logos; they commonly contain other substances such as caffeine (Figure 16.6f), amphetamine (Figure 16.6g), and lidocaine (Figure 16.6h), as well as other adulterants.

Normally, the identification of ecstasy-like drugs is carried out in laboratories using ecstasy pill testing kits, which often make use of the Marquis, Nitroprusside, or Scott tests. In the Marquis test, the drug is tested using a reagent kit producing a dark blue or black color [22]. However, these are nonspecific analyses, and false-positive results can occasionally occur [30]. Other techniques have been used to confirm the results of these tests such as gas chromatography–nitrogen-phosphorous detection (GC–NPD) [31], gas chromatography coupled with mass spectrometry (GC–MS) [32], high-performance liquid chromatography with fluorometric detection [33], and liquid chromatography coupled with mass spectrometry (LC–MS) [34]; however, these instrumental techniques require sophisticated analytical setups, are expensive, and time-consuming [22].

TLC is a low-cost and versatile technique owing to the availability of a wide range of possible developing systems [35]. A great variety of visualizing reagents for the detection of amphetamines in TLC has been reported. Apart from the observation of spots under UV light (254 nm), ninhydrin and Marquis reagents are commonly applied [36].

Several standards (MDMA, MDA, MDME, caffeine, ketamine, methamphetamine, and amphetamine) and ecstasy tablets were analyzed using TLC [23]. We developed a TLC/EASI–MS system (Figure 16.6) for the rapid and direct analysis of ecstasy tablets. The TLC results could be validated with EASI/MS, via identification of the spots observed in TLC [23].

In order to demonstrate the practical applicability of TLC/EASI–MS in the analysis of ecstasy tablets, we evaluated the $R_f$ of standard solutions and ecstasy samples obtained using four different solvent systems. The composite chromatograms are presented in Figure 16.7a–d. The $R_f$ values of each compound are shown in Table 16.4 [23].

The chromatogram obtained using the $CHCl_3$:$CH_3OH$ (50:50 v%) system, shown in Figure 16.7a, exhibited spot tailing for most ecstasy samples and for the main standards, suggesting that this routinely used mobile phase was not viable. Using $CHCl_3$:$CH_3OH$:$CH_3COOH$ (20:75/5 v%) (Figure 16.7b), we obtained defined spots corresponding to the samples and standards; nevertheless, MDMA, methamphetamine, amphetamine, and ketamine standards presented similar $R_f$ values (0.62–0.71). Therefore, this system was also rejected. The best results were obtained with $CH_3OH$:$NH_4OH$ (98/2 v%) and $CH_3CH(CH_3)OH$:$CH_3OH$ (95:5 v%) as mobile phases; the chromatograms are shown in Figure 16.7c and d. Although we

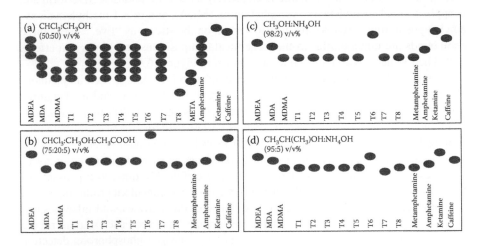

**FIGURE 16.7** Chromatograms of MDEA, MDA, MDMA, metamphetamine, amphetamine, ketamine, and caffeine standards; and ecstasy tablets (tablets from T1 to T8). (From Sabino, B.D. et al. 2010. *J. Anal. Chem.*, 1: 6–11. With permission.)

**TABLE 16.4**

$R_f$ **Values of Standards Using Thin-Layer Chromatography**

| Compound | CHCl$_3$:CH$_3$OH (50:50) v/v% | CHCl$_3$:CH$_3$OH: CH$_3$COOH (75:20:5) v/v% | CH$_3$OH: NH$_4$OH (98:2) v/v% | CH$_3$CH(CH$_3$) OH:NH$_4$OH (95:5) v/v% |
|---|---|---|---|---|
| MDEA | 0.62 | 0.74 | 0.71 | 0.87 |
| MDA | 0.48 | 0.60 | 0.67 | 0.81 |
| MDMA | 0.37 | 0.64 | 0.56 | 0.62 |
| Metamphetamine | 0.35 | 0.62 | 0.57 | 0.62 |
| Amphetamine | 0.71 | 0.66 | 0.66 | 0.70 |
| Ketamine | 0.86 | 0.71 | 0.84 | 0.80 |
| Caffeine | 0.84 | 0.94 | 0.77 | 0.70 |

*Source:* From Sabino, B.D. et al. 2010. *Braz. J. Anal. Chem.*, 1: 6–11. With permission.

observed similar $R_f$ values for MDMA (main active substance present in ecstasy tablets) and methamphetamine in all mobile phases tested, CH$_3$OH:NH$_4$OH (98:2 v%) and CH$_3$CH(CH$_3$)OH:NH$_4$OH (95:5 v%) facilitated the separation and resolution of the other compounds (MDA, MDEA, amphetamine, ketamine, and caffeine). The $R_f$ values are presented in Table 16.4 [23]. For the TLC/EASI–MS measurements, we used CH$_3$OH:NH$_4$OH (98:2 v%) (Figure 16.7c), which resulted in the best separation factor among the studied substances.

Figure 16.8a–g shows that the TLC/EASI–MS results corresponded to the spots of the standards: MDEA molecule protonated ([M+H]$^+$: $m/z$ 208) and Na$^+$ adduct ([M+Na]$^+$: $m/z$ 230), Figure 16.8a; MDA ([M+H]$^+$: $m/z$ 180) Figure 16.8b; MDMA (M+H]$^+$: $m/z$ 194) together with its characteristic fragments ($m/z$ 163 and 135) Figure 16.8c; methamphetamine (M+H]$^+$: $m/z$ 150) together with its characteristic fragment ($m/z$ 91) that corresponds to a tropylium ion, Figure 16.8d; amphetamine (M+H]$^+$: $m/z$ 136), Figure 16.8e; ketamine (M+H]$^+$: $m/z$ 237), Figure 16.8f; and caffeine (M+H]$^+$: $m/z$ 195), Figure 16.8g. Notably, caffeine exhibited lower ionization efficiency due to the low signal-to-noise ratio. The polarity of caffeine increased its interaction with the TLC system, making the desorption/ionization process more difficult [23].

Figure 16.9a shows the TLC/EASI–MS results for the spot corresponding to tablet 1 (T1), which was positive for MDMA ($m/z$ 194 and $m/z$ 423 [24]) and thus confirms that MDMA and methamphetamine exhibited the same $R_f$ in this solvent system (see Figure 16.7c). These results highlight the importance of coupling TLC and EASI–MS for a fast and conclusive analysis. Similar results were obtained for all other tablets (T2–T5 and T7–T8), except for T6, which showed an $R_f$ value that was similar to those of caffeine and ketamine.

On analysis of T6 by TLC/EASI–MS, it was revealed that no signal corresponded to MDMA, caffeine, or ketamine (Figure 16.9b). However, GC–MS revealed the presence of caffeine, as was indicated in the TLC. The retention time and respective mass spectrum characteristic of caffeine compound corresponded to those obtained for the caffeine standard solution (data not shown) [23].

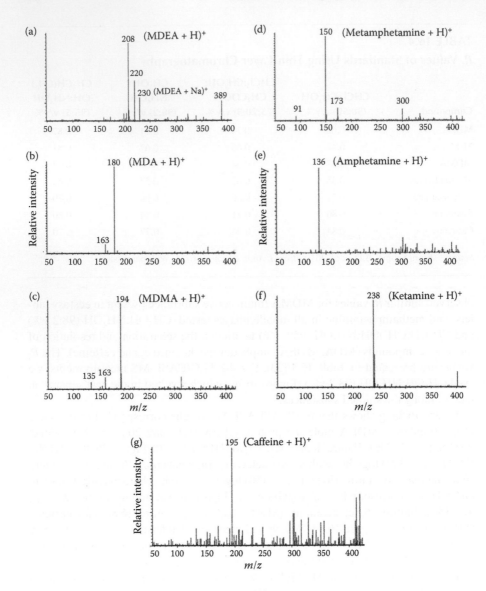

**FIGURE 16.8**   EASI–MS/TLC system using $NH_4OH:CH_3OH$ (98:2 v%) mobile phase for standards: (a) MDEA, (b) MDA, (c) MDMA, (d) metamphetamine, (e) amphetamine, (f) ketamine, and (g) caffeine. (From Sabino, B.D. et al. 2010. *Braz. J. Anal. Chem.*, 1: 6–11. With permission.)

### 16.5.2   QUALITATIVE THIN-LAYER CHROMATOGRAPHY–EASY AMBIENT SONIC SPRAY IONIZATION ANALYSIS OF SEIZED COCAINE AND CRACK COCAINE

Whole cocaine, which is available in the clandestine market, can be obtained from the leaves of *Erithroxylumcoca*, via extraction with organic solvents followed by various treatments including potassium permanganate, liquid–liquid extraction, and

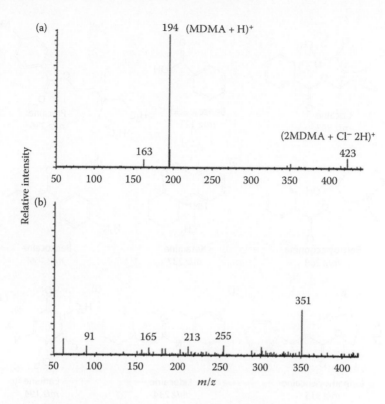

**FIGURE 16.9** EASI–MS/TLC for spots of ecstasy tablets: (a) T1 and (b) T6. (From Sabino, B.D. et al. 2010. *Braz. J. Anal. Chem.*, 1: 6–11. With permission.)

a final conversion from the freebase form to hydrochloride cocaine. Crack is a combination of cocaine hydrochloride, baking soda, and other adulterants, which produce a rock-like substance [25].

Adulterants are compounds with similar pharmacological, sensorial, and physical/chemical properties of the drug to which they are added, in order to simulate its effects. On the other hand, diluents are organic or inorganic compounds with no significant pharmacological properties, which are intentionally added to the street drug to dilute the active ingredient and increase the volume and weight of the product to be trafficked [25]. Illicit samples of cocaine are rarely pure. Figure 16.10a–i shows the chemical structure of cocaine (Figure 16.10a), impurities that may arise during manufacturing (benzoylecgonine [Figure 16.10b], cinnamoylcocaine [Figure 16.10c], and benzoic acid [Figure 16.10d]), adulterants including local anesthetics (lidocaine [Figure 16.10f], procaine [Figure 16.10g], and benzocaine [Figure 16.10h]), and other central nervous system (CNS) active drugs such as ketamine (Figure 16.10e) and caffeine (Figure 16.10i), which are usually sold in addition to or in place of cocaine in illicit markets [25,37].

Normally, the identification of cocaine and crack cocaine is accomplished in a laboratory using cocaine-testing kits, which often make use of the Scott Ruybal test [25].

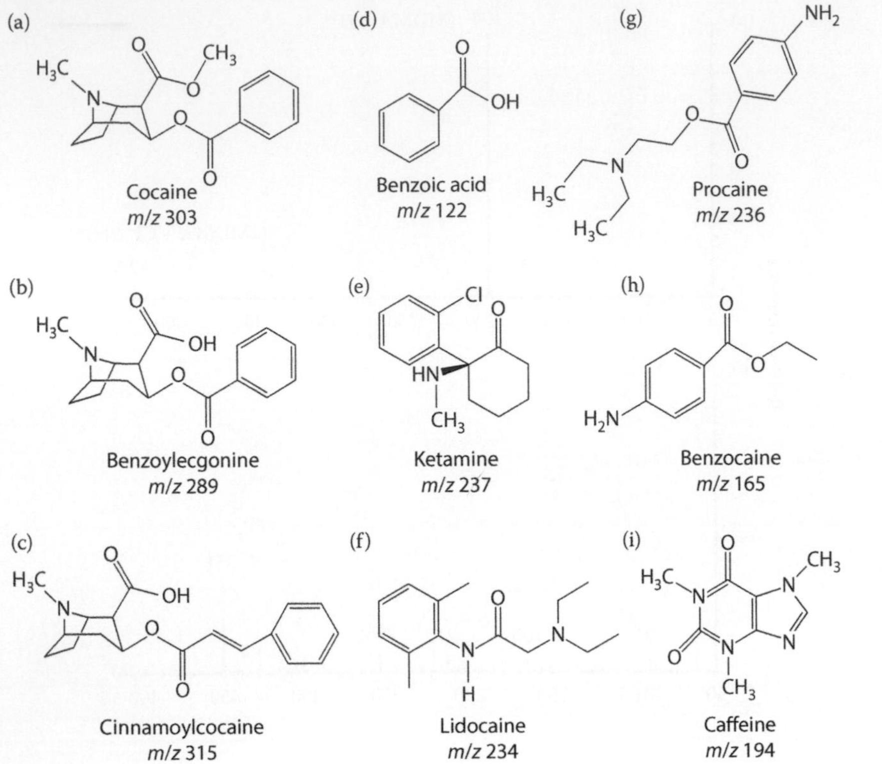

**FIGURE 16.10** Structures of compounds normally found in cocaine samples: (a) cocaine, (b) benzoylecgonine, (c) cinnamoylcocaine, (d) benzoic acid, (e) ketamine, (f) lidocaine, (g) procaine, (h) benzocaine, and (i) caffeine. (From Sabino, B.D. et al. 2011. *Am. J. Anal. Chem.*, 2: 658–664. With permission.)

In order to demonstrate the practical applicability of TLC/EASI–MS in the analysis of cocaine, we evaluated the $R_f$ values of the standard solutions and cocaine samples obtained with two different solvent systems (Figure 16.11a and b). Specifically, we analyzed the spots generated with the standard solutions, three cocaine samples (coc 1, coc 3, and coc 6), and four crack cocaine samples (crack 2, crack 4, crack 5, and crack 7). The $R_f$ values are shown in Table 16.5 [25].

The TLC system using acetone as the mobile phase (Figure 16.11a) resulted in spot tailing for most powder-cocaine and crack cocaine samples and for some standard solutions (cocaine and procaine). Additionally, cocaine and procaine showed similar $R_f$ values ($R_f \approx 0.45$ and 0.36, respectively). Therefore, this system could not be used as the mobile phase in the identification of cocaine [25].

Using methanol:chloroform:acetic acid (20:75:5 v%) as the mobile phase (Figure 16.11b), we observed defined spots for most of the samples and new spots with higher $R_f$ values, which were owing to the separation of impurities from the cocaine and crack cocaine samples. Additionally, this TLC system facilitated the separation and resolution of the cocaine standard from other standards (see $R_f$ values in Table 16.5).

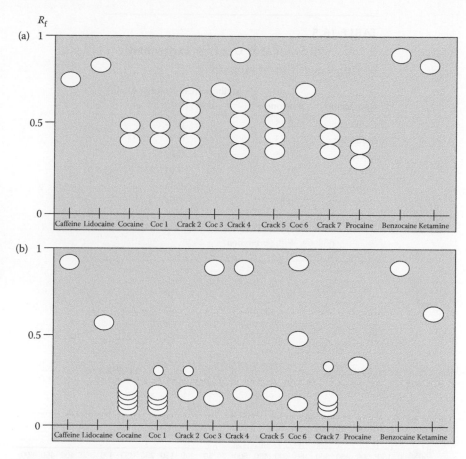

**FIGURE 16.11** TLC of standards used and cocaine and crack samples using (a) methanol:chloroform:acetic acid (20:75:5 v%), and (b) acetone-like mobile phase. (From Sabino, B.D. et al. 2011. *Am. J. Anal. Chem.*, 2: 658–664. With permission.)

Hence, in the TLC/EASI–MS measurements, we used methanol:chloroform:acetic acid (20:75:5 v%) as the mobile phase (Figure 16.11b) [25].

Figure 16.12a–f shows that the TLC/EASI–MS results corresponded to the standards: benzocaine ([M+H]$^+$: $m/z$ 166); caffeine ([M+H]$^+$: $m/z$ 195); lidocaine ([M+H]$^+$: $m/z$ 235, [2M+H]$^+$: $m/z$ 469, and [2M+Na]$^+$: $m/z$ 491); procaine ([M+H]$^+$: $m/z$ 237); ketamine ([M+H]$^+$: $m/z$ 238 and [2M+Na]$^+$: $m/z$ 497); and cocaine ([M+H]$^+$: $m/z$ 304) [25].

Among the identified standards, caffeine and benzocaine showed lower ionization efficiencies due to low signal-to-noise ratios. The high polarity and lower molar mass of these molecules increased their interactions with the TLC system, increasing the difficultly of the desorption/ionization process. Similar results were observed in the TLC analysis of ecstasy tablets using EASI–MS [23].

Figure 16.13a and b shows the TLC/EASI–MS results for two spots corresponding to a cocaine sample (coc-1). The first spot showed a similar $R_f$ value to that of the cocaine standard. The sample was confirmed to be cocaine using EASI–MS analysis

**TABLE 16.5**

**$R_f$ Values of Standards Used for Experiments of Thin-Layer Chromatography**

| Compound | Acetone | Methanol:Chloroform:Acetic Acid (20:75:5 v%) |
|---|---|---|
| Caffeine | 0.75 | 0.94 |
| Lidocaine | 0.83 | 0.47 |
| Cocaine | 0.45 | 0.15 |
| Procaine | 0.36 | 0.36 |
| Benzocaine | 0.92 | 0.89 |
| Ketamine | 0.80 | 0.64 |

*Source:* From Sabino, B.D. et al. 2011. *Am. J. Anal. Chem.*, 2: 658–64. With permission.

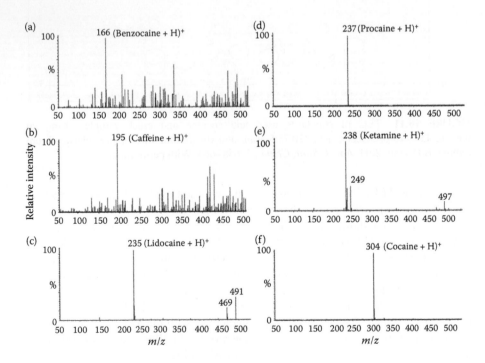

**FIGURE 16.12** TLC/EASI–MS for the standards of (a) benzocaine, (b) caffeine, (c) lidocaine, (d) procaine, (e) ketamine, and (f) cocaine. (From Sabino, B.D. et al. 2011. *Am. J. Anal. Chem.*, 2: 658–664. With permission.)

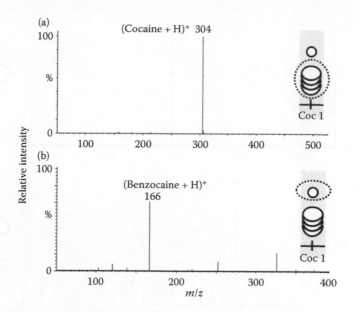

**FIGURE 16.13** EASI–MS/TLC for spots of coc-1 sample. (From Sabino, B.D. et al. 2011. *Am. J. Anal. Chem.*, 2: 658–664. With permission.)

(Figure 16.13a; [M+H]: *m/z* 304). These results were also obtained for all other cocaine samples. The second spot of the coc-1 sample exhibited a similar $R_f$ value to the procaine standard ($R_f \approx 0.32$). Surprisingly, EASI–MS (Figure 16.13b) confirmed the presence of benzocaine ([M+H]+ *m/z* 166), although the standard solution of this substance exhibited an $R_f$ value of 0.89. These results were in agreement with those obtained using CG–MS analysis, and similar results were also found in the second spot of the crack 2 and crack 7 samples ( Figure 16.13b) [25].

Figure 16.14a,b shows the EASI–MS results for the coc-3 sample that had two spots, which exhibited distinct $R_f$ values ($R_f = 0.17$ and 0.90, respectively). Cocaine ([M+H]+ *m/z* 304) was identified in the first spot (Figure 16.14a). The second spot had an $R_f$ value that was similar to that of caffeine and benzocaine. EASI–MS confirmed the presence of caffeine ([M+H]: *m/z* 195), thus clearly revealing the identity of the species. Similar results were found in the crack 4 sample [25].

### 16.5.3 QUALITATIVE THIN-LAYER CHROMATOGRAPHY–EASY AMBIENT SONIC SPRAY IONIZATION ANALYSIS OF LYSERGIC ACID DIETHYLAMIDE AND 9,10-DIHYDRO-LYSERGIC ACID DIETHYLAMIDE IN STREET DRUG BLOTTER SAMPLES

LSD is a generic name for the hallucinogen lysergic acid diethylamide. Discovered by Hofmann in 1938, LSD is one of the most potent mind-altering chemicals. LSD generally comes in small squares of paper that have been soaked in solutions of LSD, which are known as "blotters." LSD is typically utilized by people in their teens and twenties [38,39]. Although the main hallucinogen in blotters is LSD,

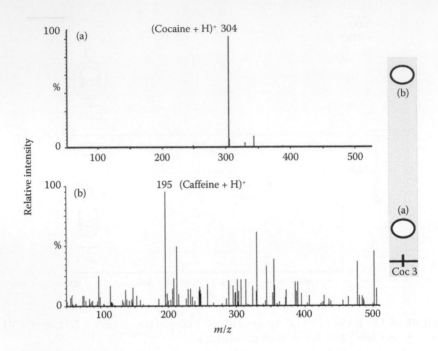

**FIGURE 16.14**   EASI–MS/TLC for spots of coc 3 sample. (From Sabino, B. et al. 2011. *Am. J. Anal. Chem.*, 2: 658–664. With permission.)

other substances have also been identified in these matrices, such as 4-bromo-2,5-dimethoxyamphetamine (DOB) [40] and bromobenzodifuranylisopropylamine (bromo-DragonFLY, ABDF) [41]. ABDF is also an extremely potent hallucinogen with a longer duration than LSD [24].

In 2009, the Brazilian Federal Police identified a new compound in seized blotters: 9,10-dihydro-LSD, an uncontrolled drug [42]. The structure of 9,10-dihydro-LSD (325 Da) differs from that of LSD (323 Da) in the hydrogenation of the 9,10 double bond (Figure 16.15). Clare [43] studied the activity of a series of hallucinogenic tryptamines as a function of various parameters such as lipophilicity, amine substituents, and orientation of nodes of occupied $\pi$-like orbitals. The author reported that 9,10-dihydro-LSD is an inactive substance (activity = 0 MU), while LSD is a potent hallucinogen with an activity of 4000 MU. The results obtained for 9,10-dihydro-LSD were consistent with those of other investigated tryptamines [24].

Separation of the soluble constituents of eight seized blotter samples containing LSD (blotter 2, 3, 4, 6, 7, and 8) and 9,10-dihydro-LSD (blotter 1 and 5) as well as standard LSD were analyzed by TLC using two different eluents: $CHCl_3$:$CH_3OH$ (90:10 v/v%) (Figure 16.16a) and $CHCl_3$:$CH_3COCH_3$ (20:80 v/v%) (Figure 16.16b). The best resolution was achieved using $CHCl_3$:$CH_3COCH_3$ ($R_f$ = 0.44 for 9,10-dihydro-LSD and $R_f$ = 0.69 for LSD). With $CHCl_3$:$CH_3OH$ as the eluent, the $R_f$ values for 9,10-dihydro-LSD and LSD were quite similar ($R_f$ = 0.78 and 0.83, respectively) [24].

Figure 16.17a–c shows the "on-spot" EASI(+)–MS data acquired directly from the surface of the TLC spots of blotters 1 and 2 and for the LSD standard. The

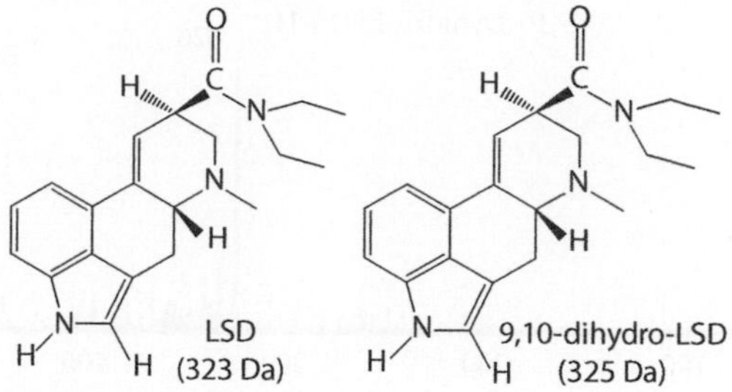

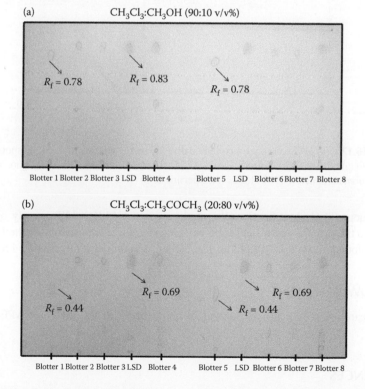

**FIGURE 16.15**   LSD and 9,10-dihydro-LSD structures. (From Romão, W. et al. 2012. *J. Forensic Sci.*, 57: 1307–1312. With permission.)

unambiguous characterization of each drug is evident, mostly as a single ion (and its natural and characteristic isotopologue profile), which facilitates spectra interpretation and analyte characterization. These ions correspond to the protonated molecules [M+H]$^+$ of each identified drug. It is also clear that even when two components elute with very similar $R_f$ values (as Figure 16.16a exemplifies), which could hamper the

**FIGURE 16.16**   TLC data for LSD standard solution and eight common seized blotters used as eluents: (a) CHCl$_3$:CH$_3$OH (90:10) v/v% and (b) CHCl$_3$:CH$_3$COCH$_3$ (20:80) v/v%. Spots developed by UV are represented by gray ellipses. (From Romão, W. et al. 2012. *J. Forensic Sci.*, 57: 1307–1312. With permission.)

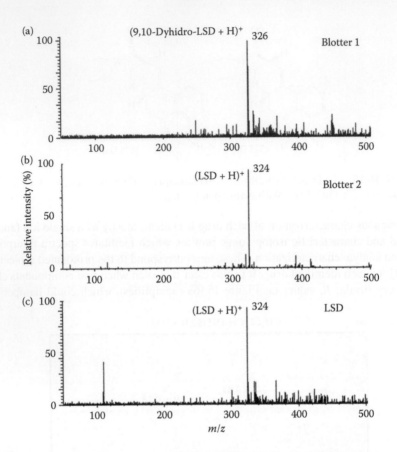

**FIGURE 16.17**    (a) EASI(+) spectra collected directly on the surface of the TLC spots corresponding to (a) blotter 1, (b) blotter 2, and (c) LSD standard samples. (From Romão, W. et al. 2012. *J. Forensic Sci.*, 57: 1307–1312. With permission.)

unambiguous TLC identification, the application of EASI(+)–MS directly on each spot led to the prompt and reliable characterization of each spot. Finally, the LOD of LSD was found to be of 0.1-µg blotter 1 at 365 nm and 0.5-µg blotter 1 at 254 nm [24].

## ACKNOWLEDGMENT

This research was generously funded by FAPES, FAPERJ, CNPq, CAPES, and FINEP.

## REFERENCES

1. Yukiko, M. 1998. *Manual for Identification of Abused Drugs*, 2nd Edition, Pharmaceutical and Medical Safety Bureau, Ministry of Health and Welfare, Japan.
2. Ojanperä, I. 1992. Toxicological drug screening by thin-layer chromatography, *Trends Anal. Chem.*, 11: 222.

3. United Nations Office on Drugs and Crimes (UNODC). 1998. Recommended methods for testing opium, morphine and heroine, *Manual for Use by National Drug Testing Laboratories*.

4. Morlock, G. and Schwack, W. 2010. Coupling of planar chromatography to mass spectrometry, *Trends Anal. Chem.*, 10: 1157–1171.

5. Kauppila, T.J., Talaty, N., Kuuranne, T., Kotiaho, T., Kostiainen, R., and Cooks, R.G. 2007. Rapid analysis of metabolites and drugs of abuse from urine samples by desorption electrospray ionization–mass spectrometry, *Analyst*, 132: 868–875.

6. Miao, Z. and Chen, H. 2009. Direct analysis of liquid samples by desorption electrospray ionization–mass spectrometry (DESI–MS), *J. Am. Soc. Mass Spectrom.*, 20: 10–19.

7. Nielen, M.W.F., Nijrolder, A.W.J.M., Hooijerink, H., and Stolker., A.A.M. 2011. Feasibility of desorption electrospray ionization mass spectrometry for rapid screening of anabolic steroid esters in hair, *Anal. Chim. Acta*, 700: 63–69.

8. Leuthold, L.A., Mandscheff, J.F., Fathi, M., Giroud, C., Augsburger, M., Varesio, E., and Hopfgartner, G. 2006. Desorption electrospray ionization mass spectrometry: Direct toxicological screening and analysis of illicit ecstasy tablets, *Rapid Commun. Mass Spectrom.*, 20: 103–110.

9. Stojanovska, N., Tahtouh, M., Kelly, T., Beavis, A., and Fu, S. 2014. Qualitative analysis of seized cocaine samples using desorption electrospray ionization—Mass spectrometry (DESI–MS), *Drug Test. Anal.*, 7(5): 393–400. doi: 10.1002/dta.1684.

10. Van Berkel, G.J., Ford, M.J., and Deibel, M.A. 2005. Thin layer chromatography and mass spectrometry coupled using desorption electrospray ionization, *Anal. Chem.*, 77: 1207–1215.

11. Steiner, R.R. and Larson, R.L. 2009. Validation of the direct analysis in real time source for use in forensic drug screening, *J. Forensic Sci.*, 54: 617–622.

12. Ropero-Miller, J.D., Stout, P.R., and Bynum, N.D. 2007. Comparison of the novel direct analysis in real time time-of-flight mass spectrometer (AccuTOF-DART™) and signature analysis for the identification of constituents of refined illicit cocaine, *Microgram J.*, 5: 34–40.

13. Fernández, F.M., Cody, R.B., Green, M.D., Hampton, C.Y., McGready, R., Sengaloundeth, S., White, N.J., and Newton, P.N. 2006. Characterization of solid counterfeit drug samples by desorption electrospray ionization and direct-analysis-in-real-time coupled to time-of-flight mass spectrometry, *Chem. Med. Chem.*, 1: 702–705.

14. Morlock, G. and Schwack, W. 2006. Determination of isopropylthioxanthone (ITX) in milk, yoghurt and fat by HPTLC–FLD, HPTLC–ESI/MS and HPTLC–DART–MS, *Anal. Bioanal. Chem.*, 385: 586–595.

15. Morlock, G. and Chernetsov, E.S. 2012. Coupling of planar chromatography with direct analysis in real time mass spectrometry, *Cent. Eur. J. Chem.*, 10: 703–710.

16. Kiguchi, O., Oka, K., Tamada, M., Kobayashi, T., and Onodera, J. 2014. Thin-layer chromatography/direct analysis in real time time-of-flight mass spectrometry and isotope dilution to analyze organophosphorus insecticides in fatty foods, *J. Chromatogr. A*, 1370: 246–254.

17. Rodriguez-Lafuente, A., Mirnaghi, F.S., and Pawliszyn, J. 2013. Determination of cocaine and methadone in urine samples by thin-film solid-phase microextraction and direct analysis in real time (DART) coupled with tandem mass spectrometry, *Anal. Bioanal. Chem.*, 405: 9723–9727.

18. Jagerdeo, E. and Abdel-Rehim, M. 2009. Screening of cocaine and its metabolites in human urine samples by direct analysis in real-time source coupled to time-of-flight mass spectrometry after online pre concentration utilizing microextraction by packed sorbent, *J. Am. Soc. Mass Spectrom.*, 20: 891–899.

19. Horsley, A.B. 2014. *High-Throughput Analysis of Contrived Cocaine Mixtures by Direct Analysis in Real Time/Single Quadrupole Mass Spectrometry and Post Acquisition Chemometric Analysis*, Boston University, Boston, MA, USA.

20. Musah, R.A., Domin, M.A., Walling, M.A., and Shepard, J.R. 2006. Rapid identification of synthetic cannabinoids in herbal samples via direct analysis in real time mass spectrometry, *Rapid Commun. Mass Spectrom.*, 26: 1109–1114.

21. Haddad, R., Sparrapan, R., and Eberlin, M.N. 2006. Desorption sonic spray ionization for (high) voltage-free ambient mass spectrometry, *Rapid Commun. Mass Spectrom.*, 20: 2901–2905.

22. Romão, W., Lalli, P.M., Franco, M.F., Sanvido, G., Schwab, N.V., Lanaro, R., Costa, J.L. et al. 2011. Chemical profile of meta-chlorophenylpiperazine (m-CPP) in ecstasy tablets by easy ambient sonic-spray ionization, X-ray fluorescence, ion mobility mass spectrometry and NMR, *Anal. Bioanal. Chem.*, 400: 3053–3064.

23. Sabino, B.D., Sodré, M.L., Alves, E.A., Rozembaum, H.F., Alonso, F.O.M, Correa, D.N., Eberlin, M.N., and Romão, W. 2010. Analysis of street Ecstasy tablets by thin layer chromatography coupled to easy ambient sonic-spray ionization mass spectrometry, *Braz. J. Anal. Chem.*, 1: 6–11.

24. Romão, W., Sabino, B.D., Bueno, M.I.M.S., Vaz, B.G., Júnior, A.C., Maldaner, A.O., Castro, E.V.R. et al. 2012. LSD and 9,10-dihydro-LSD Analyses in street drug blotter samples via easy ambient sonic-spray ionization mass spectrometry (EASI–MS), *J. Forensic Sci.*, 57: 1307–1312.

25. Sabino, B.D., Romão, W., Sodré, M.L., Correa, D.N., Alonso, F.O.M., and Eberlin, M.N. 2011. Analysis of cocaine and crack cocaine via thin layer chromatography coupled to easy ambient sonic-spray ionization mass spectrometry, *Am. J. Anal. Chem.*, 2: 658–664.

26. Eberlin, L.S., Haddad, R., Sarabia Neto, R.C., Cosso, R.G., Maia, D.R.J., Maldaner, A.O., Zacca, J.J. et al. 2010. Instantaneous chemical profiles of bank notes by ambient mass spectrometry, *Analyst*, 135: 2533–2539.

27. Haddad, R., Catharino, R.R., Marques, L.A., and Eberlin, M.N. 2008. Perfume fingerprinting by easy ambient sonic-spray ionization mass spectrometry: Nearly instantaneous typification and counterfeit detection, *Rapid Commun. Mass Spectrom.*, 22: 3662–3666.

28. Saraiva, S.S., Abdelnur, P.V., Catharino, R.R., Nunes, G., and Eberlin, M.N. 2009. Fabric softeners: Nearly instantaneous characterization and quality control of cationic surfactants by easy ambient sonic-spray ionization mass spectrometry, *Rapid Commun. Mass Spectrom.*, 23: 357–362.

29. Abdelnur, P.V., Eberlin, L.S., Sá, G.F., Souza, S.V., and Eberlin, M.N. 2008. Single-shot biodiesel analysis: Nearly instantaneous typification and quality control solely by ambient mass spectrometry, *Anal. Chem.*, 80: 7882–7886.

30. Jeffrey, W. 2004. In: Moffat, A., Osselton, M., Widdop, B., Galichet, L. (Eds.), *Clarke's Analysis of Drugs and Poisons in Pharmaceuticals, Body Fluids and Postmortem Material*, Pharmaceutical Press, London, UK, pp. 20–100.

31. Bossong, M., Brunt, T., Van Dijk, J., Rigter, S., Hoek, J., and Goldschmidt, H. 2010. mCPP: An undesired addition to the ecstasy market, *J. Psychopharmacol.*, 24: 1395–1401.

32. Sherlock, K., Wolff, K., Hay, A.W., and Conner, M. 1999. Analysis of illicit ecstasy tablets: Implications for clinical management in the accident and emergency department, *J. Accid. Emerg. Med.*, 16: 194–197.

33. Sadeghipour, F. and Veuthey, J.L. 1997. Sensitive and selective determination of methylenedioxylated amphetamines by high-performance liquid chromatography with fluorimetric detection, *J. Chromatogr. A*, 787: 137–143.

34. Bogusz, M.J. 2000. Liquid chromatography–mass spectrometry as a routine method in forensic sciences: A proof of maturity, *J. Chromatogr. B: Biomed. Sci. Appl.*, 748: 3–19.
35. Kato, N., Pharm, B., Fujita, S., Pharm, B., Ohta, H., Fukuba, M., Pharm, M., Toriba, A., and Hayakawa, K. 2008. Thin layer chromatography/fluorescence detection of 3,4-methylenedioxy-methamphetamine and related compounds, *J. Forensic Sci.*, 53: 1367–1371.
36. Zakrzewska, A., Parczewski, A., Kazmierczak, D., Ciesielski, W., and Kochanaa, J. 2007. Visualization of amphetamine and its analogues in TLC, *Acta Chim. Slov.*, 54:106–109.
37. Romão, W., Schwab, N.V., Bueno, M.I.M.S., Sparrapan, R., Eberlin, M.N., Martyni, A., Sabino, B.D., and Maldaner, A.O. 2011. Química Forense: Perspectivas sobre novos métodos analíticos aplicados à Documentoscopia, Balística e Drogas de Abuso, *Química Nova*, 34: 1717–1728.
38. Fester, U. 1995. *Practical LSD Manufacture*, Loompanics Unlimited. São Paulo, Brasil.
39. Clarkson, E.D., Lesser, D., and Paul, B.D. Effective GC–MS procedure for detecting iso-LSD in urine after base-catalyzed conversion to LSD, *Clin. Chem.*, 44: 287–292.
40. Costa, J.L., Wang, A.Y., Micke, G.A., Maldaner, A.O., Romano, R.L., and M-Júnior, H.A. 2007. Chemical identification of 2,5-dimethoxy-4-bromoamphetamine (DOB), *Forensic Sci. Int.*, 173: 130–136.
41. Kauppila, T.J., Arvola, V., Haapala, M., Pol, J., Aalberg, L., and Saarela, V. 2008. Direct analysis of illicit drugs by desorption atmospheric pressure photoionization, *Rapid Commun. Mass Spectrom.*, 22: 979–985.
42. Maldaner, A.O., Souza, D.L., Botelho, E.D., and Talhavini, M. 2009. 9,10-Dihidro-LSD: Uma nova substância encontrada em selos e micropontos, *32a Reunião Anual da Sociedade Brasileira de Química*, Fortaleza, Brazil.
43. Clare, B.W. 2004. A novel quantum theoretic QSAR for hallucinogenic tryptamines: A major factor is the orientation of π orbital nodes, *J. Mol. Struct. Theochem.*, 712: 143–148.

# 17 TLC–MS Analysis of Carotenoids, Triterpenoids, and Flavanols in Plant Extracts and Dietary Supplements

*Irena Vovk and Alen Albreht*

## CONTENTS

## 17.1 INTRODUCTION

The purpose of this chapter is to highlight the utilization of offline and online thin-layer chromatography/mass spectrometry (TLC–MS) approaches in the field of carotenoid, triterpenoid, and flavanol analysis. These compounds display many beneficial effects on human health and are found in plants and bacteria, as well as animals. Apart from the analytes of interest, these raw material extracts and multi-ingredient dietary supplements contain several interfering compounds, to which special attention should be given. TLC is a complementary analytical technique to other common separation techniques such as high-performance liquid chromatography (HPLC), gas chromatography (GC), capillary electrophoresis (CE), and others. In contrast to the latter, TLC allows for a larger degree of analytical freedom because in addition to the substantial variety of stationary phases, the choice of developing solvents seems limitless. This often enables the separation of compounds that cannot be resolved by HPLC or GC [1]. Coupling TLC with MS strengthens the analysis with an additional dimension, which enables higher specificity, sensitivity, and more detailed analyte information. The hyphenation can be achieved by an offline or online approach, respectively. The advantages and disadvantages of both approaches, relevant to the analyses of carotenoids, triterpenoids, and flavanols, will be described.

TLC–MS is progressively becoming a part of the instrumental planar chromatography platform along with image analysis, densitometric scanning of chromatograms, and *in situ* absorption spectra. TLC–MS can provide additional information in chemical fingerprinting of plant materials, analysis and structural elucidation of bioactive compounds in plant materials and dietary supplements, analysis of raw materials for dietary supplement products, and detection of adulterants in plant raw materials and dietary supplement products [2,3]. However, this can be a very challenging task as there are endless possible combinations of bioactive ingredients and excipients, chemically undefined plant ingredients and adulterants.

## 17.2  OFFLINE VERSUS ONLINE TLC–MS

An offline TLC–MS approach has been used for a long time in organic synthesis, phytochemical analysis, food analysis, pharmaceutical and medical analysis, life sciences, and related areas. As a rule, in offline TLC–MS, the adsorbents on the preparative plates are fairly thick (0.5–2 mm) so that larger amounts of samples can be applied. This compensates for potential losses due to degradation of compounds and low purification yields. Samples are usually applied as wide bands, ranging from the left-hand side to the right-hand side of the plate, and compounds are then separated by a single or multiple consecutive TLC developments. The bands representing compounds of interest are scraped from analytical or preparative TLC plates afterward, reextracted with a suitable solvent system, and subjected to MS analysis.

This can be a very tedious procedure during which labile analytes, such as carotenoids, are exposed to detrimental external influences such as acids, light, heat, and oxidants (especially oxygen from air). This may result in pigment oxidation, degradation, and isomerization into their Z isomers, which are formed mostly under acidic conditions by the reorganization around the double bonds of the conjugated carotenoid chain. The limited analyte amount can have a detrimental effect on MS sensitivity, and in the worst case, the concentration of carotenoids can fall under the detection limit. This is usually tackled either by addition of a base to the water-silica slurry during the preparation of the TLC plate, or by exposure of the TLC plate to ammonia vapors prior to plate development, or by addition of a base to the predevelopment solvent and an antioxidant to the developing solvent [4–6].

On the other hand, an obvious advantage of offline TLC–MS is the broad list of chemicals, which can be used in the course of the analysis. For example, there are practically no limitations to the solvents that are used for reextraction of analytes from the chromatographic adsorbent. Many MS noncompatible solvents and buffers (phosphate buffer and triethylammonium acetate, for instance) can readily be used for optimal extraction and stability of analytes, as long as they are removed prior to MS analysis. This way, and if care is exercised, labile compounds can be transferred from the TLC plate to the MS with negligible analyte loss, although the overall TLC–MS analysis can still be time consuming. Additionally, analytes extracted from the plates can be redissolved in a minimal amount of solvent used for MS analysis, which results in a concentrated sample solution. In both cases, a significant increase in sensitivity can be achieved.

With the development of MS ion source technology and TLC–MS interfaces, the online approach to TLC–MS analysis has become more and more frequent. Here, the developed chromatographic plate is directly inserted into the MS ion source, or alternatively, the compounds are extracted from the plate and introduced into the MS in a simultaneous fashion. Different techniques have been brought forward, which render TLC amenable for online coupling with MS. Analytes can be eluted from the plates by a solvent using a TLC–MS interface, they can be thermally desorbed, or they can be ionized directly on the plate by using a wide variety of ionization methods such as desorption electrospray ionization (DESI), fast atom bombardment (FAB), secondary ion mass spectrometry (SIMS), and matrix-assisted laser desorption ionization (MALDI), just to name a few. There are numerous advantages of online over offline TLC–MS. The transfer of analytes from the plates to the MS is usually very fast, which minimizes unwanted transformations of labile compounds such as carotenoids and others. Sample test solutions can be applied as narrow bands and high-resolution chromatographic media can also be employed, such as high-performance thin-layer chromatographic (HPTLC) and ultrathin-layer chromatographic (UTLC) plates, and adequate sensitivity is still achieved. Thus, online coupling is very convenient, although some potential nuisances can be encountered. For example, in TLC–MALDI–MS bands on the developed plate can diffuse on addition of the matrix, which is essential for the ionization of analytes. However, the area surrounding the band can be carefully scratched off beforehand, thus preventing the diffusion of compounds and loss of MS sensitivity [7]. Another issue in online coupling when using an elution technique is the restricted selection of eluents, which are acceptable for the TLC–MS analysis. A poorly chosen solvent can produce a high MS background, which can cause some serious frustration. This can result from contaminants, which originate from solvents and solvent mixtures used for the predevelopment and development of the plates, or even from the elution solvent. Intense background ions can also stem from the TLC plate itself and can vary from batch to batch. Therefore, proper analytical approaches need to be considered and TLC–MS data have to be evaluated with extreme caution to get an accurate result. Such inconveniences may be circumvented in the offline approach by additional purification steps, which diminish the influence of such contaminants and interfering compounds, respectively.

An additional challenge of online TLC–MS, using solvent elution, was shown to be the analysis of flavanols [8]. This is an example where inferior resolution of TLC in principle can pose a problem. The flavanol isomers within the group with the same degree of polymerization (dimers, trimers, etc.) are difficult to separate using only TLC and the result is a chromatogram with stretched bands, which are reminiscent of a severe tailing effect. A conventional elution head with the dimensions of 4 mm × 2 mm is unable to individually elute and transfer all of these bands to the MS due to the insufficient resolution between the individual compounds (Figure 17.1). A simple solution to this issue is either an alternating sampling technique of two neighboring chromatograms from the TLC plate, also known as comprehensive TLC × MS, or meticulous scraping of the adsorbent from the support

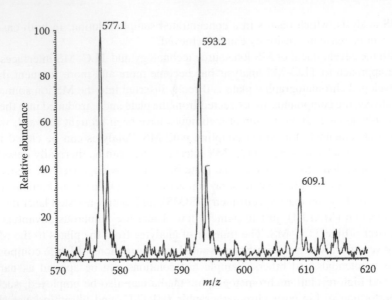

**FIGURE 17.1**  TLC–MS spectrum of pomegranate fruit peel sample test solution, showing proanthocyanidin dimers composed of two (+)-catechin units ($m/z = 577$), one (+)-catechin and one (+)-gallocatechin unit ($m/z = 593$), and two (+)-gallocatechin units ($m/z = 609$). HPTLC cellulose plate was developed with $n$-propanol–water–acetic acid (4:2:1, v/v) as a developing solvent. (From Smrke, S. and Vovk, I. 2013. *J. Chromatogr. A*, 1289: 119–126. With permission.)

with reextraction and subsequent offline MS analysis. This way, reconstructed chromatograms for the individual analyte can be obtained, although some may overlap (Figure 17.2). The oversampling in this and related cases could also be circumvented by use of laser ionization or similar techniques, which can target the analyte zone very accurately in a narrow range of the TLC plate. A related issue was also encountered in the analysis of triterpenoids from the epicuticular waxes of vegetables [9]. The authors approached the problem by rotating the 20 cm × 10 cm TLC plate by 90°, extending the developing distance and, hence, the interband space, which enabled a selective analyte sampling.

In some cases, an online combination of cellulose-coated TLC plates and MALDI–MS produces higher quality MS spectra with no or little background compared to an offline approach. In the latter case, pure sample test solution and matrix are crystallized on a conventional metal MALDI plate and several interfering signals are observed in the MS, which originate from matrix ions and cluster ions, respectively. This concept was readily presented in the analysis of triterpenoids [10].

To sum up, each approach—either offline or online TLC–MS—has its advantages and disadvantages. The technique that will be most suitable to our needs will largely depend on the type of application at hand. Today, several shortcomings of a particular technique can be overcome by some elegant tricks and these seem to be limited only by our own imagination.

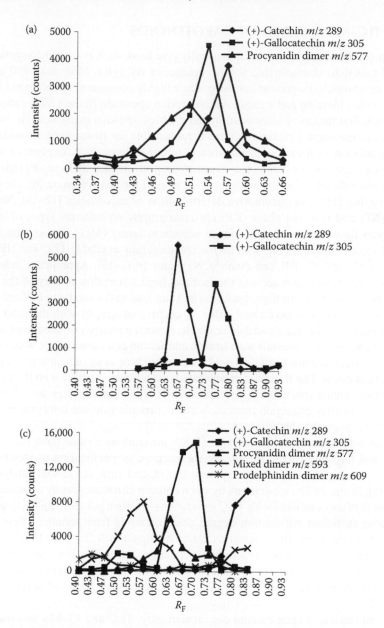

**FIGURE 17.2** TLC × MS chromatograms of pomegranate fruit peel test solutions developed on cellulose HPTLC plates using water (a) or *n*-propanol–water–acetic acid (4:2:1, v/v) as developing solvent (b and c). In the case of (c), the amount of applied sample was four times the amount in (b), hence, oligomeric flavanols could be detected on the expense of (+)-catechin and (+)-gallocatechin coelution. (From Smrke, S. and Vovk, I. 2013. *J. Chromatogr. A*, 1289: 119–126. With permission.)

## 17.3   TLC–MS ANALYSIS OF CAROTENOIDS

Carotenoids are natural pigments that usually give food, such as fruit and vegetables, and animals their characteristic yellow, orange, or red color. More than 600 carotenoids are known to be present in nature. Their highly conjugated double-bond backbone is both a blessing and a curse. An absorption spectrum in the visible range is a convenient first means of identification and enables sensitive quantification. On the other hand, the same structural feature is responsible for isomerization, oxidation, and degradation of these pigments when exposed to light, heat, oxygen, or acids. Carotenoids are also unstable on a chromatographic sorbent and can degrade during and immediately after the analysis. TLC is used for fast screening [6], chemical fingerprinting [11], and quantitative determination of carotenoids [12–14]. Normal phase (NP) and reversed phase (RP) chromatography on different types of adsorbent layers have been used. Homemade adsorbent layers (MgO, Kieselguhr, silica gel) [11,15] are nowadays replaced by the commercially available TLC and HPTLC silica gel, $C_{18}$ RP, $C_8$ RP, and ciano (CN) plates [6,11–15]. Appropriate selection must be made taking into account the fact that high adsorption activity of the layer is not always favorable for high resolution and can lead to the production of artifacts. Analysis of a sample is performed either by cochromatography with the most common carotenoid reference standards available, or with standards isolated from different plant and animal materials with known carotenoid compositions, or with known standard extract as a marker for particular carotenoids or as an indicator of the polarity of an unknown. The $R_F$ values of separated carotenoids, together with their *in situ* scanned absorption spectra ($\lambda_{max}$ and fine structure) and mass spectra (also fragmentation pattern) after extraction from the sorbent, provide valuable information in the process of compound identification.

In the field of carotenoids, most TLC–MS utilizations to date have been made offline and have used TLC merely for the purpose of purification or isolation of these pigments. Mass spectrometry was introduced into carotenoid analysis in 1965 [16]. In the 1970s, separations by open column chromatography on aluminum oxide were often combined with TLC separations on silica gel and MgO/Kieselguhr to achieve sufficient purification degree of carotenoids from tomato. These were analyzed afterward by direct-insertion electron impact–MS (EI–MS) [17–19]. Such isolation procedures, applied reactions (acetylation, saponification, and reduction), $R_F$ values, absorption, and MS spectra enabled identification of phytoene 1,2-oxide, and related compounds as the first naturally occurring epoxides of acyclic carotenoids [17].

A combination of open column chromatography, TLC and EI–MS was used for isolation and identification of carotenoids from a complex extract obtained from the fruit of sea buckthorn (*Hippophae rhamnoides*) [5]. Using alumina column, three fractions were obtained, and were further purified on homemade silica gel $GF_{254}$ plates. These were made neutral by adding a pellet of potassium hydroxide to the slurry, intended for plate preparation. Selected zones were scraped from the plates and further purified on homemade MgO plates and additionally on $Al_2O_3$ in Pasteur pipettes, before EI–MS analysis was utilized. It was demonstrated that by combining open column chromatography and TLC, very pure pigments, needed for MS analysis, could be isolated from the extract containing more than 50 carotenoids. The identity confirmation of the isolated β-carotene, γ-carotene, δ-carotene, β-cryptoxanthin, and zeaxanthin was based on the chromatographic properties, ultraviolet–visible (UV–vis), MS, and tandem MS spectra, without using any reference standards.

An offline TLC–MS approach was used to determine the carotenoid constituents of halophilic bacteria *Haloferax volcanii* and *Halobacterium salinarium* [20]. Alkaline TLC plates and ordinary silica TLC plates were used for the isolation of carotenoids, which were then subjected to further spectroscopic analyses. The plates were developed using different combinations of developing solvents, each optimized for a particular compound. The developing solvents were acetone–1,1,1-trichloroethane (2:3, v/v), acetone–propanol–chloroform (5:1:9, v/v), and acetone–hexane in different ratios, ranging from 1:1 (v/v) to 3:7 (v/v). In this study, the obtained MS data played a crucial role in the structure elucidation of three new pigments: 3′,4′-dihydromonoanhydrobacterioruberin, 3′,4′-epoxymonoanhydrobacterioruberin, and 3′,4′-dihydro monohydrobacterioruberin, since the isolated carotenoid fractions contained a mixture of geometrical isomers which made it very difficult to interpret their nuclear magnetic resonance (NMR) spectra. Analogs of these carotenoids were also studied in psychrotrophic bacterium *Micrococcus roseus* [21]. For preparative isolation of pigments, the crude extract was chromatographed on silica gel TLC plates by using acetone–heptane (1:1, v/v) as a developing solvent. The resulting fractions were analyzed by EI–MS to identify seven carotenoids: (2S, 2′S)-bacterioruberin (68% of total), bacterioruberin monoglycoside (21%), monoanhydrobacterioruberin (6%), an unidentified polar tridecaene carotenoid (3%), haloxanthin (2%), and β,β-carotene (0.4%). Subsequent HPLC analysis of the main (bacterioruberin) TLC fraction revealed a number of geometrical isomers: all-*E*-(75%), 5Z-(5%), 9Z-(5%), and 13Z-bacterioruberin (15%).

Carotenoid pigments from the red tide dinoflagellate *Karenia brevis* were reexamined using a more powerful set of analytical tools, including MS and NMR [22]. The pigments were isolated by using a two-stage preparative TLC analysis. The crude extract was chromatographed on a silica G–CaCO$_3$ (2:1, w/w) TLC plate with *n*-hexane–acetone–i-propanol (75:30:1, v/v) as a developing solvent. The resulting four fractions were subjected to an additional TLC analysis on silica G–silica guhr–Ca(OH)$_2$–MgO (14:16:9:9, w/w) plates. *n*-Hexane–i-butylmethylketone (97:3, v/v) was used as a developing solvent for fraction 1 (β,ε- and β,β-carotene), and appropriate mixtures of *n*-hexane, acetone, and i-propanol for fractions 2 (gyroxanthin diester and diatoxanthin), 3 (19-hexanoyloxyparacentrone 3-acetate and diadinoxanthin), and 4 (fucoxanthin, 19′-hexanoyloxyfucoxanthin and 19′-butanoyloxyfucoxanthin). The final fractions from repeated TLC analyses were subjected to EI–MS, which aided in structure elucidation of nine colored compounds. As concluded, MS and NMR results showed the absence of some class-characteristic xanthophylls such as peridinin, which confirmed the assumed anomaly within the class.

Carotenoids from orange juice were isolated from the developed silica gel 60 GF$_{254}$ plate and additionally passed through alumina microcolumns prior to EI-MS analysis [23]. Light petroleum ether (bp 65–95°C)–acetone–diethylamine (10:4:1, v/v) were used as a developing solvent for isolation of β-cryptoxanthin, and diethyl ether for lutein and monohydroxycarotenoid fraction. Despite the generally accepted concept that orange juice contains provitamin A α-cryptoxanthin, this work revealed that nonprovitamin A carotenoid zeinoxanthin, a pigment with similar chemical and physical characteristics, is present instead. In a later work [4], the same group studied the geometrical isomers of violaxanthin in orange juice as well. The saponified juice extract was first analyzed on silica gel 60 $GF_{254}$ TLC plate prepared in-house. The water-silica slurry contained sodium hydroxyde and the TLC plate was additionally exposed to ammonia vapor to reduce the intrinsic acidity of silica and, therefore, reduce the isomerization of 5,6-epoxycarotenoids. The developing solvent used was diethyl ether. The band representing violaxanthin geometrical isomers was scraped off and rechromatographed on laboratory-made aluminum G-type E plates, by use of acetone–petroleum ether (40–60°C) (3:7, v/v). The band was also subjected to EI–MS analysis. The fragmentation pattern revealed neutral losses of 18 and 36, corresponding to mono- and di-hydroxy groups, and 80 and 160, which is indicative of mono- and di-epoxy functionality. Fragment ions at $m/z$ 352, 221, and 181 further confirmed the close proximity of hydroxy and epoxy groups within the terminal rings of violaxanthin isomers.

Offline TLC–MS was also shown to be a powerful tool for the purification and identification of yellow pigments of *Cronobacter sakazakii* BAA894, which led to the reconstruction of their biosynthetic pathway using *Escherichia coli* [24]. Silica gel 60 TLC plates were developed with different developing solvents: chloroform–methanol (65:25, v/v) and hexane–acetone (4:1, v/v) for a general isolation of carotenoids, and hexane–dichloromethane (9:1, v/v) for the isolation of lycopene and β-carotene. Yellow bands of interest were scraped off from preparative silica TLC plates, reextracted with methanol, and the resulting carotenoid solutions were subjected to MS and tandem MS analysis using electrospray ion source in positive ion mode. Based on UV–vis spectral characteristics, $m/z$ values of the molecular ions in the MS spectra, and their fragmentation patterns, the two major yellow constituents of *Cronobacter sakazakii* were shown to be zeaxanthin-monoglycoside and zeaxanthin-diglycoside. Additionally, when seven genes *crtE-idi-crtXYIBZ* were overexpressed in *Escherichia coli*, the same two pigments were synthesized, which was again confirmed by offline TLC–MS. Thus, these results suggested that this gene cluster is responsible for the yellow pigmentation of *Cronobacter sakazakii*. By expression of four, five, six, or all seven genes, respectively, different carotenoids were synthesized (lycopene, β-carotene, zeaxanthin, cryptoxanthin, and zeaxanthin-diglycoside). Based on these results, the carotenoid biosynthetic pathway was proposed.

The first online coupling of TLC and MS for the analysis of carotenoids was applied for detection of neoxanthin, violaxanthin, lutein, and β-carotene in spinach extract. Separation on $C_{18}$ RP HPTLC plate was followed by extraction of the carotenoids by means of CAMAG TLC–MS interface. After the elution of compounds from the sorbent with methanol, 1% acetic acid was added to the effluent to augment the ionization in the atmospheric pressure chemical ionization (APCI) source, which operated in positive mode [25].

The second online TLC–MS was done by the same group [6]. Their focus was directed toward stability of carotenoids on $C_{18}$ RP HPTLC plates. Instability of these yellow pigments, especially on acidic stationary phases such as bare silica, is in fact the prevailing reason why TLC, and consequently TLC–MS, are not two techniques frequently used in the qualitative and quantitative analysis of carotenoids. In this study, the stability of lutein, lycopene, and β-carotene was enhanced considerably by plate predevelopment with methanol–dichloromethane (1:1, v/v) and more importantly by the addition of 0.1% of antioxidant tert-butylhydroquinone to the developing solvent methanol–acetone (1:1, v/v). This enabled densitometric scanning of *in situ* absorption spectra and identification of carotenoids with MS (Figure 17.3) within 1 h after the development. TLC–MS analysis was carried out using $C_{18}$ RP HPTLC plates from which the yellow bands were transferred directly to the MS by means of CAMAG TLC–MS interface. The compounds were eluted from the plates using methanol–ethyl acetate (3:1, v/v). Methanolic 0.2% acetic acid was added to the effluent before it was introduced into an APCI source, which operated in positive-ion mode.

The third and the only other online TLC–MS approach in carotenoid analysis was presented in the study of the introduction of $TiO_2$ nanoparticles on increase of carotenoid production by the extremophilic haloarchea *Haloferax mediterranei* [7]. The carotenoids were extracted from bacteria and chromatographed on silica gel TLC plates developed by acetone–*n*-heptane (1:1, v/v). To prevent the diffusion of bands on the developed silica gel TLC plate, the area surrounding the bands was carefully scraped off prior to the addition of MALDI matrix. Based on the high-resolution mass spectra, the four colored pigments were identified as bisanhydrobacterioruberin, monoanhydrobacterioruberin, 2-isopentenyl-3,4-dehydrorhodopin, and

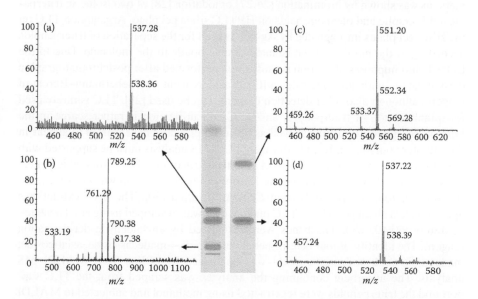

**FIGURE 17.3** Mass spectra of lycopene (a), lutein dipalmitate (b), lutein (c), and β-carotene (d), from two dietary supplement samples, obtained after elution of the zones from $C_{18}$ RP HPTLC plate developed in methanol–acetone (1:1, v/v) + 0.1% TBHQ. (From Rodić, Z. et al. 2012. *J. Chromatogr. A*, 1231: 59–65. With permission.)

bacterioruberin. TLC–MALDI–MS proved to be a very sensitive method for carotenoid detection and fast enough to avoid their degradation. For the acquisition of high-resolution mass spectra, a time-of-flight (TOF) mass analyzer was used, which operated in positive-ion mode.

## 17.4  TLC–MS ANALYSIS OF TRITERPENOIDS

Triterpenoids are a group of secondary metabolites widely distributed in nature. Their relatively complex cyclic carbon structures, based on six isoprene units, can be heavily substituted with different functional groups, which may be esterified or glycosylated, for instance. As a result, over 20,000 different natural triterpenoids are known to humans. Among the most widely spread are pentacyclic triterpenoids ($C_{30}$), which can be divided into several structural subgroups based on their skeleton. Many of these compounds show important pharmacological activities. Reported beneficial effects of various triterpenoids on human health indicate the nutritional importance of these compounds.

Analytical and preparative TLC are frequently used in the analysis of triterpenoids. Fast screening and fractionation (sample purification, isolation of standard compounds) is usually performed on TLC or HPTLC silica gel plates with or without fluorescent indicator $F_{254}$. However, RP $C_2$ and $C_{18}$ TLC and HPTLC plates are also used for analytical separations. The power of complementary NP and RP separations is especially important [1,9,26,27]. Prechromatographic derivatization on the start position before the development can be used for improving the separation of the isomers, as was shown by bromination [26,27] or iodation [28] of two isomeric triterpenic acids ursolic and oleanolic acids on HPTLC silica gel plate. Argentation TLC on the silica gel plates impregnated by $AgNO_3$ is used for the separation of triterpenoids according to the number of the isolated double bonds in the molecule. Due to the lack of chromophores, detection is most often performed after postchromatographic derivatization with anisaldehyde–sulfuric acid reagent or Liebermann–Burchard reagent, although also other detection reagents can be used [29]. TLC is rarely used for quantification of triterpenoids and TLC–MS utilization is rather scarce in the field of triterpenoids. Offline as well as online approaches have started to appear in the literature only recently. In both cases, TLC–MS analysis must be supported with postchromatographic derivatization of selected parts of the chromatographic plate.

A modified TLC method from the European Pharmacopoeia was used for identification of four triterpenoids from *Centella asiatica* [30]. The plant extract was applied onto a silica gel 60 $F_{254}$ TLC plate, which was developed using ethyl acetate–methanol (60:40, v/v). The bands were visualized by anisaldehyde derivatization reagent. The identity of four determined triterpenoids—madecassoside, asiaticoside, madecassic acid, and asiatic acid—was confirmed by offline TLC–MALDI–MS analysis. The adsorbent containing the analytes was scraped from the TLC support and the triterpenoids were reextracted using methanol and subjected to MALDI plates, along with the matrix, for MS analysis.

Preparative TLC and high-resolution (HR) EI–MS were used for isolation of santolinoic acid, a new ursane-type triterpenoid, from *Salvia santolinifolia* [31]. Partitioning of the ethanolic extract with different solvents was followed by column chromatography of the chloroform fraction over silica gel eluting with hexane–chloroform, chloroform, chloroform–methanol, and methanol in increasing order of polarity. The fraction obtained from chloroform–methanol (9.6:0.4, v/v) was further purified on the same column using a solvent system chloroform–methanol (9.3:0.7, v/v). Final purification by preparative TLC plates developed in chloroform–methanol (8.8:1.2, v/v) resulted in santolinoic acid, the identity of which was confirmed by HR-EIMS, $^1$H-NMR, $^{13}$C-NMR, and infrared (IR) spectroscopy.

In addition to $^1$H and $^{13}$C NMR analysis, TLC coupled in an offline manner with electrospray mass spectrometry (ESI–MS) and high-resolution ESI Fourier transform ion cyclotron resonance (FTICR) MS for isolation and characterization of two novel lupane triterpenoids from *Paullinia pinnata* L.: 6β-(3′-methoxy-4′-hydroxybenzoyl)-lup-20(29)-ene-one and 6β-(3′-methoxy-4′-hydroxybenzoyl)-lup-20(29)-ene-ol, which are suspected to play a crucial role in the plant's wound healing effects [32]. The extract from *Paullinia pinnata* L. was subjected to an exhaustive isolation procedure starting with two consecutive column chromatography purifications on silica gel; different ratios of chloroform–methanol were used as eluent. The triterpenoid-containing fraction was purified on preparative silica gel TLC plate with chloroform–methanol (9:1, v/v) as a developing solvent. The two resulting lupane bands were finally submitted to MS analyses.

Another example of offline TLC–MS analysis was demonstrated in a study by Srivastava et al. [33]. A quality by design concept was put into practice for the optimization of extraction of taraxasterol, taraxasterol acetate, and stigmasterol from *Pluchea lanceolata*. Three distinct procedures were assessed: microwave-assisted, pulsed ultrasonication-assisted, and continuous ultrasonication-assisted extraction. The extraction yields of a particular extraction attempt were determined by TLC method with densitometric evaluation after postchromatographic derivatization with anisaldehyde/sulfuric acid reagent. TLC–MS analyses were undertaken to provide additional specificity by confirming the identity of the isolated triterpenoids. The separation was carried out using silica gel $F_{254}$ HPTLC plates, which were developed in *n*-hexane–ethyl acetate (88:12, v/v). The analyte-containing bands were scraped off the plates and after that introduced into the ESI–MS system to compare their MS spectra with that of a standard compound. The pulse ultrasonic-assisted extraction utilizing organic solvents (ethyl acetate–methanol 75:25, v/v) resulted in optimum extraction of all three studied triterpenoids.

The first online TLC–MS attempt in the field of triterpenoids was done only in 2005 in the study of the photo-oxidation of natural di- and triterpenoid resins used as paint varnishes [10]. The resinous samples were applied onto a cellulose-coated TLC plate, which afterward was subjected to direct MALDI-TOF–MS analysis without any development. The plates were only sprayed with a saturated ethanol solution of 2,5-dihydroxybenzoic acid as matrix to assist the ionization of compounds. Triterpenoids were observed as protonated molecules or as sodium clusters. Dammaradienone, dammaradienol, nor-α-amyrone, and dammarenolic, oleanonic, and ursonic acid were detected in dammar resin; moronic acid, masticadienonic acid, and 3-*O*-acetyl-3-epi(iso)masticadienonic acid were found in mastic resin; and diterpenoid abietane and pimarane acids were present in colophony. The induced aging process produced oxidized triterpenoids, which were observed in the MS spectra as ions corresponding to triterpenoids from the unaged samples with multiple mass increments of 16 Da. Uptake of up to six oxygen atoms was found in individual cases, which indicates extensive oxidation of these resins. In this quasi-TLC–MS analysis, no interferences due to matrix ions or cluster ions were observed, which is usually a common problem in MALDI-TOF–MS. However, a high MS background was encountered when conventional MALDI metal plates were used instead of cellulose TLC plates. This highlights the effectiveness of the latter as a support for the matrix/sample solution in MALDI experiments. Thus, to some extent, this work underlies the foundation for online TLC–MALDI–MS analysis of triterpenoids by taking advantage of cellulose-coated TLC plates.

A comparison of one-dimensional low temperature TLC–MS (1D LT TLC–MS) and two-dimensional LT TLC LC–MS system with the purpose of *Salvia lavandulifolia* fingerprinting was made [34]. Essential oil samples were applied on silica gel 60 $F_{254}$ plates, which were developed using toluene–ethyl acetate (95:5, v/v) at −10°C. TLC–MS interface (CAMAG) was used for the elution of compounds with methanol from TLC plates to either MS or HPLC–MS system. While the 1D approach separated the constituents of *Salvia lavandulifolia* into three groups on the basis of their polarity, the 2D approach enabled further resolution of compounds into subgroups, but neither enabled baseline resolution of all analytes. This is due to the complexity of *Salvia lavandulifolia* essential oil composition, which contains different monoterpenes, sesquiterpenes, monoterpenoids, sesquiterpenoids, diterpenoids, and triterpenoids.

To estimate the content of dihydro-2,5-dihydroxy-6-methyl-4*H*-pyran-4-one (DDMP) saponin and saponin B in selected pea cultivars, an HPTLC method was developed [35]. Silica gel 60 $F_{254}$ plates were prewashed with methanol and activated at 100°C prior to development in automated multiple development chamber AMD2 using chloroform–methanol–water (55:37:8, v/v). Densitometry, after postchromatographic derivatization with anisaldehyde–sulfuric acid, revealed the prevalence of saponin B over DDMP saponin in all pea cultivars. The identities of the two compounds were determined by coupling HPTLC directly to ESI–MS and additionally by offline MALDI-TOF/TOF–MS by application of a purified extract/matrix mixture onto a standard steel MALDI plate. HPTLC plates intended for MS analysis were developed with a modified developing solvent chloroform–methanol–water (6.5:3.5:0.9, v/v). The analytes were eluted from the plates with 0.1% formic acid–acetonitrile (40:60, v/v) by means of TLC–MS interface (CAMAG) and transferred into the ESI–MS system, which operated in positive-ion mode.

Recently, a new TLC method and online TLC–MS were used for screening of isomeric triterpenoid acids (ursolic, oleanolic, and betulinic acids) in epicuticular waxes of different vegetables [26]. Separation of compounds on $C_{18}$ RP HPTLC plates, predeveloped in acetone and developed in a horizontal developing chamber using *n*-hexane–ethyl acetate (5:1, v/v) as a developing solvent, was followed by postchromatographic derivatization with anisaldehyde detection reagent. No interference from other plant triterpenoids (lupeol, α-amyrin, β-amyrin, cycloartenol, lupenone, friedelin, lupeol acetate, or cycloartenol acetate) and phytosterols (β-sitosterol, stigmasterol) was observed. The presence of ursolic, oleanolic, and betulinic acids, detected in some of the studied vegetable extracts, was additionally confirmed by

TLC–MS. Each of the sample zones with $R_F$ equal to the $R_F$ of the cochromato-graphed standards was transferred into the APCI source (operated in negative-ion mode) of the MS detector by means of TLC–MS interface (CAMAG) using ace-tonitrile. The isomeric acids were well separated from each other, but they showed similar first-order mass spectra, while the product ion (MS$^2$) spectra are more useful for their differentiation. By the use of this TLC–MS method, ursolic and oleanolic acids were found for the first time in radicchio "Leonardo" and white-colored radic-chio "di Castelfranco" extracts. Additionally, TLC detection of betulinic acid in the eggplant extract was proved a false-positive as it was denied by TLC–MS.

In another study, a survey of triterpenoids and phytosterols in epicuticular waxes of various vegetables (zucchini, eggplant, tomato, red pepper, mangold, spinach, lettuce, white-colored radicchio "di Castelfranco," radicchio "Leonardo," white cabbage, red cabbage, and savoy cabbage) was executed by online TLC–MS$^2$ [9]. The samples were screened for eight triterpenoids (lupeol, α-amyrin, β-amyrin, cycloartenol, cycloartenol acetate, lupeol acetate, lupenone, and friedelin) and two phytosterols (β-sitosterol and stigmasterol). These are structurally highly simi-lar compounds, and therefore, separation and differentiation of these compounds can be a demanding task. In this study, HPTLC silica gel 60 and HPTLC C$_{18}$ RP plates were used and they were predeveloped with chloroform–methanol (1:1, v/v) and acetone, respectively. Silica gel plates were developed by using $n$-hexane–ethyl acetate (5:1, v/v) and RP plates by using acetone–acetonitrile (5:1, v/v) and ethyl acetate–acetonitrile (3:2, v/v). The use of three TLC methods was necessary in order to achieve distinction between all studied compounds. Silica gel plates enabled separation of compounds according to their functional groups, while RP plates completely, or in some cases, partly resolved positional isomers. The authors discriminated between various triterpenoids and phytosterols based on $R_F$ values and characteristic colors of TLC bands after postchromatographic derivatization with anisaldehyde reagent. Unambiguous confirmation of compounds was achieved through investigation of their product ion spectra (MS$^2$), which were correlated with those of standards (Figure 17.4). For TLC–MS$^2$ analyses, a modified method using RP plates was employed with the developing solvent ethyl acetate–acetonitrile (3:2, v/v); the plates were rotated 90° (10 cm × 20 cm) and developed to a distance of 18 cm to dissociate the adjoining bands even further apart than in the original method. This enabled elution of compounds from the adsorbent by means of TLC–MS interface (CAMAG). The effluent (acetonitrile) was directed into an APCI ion source, which operated in positive-ion mode. Online TLC–MS$^2$ was shown to be a powerful tool in qualitative analysis of triterpenoids and phytosterols, and some of these compounds were confirmed in the epicuticular waxes of particular vegetables for the first time (Figure 17.5).

## 17.5 TLC–MS ANALYSIS OF FLAVANOLS

Flavanols are secondary metabolites found in different parts of plants where they serve as a natural barrier against oxidation and pathogens as well as protectors against herbivores. Apart from their protective role against the development of car-diovascular diseases and type 2 diabetes, suggested by epidemiological studies,

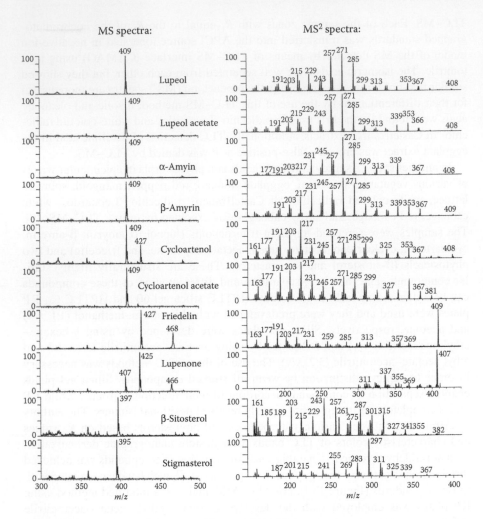

**FIGURE 17.4** MS and MS$^2$ spectra of some triterpenoid and phytosterol standards eluted with acetonitrile from C$_{18}$ RP HPTLC plates and injected directly into MS. (From Naumoska, K. and Vovk, I. 2015. *J. Chromatogr. A*, 1381: 229–238. With permission.)

antimicrobial and antioxidant activity were also reported. These are the main reasons why these compounds attracted considerable attention of researchers and also producers of dietary supplement products containing these compounds as the active ingredients.

Flavanols (or flavan-3-ols) are a class of flavonoids with a backbone structure composed of three rings. Individual flavanol monomeric units can be linked together via interflavanol bonds, merging into larger building blocks by oxidative polycondensation, thus forming oligomeric or polymeric proanthocyanidins. There is no key by which the monomeric units bind together and can be done through various carbon atoms, which increases the number of possible structural isomers. In addition, flavanols have two chiral carbon atoms. The structural complexity of flavanols is a

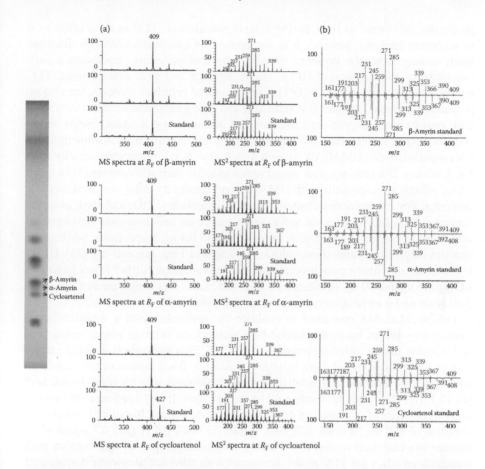

**FIGURE 17.5** Confirmation and disproof of identity of some compounds extracted from red pepper epicuticular wax. (a) Parallel mass spectra comparison: the upper two spectra in each MS and MS² comparison section belong to the eluted sample test solution zones (from two neighboring tracks) from the C₁₈ RP HPTLC plate developed with ethyl acetate–acetonitrile (3:2, v/v), while the third represents the corresponding standard. (b) Head to tail comparison of the MS² spectra obtained from the eluted sample test solution zones and the corresponding standards, represented by the upward and downward pointed mass spectra, respectively. (From Naumoska, K. and Vovk, I. 2015. *J. Chromatogr. A*, 1381: 229–238. With permission.)

major challenge in qualitative and quantitative analysis of these compounds in plant materials, food, and dietary supplements. Another issue is the absence of commercially available standards; only catechins and some of their dimers are available. Separation techniques such as TLC, HPLC, and CE are indispensable in qualitative and quantitative analysis of these compounds. The most commonly used HPLC with UV detection has weak specificity because data acquisition at relatively low wavelengths must be used due to the lack of a suitable chromophore. This increases unwanted interferences by phenolic acids, stilbenes, and others, which are usually present in flavanols' test solutions, given their similar chemical and physical properties that come to light during sample preparation. TLC is most often used in screening analyses; however, it is also applied for quantitative analysis. Baseline shift, arising from the presence of oligomers and polymers, represents a serious problem in evaluation of HPLC chromatograms and TLC densitograms. TLC analysis mostly carried out on HPTLC silica gel and cellulose sorbents, but also on polyamide sorbents, enables fast screening and also quantification when combined with postchromatographic derivatization and densitometry. Reagents based on the combination of strong acids and aldehydes (vanillin, anisaldehyde, 4-dimethylaminocinnamaldehyde [DMACA]), as well as fast blue B salt reagent are usually used for detection. The reason is that postchromatographic derivatization results in much better selectivity (especially with DMACA) and sensitivity compared to direct UV detection. For example, densitometric limit of detection (LOD) and limit of quantitation (LOQ) for (+)-catechin and (−)-epicatechin on cellulose plate developed in water and derivatized by DMACA were 0.2 ng and 0.4 ng, respectively, while using vanillin reagent increases these values to 0.5 ng and 1 ng, respectively [36]. Direct UV evaluation without postchromatographic derivatization further raises LOD and LOQ to 18 ng and 40 ng. In the case of TLC–MS, LOD for (−)-epicatechin was 17 ng (full scan) and 5 ng (single reaction monitoring [SRM]) [8].

Offline TLC–MS was used to evaluate the applicability of a multifunctional instrument—ExtraChrom for forced-flow techniques, rotation planar extraction, and rotation planar chromatography (RPC) [37]. This instrument enabled extraction of flavanols from oak bark (*Quercus robur* L.), fractionation of the extract on silica gel H for TLC using three different eluents (toluene–ethyl acetate–formic acid [35:15:1,v/v]; ethyl acetate–methanol [1:1,v/v]; methanol) and confirmed the unambiguous presence of (+)-catechin directly in the crude extract. Rotational planar fractionation of 840 mg of crude oak bark extract on silica gel H gave 6.7 mg of white powder ((+)-catechin) in one run. Further cochromatography of this fraction with standards on silica gel TLC plates, developed with ethyl acetate–water–formic acid (85:15:10, v/v) and detected with vanillin–phosphoric acid reagent, pointed toward (+)-catechin or (−)-epicatechin. A direct injection of the isolated compound solution into the APCI–MS, operating in negative-ion mode, confirmed the assumption. Finally, planar chromatography on the cellulose plates developed with pure water in two developing modes, linear using normal developing chamber and circular using ultramicro chamber rotation planar chromatography (U-RPC), served for distinguishing between both possible epimeric flavan-3-ols and final identification of the isolated compound as (+)-catechin.

Recently, TLC–MS was used for quality control of 21 dietary supplement products containing grape seed extracts [38]. The separation on TLC silica gel $F_{254}$ plates developed in acetone–acetic acid–toluene (3:1:3, v/v) [39] was followed by postchromatographic derivatization with vanillin–HCl detection reagent. Chromatograms of authentic grape seed, peanut skin, and pine bark extracts, procyanidin B2 reference standard and 21 grape seed extract containing dietary supplements were compared. Authentic grape seed samples contain only procyanidin B dimers; however, unexpected procyanidin A dimers were also found in some dietary supplement samples. Those samples were rechromatographed using the same system. Zones were visualized by UV light and the zone corresponding to procyanidin A2 was subsequently scraped off, extracted by 0.1% acetic acid in methanol and injected directly into ESI–MS to confirm its identity. The MS system operated in positive ion mode. The obtained results, in combination with HPLC–UV–MS results, confirmed adulteration of nine dietary supplement products with peanut skin extract. Therefore, the described TLC–MS method is a simple and inexpensive tool for distinguishing authentic grape seed extracts from its adulterants.

The first use of online coupling of TLC with MS in the analysis of flavanols was reported for their detection in chocolate [40], which is a good source of plant-derived (–)-epicatechin and its dimer procyanidin B2 (Figure 17.6). Compounds were separated on the cellulose HPTLC plate developed in a horizontal developing chamber using n-propanol–water–acetic acid (20:80:1, v/v) [41] as a developing solvent. Flavanols were eluted from the adsorbent by means of TLC–MS interface (CAMAG) using methanol. Mass spectra of (–)-epicatechin and procyandin B2 were obtained using ESI–MS in a negative-ion mode.

The only other online TLC–MS approach was applied to detect flavanols in the peel of *Punica granatum* L. fruits and in seeds of *Juniperus communis* L. [8]. TLC was performed on cellulose and silica gel 60 HPTLC plates. For cellulose plates, pure water and n-propanol–water–acetic acid (4:2:1, v/v) [41] were used as developing solvents, while silica gel plates were developed in acetone–toluene–acetic acid (6:3:1, v/v) [42]. The extraction of compounds from the plates was accomplished by means of TLC–MS interface (CAMAG) using methanol as eluent in most cases. Formic acid solution was added to the effluent prior to injection in ESI–MS (negative-ion mode), to render the ionization process more selective. A high MS background was encountered when the samples were being eluted from silica gel plates. To circumvent this nuisance, a HILIC guard column was mounted between TLC–MS interface and the ion source to retain impurities, which caused ion suppression. This simple trick enabled the detection of flavanols not only on cellulose but also on silica gel plates. As a result, flavanols and proanthocyanidin dimers and trimers were detected in *Juniperus communis* L. for the first time, using an optimized online TLC–MS method.

## 17.6 CHALLENGES FOR THE FUTURE

Utilization of TLC–MS in the analysis of secondary metabolites, such as carotenoids, triterpenoids, and flavanols, has only begun to grow in the last couple of years, which is made evident by the increasing number of publications on this topic. This is especially true for the online coupling, which is evolving alongside state-of-the-art innovations in TLC and MS instrumentation. The offline approach has been readily used for quite some time. Analyte-containing band is scraped from the chromatographic plates, the compounds of interest reextracted from adsorbent, and directed toward MS analysis. Degradation of labile carotenoids on the chromatographic media, insufficient separation of some structurally similar compounds and, therefore, their unselective transfer from TLC to MS, compromised sensitivity, high spectral background, band diffusion upon addition of MALDI matrix to the developed TLC plate, etc. are just a few current drawbacks of TLC–MS, which were already addressed at the beginning of this chapter. However, these obstacles serve as seeds of innovation

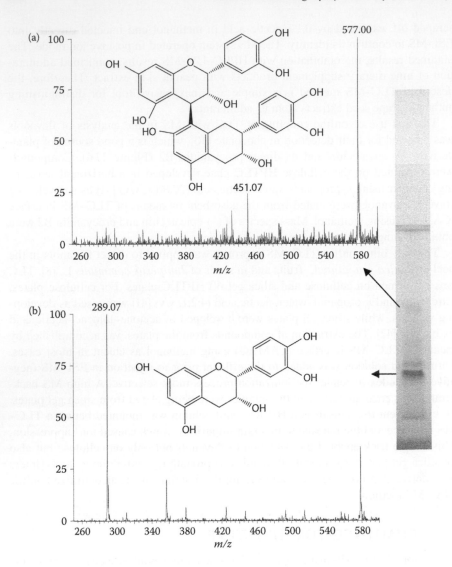

**FIGURE 17.6** Mass spectra of procyanidin B2 (a) and (−)-epicatechin (b) obtained from chocolate sample test solution after elution of zones from the HPTLC cellulose plate developed in water. Here, bands are visualized by postchromatographic derivatization with DMACA detection reagent.

and further development of both offline and online TLC–MS couplings, which results in easier and faster analysis, and more reliable, selective, and informative experimental data. Thus, there is still a lot of room for improvement in the area of TLC–MS techniques and instrumentation, as well as the quality, homogeneity, and batch-to-batch reproducibility of commercially available adsorbent layers. In this respect, even recently introduced MS grade silica gel plates, which are designed and developed for minimal background signal, do not always rise to their expectations.

We can expect an increased use of multidimensional techniques to tackle the need for a higher resolving power when dealing with complex natural materials. These include plant, animal, and bacteria samples with diverse metabolite composition, including flavanols, carotenoids, and triterpenoids. An obvious future direction in carotenoid analysis is a comprehensive 2D TLC × MS in conjunction with the parallel development of orthogonal mixed-mode TLC plates. For instance, separation of a carotenoid mixture using silica gel in the first dimension and magnesium oxide in the second dimension would enable differentiation between these pigments on account of their polarity and the length of the conjugated double bond chain, respectively. Additionally, by the use of techniques that enable very accurate localization and elution of the analyte from the TLC plate, 2D imaging is readily available. For even higher resolution, 2D techniques such as TLC–LC–MS and TLC–GC–MS will undoubtedly become more frequently used. In the circumstances that require enhanced specificity and structural information, TLC–DAD–MS should prove to be a powerful tool by enabling simultaneous acquisition and comparison of UV–vis and MS spectra. It is also expected that libraries of standard MS (and MS²) spectra obtained via TLC–MS, along with all experimental conditions, will be available online in the future. This will provide a significant support in the fast growing field of dietary supplements, where TLC and TLC–MS serve as an important tool in the development, quality control, and adulteration analyses.

## REFERENCES

1. Martelanc, M., Vovk, I., and Simonovska, B. 2009. Separation and identification of some common isomeric plant triterpenoids by thin-layer chromatography and high performance liquid chromatography, *J. Chromatogr. A*, 1216: 6662–6670.
2. Vovk, I. and Glavnik, V. 2015. Analysis of dietary supplements, In: *Instrumental Thin-Layer Chromatography*, Poole, C.F. Ed., Elsevier, Amsterdam, Chapter 21.
3. Vovk, I., Glavnik, V., Albreht, A., Naumoska, K., Simonovska, B., and Smrke, S. 2014. Planar chromatography and mass spectrometry in analysis of phytonutrients in the extracts of edible plants, *International Symposium for High-Performance Thin-Layer Chromatography*, Lyon, France, July 2–4, Abstract O-29.
4. Meléndez-Martínez, A.J., Vicario, I.M., and Heredia, F.J. 2007. Geometrical isomers of violaxanthin in orange juice, *Food Chem.*, 104: 169–175.
5. Crăpătureanu, S., Rosca, G., Neamtu, G., Socaciu, C., Britton, G., and Pfander, H. 1996. Carotenoids from seabuckthorn fruit determined by thin-layer chromatography and mass spectrometry, *Rev. Roum. Biochim.*, 33: 167–174.
6. Rodić, Z., Simonovska, B., Albreht, A., and Vovk I. 2012. Determination of lutein by high-performance thin-layer chromatography using densitometry and screening of major dietary carotenoids in food supplements, *J. Chromatogr. A*, 1231: 59–65.
7. Manikandan, M., Hasan, N., and Wu, H.F. 2013. Rapid detection of haloarchaeal carotenoids via liquid–liquid microextraction enabled direct TLC MALDI–MS, *Talanta*, 107: 167–175.
8. Smrke, S. and Vovk, I. 2013. Comprehensive thin-layer chromatography mass spectrometry of flavanols from *Juniperus communis* L. and *Punica granatum* L., *J. Chromatogr. A*, 1289: 119–126.
9. Naumoska, K. and Vovk, I. 2015. Analysis of triterpenoids and phytosterols in vegetables by thin-layer chromatography coupled to tandem mass spectrometry, *J. Chromatogr. A*, 1381: 229–238.

10. Scalarone, D., Duursma, M.C., Boon, J.J., and Chiantore, O. 2005. MALDI-TOF mass spectrometry on cellulosic surfaces of fresh and photo-aged di- and triterpenoid varnish resins, *J. Mass Spectrom.*, 40: 1527–1535.

11. Britton, G. 2008. TLC of carotenoids, In: *Thin Layer Chromatography in Phytochemistry*, Waksmundzka-Hajnos, M., Sherma, J., and Kowalska, T., Eds., CRC Press/Taylor & Francis Group, Boca Raton, FL, Chapter 21.

12. Sechrist, J., Pachuski, J., and Sherma, J. 2002. Quantification of lutein in dietary supplements by reversed-phase high-performance thin-layer chromatography with visible-mode densitometry, *Acta Chromatogr.*, 12: 151–158.

13. Vasta, J.D. and Sherma, J. 2010. Analysis of lycopene in nutritional supplements by silica gel high-performance thin-layer chromatography with visible-mode densitometry, *Acta Chromatogr.*, 20: 673–683.

14. Zeb, A. and Murkovic, M. 2010. Thin-layer chromatographic analysis of carotenoids in plant and animal samples, *J. Planar Chromatogr.*, 23: 94–103.

15. Britton, G. 1985. General carotenoid methods, *Methods Enzymol.*, 111: 113–149.

16. Schwieter, U., Bolliger, H.R., Chopard-dit-Jean, L.H., Englert, G., Kofler, M., König, A., von Planta, C., Rüegg, R., Vetter, W., and Isler, O. 1965. Synthesen in der carotinoidreihe. 19. Mittelung: Physikalische Eigenschaften der Carotine, *Chimia*, 19: 294–302.

17. Britton, G. and Goodwin, T.W. 1969. The occurrence of phytoene 1,2-oxide and related carotenoids in tomatoes, *Phytochemistry*, 8: 2257–2258.

18. Ben-Aziz, A., Britton, G., and Goodwin, T.W. 1973. Carotene epoxides of *Lycopersicon esculentum*, *Phytochemistry*, 12: 2759–2764.

19. Britton, G. and Goodwin, T.W. 1975. Carotene epoxides from delta tomato mutant, *Phytochemistry*, 14: 2530–2532.

20. Rønnekleiv, M., Lenes, M., Norgård, S., and Liaaen-Jensen, S. 1995. Three dodecaene $C_{50}$-carotenoids from halophilic bacteria, *Phytochemistry*, 39: 631–634.

21. Strand, A., Shivaji, S., and Liaaen-Jensen, S. 1997. Bacterial carotenoids 55.* $C_{50}$-Carotenoids 25. Revised structures of carotenoids associated with membranes in psychrotrophic *Micrococcus roseus*, *Biochem. Syst. Ecol.*, 25: 547–552.

22. Bjørnland, T., Haxo, F.T., and Liaaen-Jensen, S. 2003. Carotenoids of the Florida red tide dinoflagellate *Karenia brevis*, *Biochem. Syst. Ecol.*, 31: 1147–1162.

23. Meléndez-Martínez, A.J., Britton, G., Vicario, I.M., and Heredia, F.J. 2005. Identification of zeinoxanthin in orange juices, *J. Agric. Food Chem.*, 53: 6362–6367.

24. Zhang, W., Hu, X., Wang, L., and Wang, X. 2014. Reconstruction of the carotenoid biosynthetic pathway of *Cronobacter sakazakii* BAA894 in *Escherichia coli*, *PLoS one*, 9: e86739–e86739.

25. Černelič, K., Simonovska, B., Vovk, I., and Albreht, A. 2010. TLC–MS method for detection of neoxanthin, violaxanthin, lutein and beta-carotene, *28th International Symposium on Chromatography*, Valencia, Spain, September 12–16, Abstract P15–098.

26. Naumoska, K., Simonovska, B., Albreht, A., and Vovk, I. 2013. TLC and TLC–MS screening of ursolic, oleanolic and betulinic acids in plant extracts, *J. Planar Chromatogr.*, 26: 125–131.

27. Simonovska, B. and Vovk, I. 2002. TLC separation of some triterpenoids, *Planar Chromatography Today 2002*, Novo mesto, Slovenia, October 4–6, Abstract O-06.

28. Wójciak-Kosior, M. 2007. Separation and determination of closely related triterpenic acids by high performance thin-layer chromatography after iodine derivatization, *J. Pharm. Biomed. Anal.*, 45: 337–340.

29. Oleszek, W., Kapusta I., and Stochmal, A. 2008. TLC of triterpenoids (including saponins), in *Thin Layer Chromatography in Phytochemistry*, Waksmundzka-Hajnos, M., Sherma, J., and Kowalska, T., Eds., CRC Press/Taylor & Francis Group, Boca Raton, FL, Chapter 20.

30. Bonfill, M., Mangas, S., Cusidó, R.M., Osuna, L., Piñol, M.T., and Palazón, J. 2006. Identification of triterpenoid compounds of *Centella asiatica* by thin-layer chromatography and mass spectrometry, *Biomed. Chromatogr.*, 20: 151–153.
31. Ahmad, Z., Mehmood, Z., Ifzal, R., Malik, A., Afza, N., Ashraf, M., and Jahan E. 2007. A new ursane-type triterpenoid from *Salvia santolinifolia*, *Turk. J. Chem.*, 31: 495–501.
32. Annan, K. and Houghton, P.J. 2010. Two novel lupane triterpenoids from *Paullinia pinnata* L. with fibroblast stimulatory activity, *J. Pharm. Pharmacol.*, 62: 663–668.
33. Srivastava, P., Ajayakumar, P.V., and Shanker, K. 2014. Box-Behnken design for optimum extraction of biogenetic chemicals from *P. lanceolata* with an energy audit (thermal × microwave × acoustic): A case study of HPTLC determination with additional specificity using on-line/off-line coupling with DAD/NIR/ESI–MS, *Phytochem. Anal.*, 25: 551–560.
34. Sajewicz, M., Wojtal, Ł., Natić, M., Staszek, D., Waksmundzka-Hajnos, M., and Kowalska, T. 2011. TLC–MS versus TLC–LC–MS fingerprints of herbal extracts. Part I. Essential oils, *J. Liq. Chromatogr. Relat. Technol.*, 34: 848–863.
35. Reim, V. and Rohn, S. 2014. Characterization of saponins in peas (*Pisum sativum* L.) by HPTLC coupled to mass spectrometry and a hemolysis assay, *Food Res. Int.*, article in press, http://dx.doi.org/10.1016/j.foodres.2014.06.043.
36. Glavnik, V., Simonovska, B., and Vovk, I. 2009. Densitometric determination of (+)-catechin and (−)-epicatechin by 4-dimethylaminocinnamaldehyde reagent, *J. Chromatogr. A*, 1216: 4485–4491.
37. Vovk, I., Simonovska, B., Andrenšek, S., Vuorela, H., and Vuorela, P. 2003. Rotation planar extraction and rotation planar chromatography of oak (*Quercus robur* L.) bark, *J. Chromatogr. A*, 991: 267–274.
38. Villani, T.S., Reichert, W., Ferruzzi, M.G., Pasinetti, G.M., Simon, J.E., and Wu, Q.L. 2015. Chemical investigation of commercial grape seed derived products to assess quality and detect adulteration, *Food Chem.*, 170: 271–280.
39. Xu, Y.P., Simon, J.E., Welch, C., Wightman, J.D., Ferruzzi, M.G., Ho, L., Passinetti, G.M., and Wu, Q.L. 2011. Survey of polyphenol constituents in grapes and grape-derived products, *J. Agric. Food Chem.*, 59: 10586–10593.
40. Glavnik, V., Simonovska, B., Vovk, I., and Albreht, A. 2010. TLC–MS detection of lecithin and proanthocyanidins in chocolate, *28th International Symposium on Chromatography*, Valencia, Spain, September 12–16, Abstract P15–099.
41. Vovk, I., Simonovska, B., and Vuorela, H. 2005. Separation of eight selected flavan-3-ols on cellulose thin-layer chromatographic plates, *J. Chromatogr. A*, 1077: 188–194.
42. Lea, A.G.H. 1978. Phenolics of ciders-oligomeric and polymeric procyanidins, *J. Sci. Food Agric.*, 29: 471–477.

# 18 TLC/MALDI MS of Carbohydrates

*Katharina Lemmnitzer, Rosmarie Süß,
and Jürgen Schiller*

## CONTENTS

## 18.1 INTRODUCTION

Besides proteins, DNA/RNA, and lipids, carbohydrates represent another important, but thus far often neglected type of biomolecules. However, the interest in carbohydrates (and the related analysis) is continuously increasing because carbohydrates (e.g., the sulfated glycosaminoglycans) were identified to have important regulatory functions in the human body [1].

Although a comprehensive treatise of the individual carbohydrates is clearly beyond the scope of this chapter [2], it must be stated that carbohydrates are very complex molecules—much more complex as one would expect from the historical definition "hydrates of carbon," that is, the general formula $C_x(H_2O)_x$. It is important to note that some caution is needed when this simple definition is used: many typical carbohydrates such as chitin or the glycosaminoglycans (which contain nitrogen) do not agree at all with this simple definition [3]. This also applies for many glycolipids, which will be discussed in this chapter. In contrast, other molecules such as lactic acid ($C_3H_6O_3$) are identified by the formal definition as "carbohydrates," but lactic acid of course does not represent a typical carbohydrate. Some relevant carbohydrate structures are shown in Figure 18.1.

The analysis of carbohydrates is challenging due to the following aspects [4]:

1. There are many different isomers (e.g., the epimeric sugars glucose and galactose) that make separation difficult. This problem is even nowadays

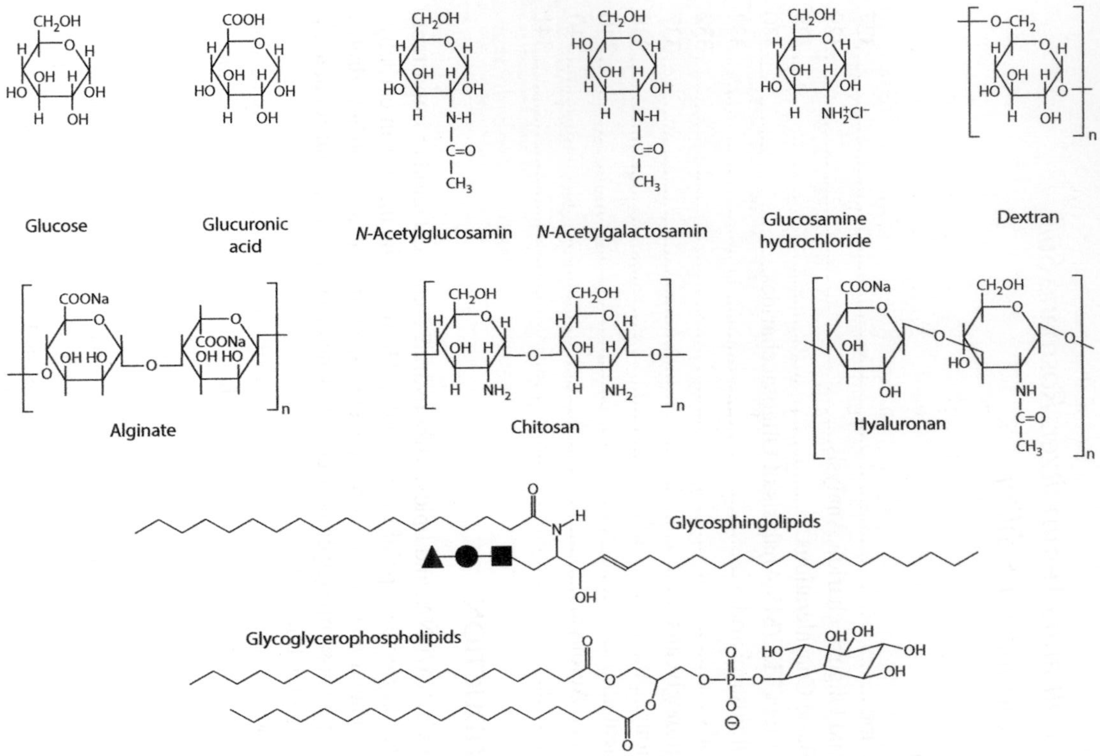

**FIGURE 18.1** Chemical structures of the compounds mentioned in this chapter. Besides monosaccharides, some selected polysaccharides, such as dextran or hyaluronan (subsequent to enzymatic or chemical degradation), will be discussed as well. Please note that alginate is actually composed of guluronic and mannuronic acid units. However, we will not differentiate the presence of both of these isomers. Finally, some simple glycolipids, such as glycosphingolipids or glycoglycerophospholipids, are also discussed. The geometrical symbols represent different sugar residues.

best overcome by gas chromatography (GC), although GC is boring and laborious because previous derivatization is necessary [5].

2. All native carbohydrates are compounds of low volatility, which minimizes the ion yields and, thus, aggravates their analysis by mass spectrometry [6].

3. The lack of UV-absorbing or fluorescent moieties prevents the application of many commonly used analytical techniques—at least they cannot be employed without prior modification of the target carbohydrate by introducing a chromo- or fluorophore [7].

These problems normally lead to the necessity of time-consuming sample derivatization to improve the detection of carbohydrates by a UV, fluorescence, or MS detector. We will focus here exclusively on the MS detection of TLC-separated carbohydrates without previous derivatization because this is a major methodological progress achieved in the last decade. Hopefully, we will be able to show that the knowledge of the $m/z$ value adds an important source of information, which may often help to identify an unknown compound. Additionally, the $m/z$ ratio is a more reliable measure in comparison to the $R_f$ values, which are affected by many different parameters and, thus, normally not well reproducible.

Although the TLC analysis of mono- and disaccharides such as glucose, fructose, or saccharose is well established and helps to identify even compounds present in small concentrations and in complex mixtures (such as diary products) [8], to our best knowledge there are no data available regarding the direct detection of these sugars by MS on a TLC plate. This is not surprising because MALDI is—despite many obvious advantages—generally not the method of choice to characterize small molecules ($m/z < 500$): the small mass range is characterized by a significant "background" stemming from the applied matrices, which normally undergo photochemical reactions [9].

## 18.2 MONO- AND OLIGOSACCHARIDE ANALYSIS

### 18.2.1 BASIC CONSIDERATIONS

It is well known that even complex carbohydrate mixtures (found in food or urine samples) can be separated by TLC [10]. Although many different stationary phases are nowadays commercially available, there are in practice only three suitable layers for the separation of carbohydrates: cellulose, silica, and aminopropyl bonded silica [3].

Cellulose was (and in fact is) widely used to separate carbohydrates because many of the solvent systems established in the past for paper chromatography (often mixtures between butanol, water, and acetic acid or acetonitrile and water) could be readily applied to cellulose plates [3]. However, the development time is shorter and there is less spot diffusion in comparison to paper chromatography when TLC on cellulose plates is used [11].

Nevertheless, silica gel is nowadays the most commonly used sorbent regarding TLC separation of carbohydrates. Silica gel layers are suitable for nearly all carbohydrates (with the exception of polysaccharides because they do not show any migration) and may result in reasonable resolution: for instance, it has been shown that oligosaccharides of the dextran type can be resolved when they contain less than 12 (glucose) monosaccharide units [12], and this resolution also can be achieved when complex carbohydrate mixtures are of interest.

Besides its commercial availability, another advantage of silica is its chemical stability against almost all solvents as well as corrosive reagents. For instance, semiconcentrated sulfuric acid is often used for the visualization of carbohydrates by charring.

Amino groups added as aminopropyl groups bonded to silica gel or simply as aminosilica gel ($NH_2$ silica gel) are particularly useful as sorbent modifications for carbohydrate analysis—particularly when combined with additives such as monosodium phosphate [13]. Similar solvent systems as in the case of unmodified silica gel can be used at these conditions. One important advantage of these layers is that there is no need of staining the analytes: the amino group of the stationary phase reacts with the aldehyde group of reducing sugars under generation of intensely fluorescing derivatives, which are very sensitively detectable [14].

As already mentioned (vide supra), the analysis of carbohydrates is very important in the context of food chemistry, for instance, honey, diary products, and chocolate [15], which have all been already successfully investigated. A lot of interest is also coming from the analysis of urine, which contains a lot of different mono- and disaccharides [16] as well as even polymeric carbohydrates, particularly glycosaminoglycans [17]. Eleven simple reference sugars, including the acidic sugar, glucuronic acid, could be successfully analyzed by means of TLC and the individual approaches compared by Zhang and coworkers [18]: based on these studies, a simple, reproducible, and quantifiable procedure was developed that permitted several sugars to be identified in normal urine samples without the need of a prior desalting or concentration step. Ethyl acetate:pyridine:water (60:25:20, v/v/v) was used in combination with a Celite adsorbent and anisaldehyde as the visualization reagent.

## 18.2.2   Direct TLC/MS Analysis of Oligosaccharides

To our best knowledge, there are thus far no reports available describing the application of modern desorption MS techniques (such as MALDI or DESI) for carbohydrate analysis directly from a developed TLC plate. This is not surprising regarding MALDI MS because the smaller $m/z$ range (where typical carbohydrates are detectable) is dominated by matrix-derived ions. This applies at least when common organic molecules (such as 2,5-dihydroxybenzoic acid [DHB]) are used as MALDI matrices [19].

However, there are some reports available where particle beam ionization methods such as FAB (fast atom bombardment) were used [20]: 2,3,4,5-bis-$O$-(methylethylidene)-β-D-fructopyranose as well as its sulfamate and the corresponding carbamate were investigated by Caldwell and coworkers [20] using an indirect approach, that is, a microtransfer method to isolate the carbohydrates of interest from the TLC plate prior to FAB MS analysis. The carbohydrates of interest could be separated by using cyclohexane and 2-propanol (5:1, v/v).

Dreisewerd and coworkers [21] performed an interesting study where native milk oligosaccharides were characterized by IR MALDI MS using glycerol as matrix. This is illustrated in Figure 18.2. The limit of detection for the MS analysis was about 10 pmol of the individual oligosaccharides spotted for chromatography.

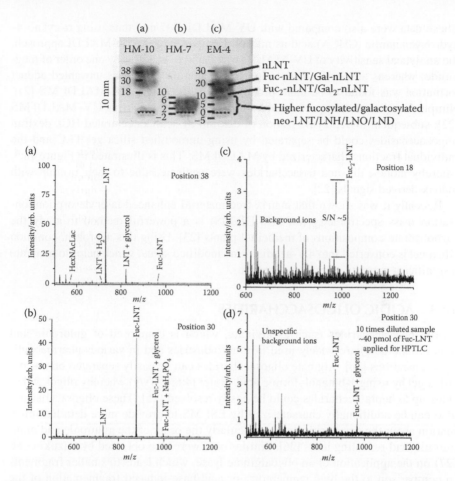

**FIGURE 18.2** Top: Orcinol-stained HPTLC chromatograms of human milk (HM) and elephant milk (EM) fractions: (a) HM-10, (b) HM-7, and (c) EM-4. The horizontal lines at the bottom of the chromatograms indicate the approximate position at which samples were applied to the HPTLC plate. The figures next to the lanes indicate the laser positions at which the mass spectra were acquired. All mass spectra were acquired from unstained lanes, which were developed in parallel on the same HPTLC plate. The center-to-center distance between two adjacent laser positions was about 300 μm for the analysis of HM-10 and about 400 μm for the experiments with the HM-7 and EM-4 samples. The assignments indicate the expected oligosaccharide species in the analyte bands for the EM-4 sample. Only fucosylated LNT (lacto-*N*-tetraose) and not Gal-LNT is expressed in human milk. Moreover, in human milk the core unit may contain both LNT and nLNT. Amounts of 6 μg of HM-10, 5 μg of HM-7, and approximately 10 μg of total EM-4 oligosaccharides, respectively, were applied for HPTLC. Bottom: Direct HPTLC/IR/MALDI/oTOF mass spectra of human milk fraction HM-10, recorded from different lateral positions on the chromatographic lanes: (a) at position 38, (b) at position 30, and (c) at position 18. An amount of 0.6 μg of HM-10 oligosaccharides was applied for HPTLC. (d) Mass spectrum acquired from Position 30 of a 10 times more diluted sample, displaying the approximate limit of detection. Here, about 60 ng of total oligosaccharide sample was applied for HPTLC corresponding to about 40 pmol of Fuc-LNT. (Reproduced from Dreisewerd, K. et al. 2006. *J. Am. Soc. Mass Spectrom.*, 17: 139–150. With permission.)

These data were also compared with UV MALDI (337 nm) data using α-cyano-4-hydroxycinnamic (CHCA) acid as matrix. Compared to the IR–MALDI approach, the analytical sensitivity of UV–MALDI was found to be lower by one order of magnitude, whereas unspecific analyte ion fragmentation as well as unwanted adduct formation was found to be more pronounced in the case of IR MALDI MS [21]. Nimptsch and coworkers performed a similar experiment by using UV–MALDI MS [22]: subsequent to depolymerization of dextran by semiconcentrated HCl, dextran oligosaccharides could be separated by using unmodified silica gel TLC and the individual fractions characterized by MALDI MS. This is illustrated in Figure 18.3, whereby mono-, di-, and trisaccharides were neglected due to their overlap with matrix-derived signals [22].

Recently it was shown that matrix-free material enhanced laser desorption/ionization mass spectrometry (mf-MELDI–MS) is a powerful method to study the carbohydrate compositions of medicinal plants [23]. Using this approach, common silica gel is converted into 4,4′-azodianiline modified silica, which helps to generate a significant quantity of carbohydrate ions.

## 18.3   ACIDIC OLIGOSACCHARIDES

Acidic polysaccharides (such as alginate, which is composed of guluronic and mannuronic acid) are widely used in food industries and in various pharmaceutical preparations [24]. Alginate oligosaccharides can be easily separated on normal silica gel by using 1-butanol–formic acid–water (4:6:1, v/v/v) whereby oligosaccharides up to heptasaccharides could be easily resolved [25]. These oligosaccharides also can be additionally characterized by ESI MS to provide more detailed information about the composition and particularly the order of the guluronic and mannuronic acid repeating units [26]. Similar data were also obtained by Suzuki et al. [27] on the application of an oligoalginate lyase, which leads to smaller fragments in comparison to the high temperature or acid/base-induced fragmentation of the alginate polysaccharide. Similar data were also obtained by using silica gel and 1-propanol/water (7:2, v/v) [28]. Although identification is presumably also possible by MALDI MS, to the best of our knowledge thus far there are no reports available dealing with this aspect.

## 18.4   GLYCOLIPIDS

Glycolipids are unequivocally the molecules of choice when applications of TLC/MS are summarized and there are already many reports available [29]. Although phospholipids such as phosphatidylinositol (PI) do also represent a "glycolipid," such (relatively simple) compounds will not be discussed here but rather in Chapter 13 of this book. Glyolipids are very abundant compounds in all mammalians and are assumed to have considerable medical relevance [30]. Therefore, an increasing number of glycolipids are nowadays assumed to be suitable as markers of many diseases. More details regarding the chromatographic aspects have been summarized by Fuchs et al. [31] and will not be discussed here to a major extent. We will focus here particularly

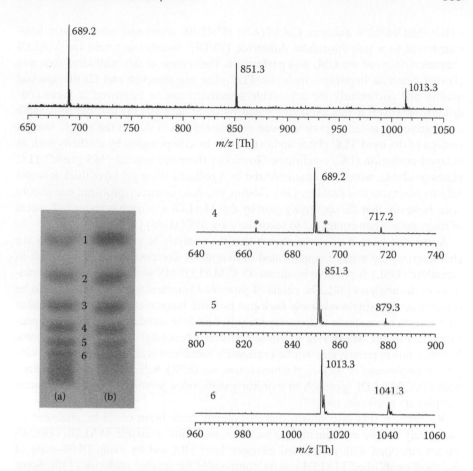

**FIGURE 18.3** HCl-induced hydrolysis of dextran: A 2 mg/mL dextran 6000 sample in water was treated with 0.7 M HCl for 20 (a) and 40 (b) min at 100°C under shaking. It is evident from the chromatogram (left) that smaller oligomers (indicated by the numbers of the glycopyranose repeating units) are generated with time. Some positive ion MALDI/TOF mass spectra of selected oligosaccharides are shown at the right. Finally, a spectrum of the total hydrolyzate (without TLC) is shown at the top to enable the comparison of the qualities of the achieved mass spectra. Impurities are marked by asterisks. (Reproduced from Nimptsch, K. et al. 2010. *J. Chromatogr. A*, 1217: 3711–3715. With permission.)

on aspects of the MALDI MS characterization while a comprehensive review about MS desorption techniques in general has recently appeared [32]. A very detailed study of the sphingolipidome of the eye lens has been recently published and gives an excellent survey of the possibilities of DESI MS [33].

An excellent, timely review regarding applications of MALDI MS to characterize glycosphingolipids (GSL) has been recently published [34] and this is the reason why we will mention here only a few selected highlights. In an early MALDI attempt [35], native GSL were separated on a conventional (silica gel 60) TLC plate by using

CHCl$_3$/MeOH/0.2% aqueous CaCl$_2$ (w/v) (55:45:10, v/v/v) and subsequently heat-transferred to a polyvinylidene difluoride (PVDF) membrane where the MALDI characterization of the GSL was performed. The reason of this additional step was (1) that potential impurities from the TLC plate are removed and (2) the spectral quality and particularly the achievable sensitivity can be improved at these conditions. However, it was explicitly stated by these authors [35] that the achievable mass accuracy is rather poor at these conditions: this is due to the rough, uneven surface of the used TLC plates and can hardly be compensated by methods such as delayed extraction (DE) conditions. Nowadays there are special "MS grade" TLC plates available, which are characterized by a reduced silica gel layer thickness and help to minimize this problem [36]. Despite the mass accuracy problem, one should note, however, that the sensitivity gain by this MALDI approach is about 1–2 orders of magnitude when compared to secondary ion MS (SIMS) [37].

Somewhat later, it could be shown that the analysis of gangliosides (which are characterized by a more complicated carbohydrate composition in comparison to "standard" GSL) is possible by direct TLC/MALDI MS without major fragmentations of the analytes [38]. The extent of unwanted fragmentation processes could be minimized by using a relatively high gas pressure (source chamber pressure about $10^{-3}$ mbar in comparison to approximately $10^{-6}$ mbar in standard MALDI mass spectrometers) in the MS device to allow collisional "cooling" of the generated ions. Notably, this approach may not be exclusively combined with TLC but as well with gel electrophoresis or surface plasmon resonance (SPR). Selected data using an antibody/TLC/MALDI approach to monitor gangliosides present in pancreatic cancer samples are available, too [39].

Recently, it was also shown that glycolipids from brain could be analyzed by using very simple equipment, that is, a commercially available MALDI/TOF/MS device equipped with a standard nitrogen laser [40] and by using DHB—one of the most established MALDI matrix compounds for smaller molecules [40]. Some selected data [41] are shown in Figure 18.4 to emphasize the resolving power.

The majority of TLC/MALDI studies of glycolipids thus far were carried out by using UV lasers with an emission wavelength of either 337 or 355 nm. These lasers are installed at the majority of commercially available MALDI instruments. However, there are also some studies where infrared (IR) lasers (instead of UV) were applied. IR lasers, of course, require completely different matrices in comparison to UV lasers: while UV lasers require compounds with an aromatic ring system (i.e., delocalized $\pi$-electrons), such compounds are useless when an IR laser is used. Here, glycerol is the matrix of choice because it absorbs perfectly the IR radiation and is stable under conditions of high vacuum. Finally, glycerol is a liquid and, thus, there is much less problem with irregular crystallizations of the matrix/analyte cocrystals. This is a serious problem when common crystalline UV–MALDI matrices are used. One disadvantage of IR–MALDI is, however, that the MALDI spectra generated with IR lasers show some unusual adducts (e.g., glycerol or NaCl), which are never seen when UV–MALDI spectra are recorded [42]. It has also been recently suggested that water is a very promising IR–MALDI matrix. This is normally done by freezing the sample and desorbing the analytes

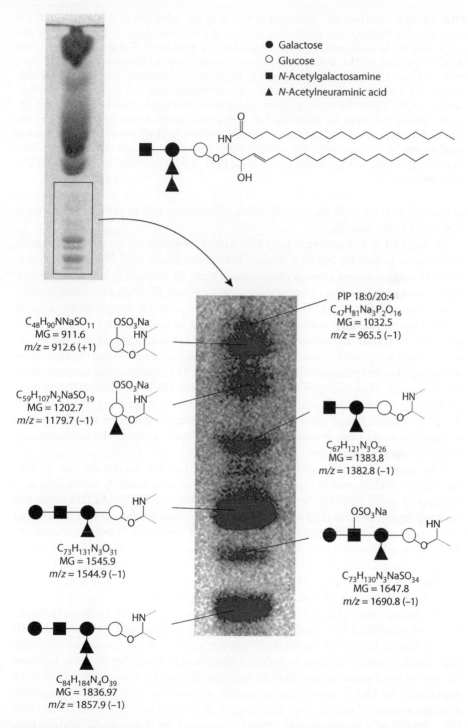

Galactose
Glucose
N-Acetylgalactosamine
N-Acetylneuraminic acid

PIP 18:0/20:4
$C_{47}H_{81}Na_3P_2O_{16}$
MG = 1032.5
m/z = 965.5 (−1)

$C_{48}H_{90}NNaSO_{11}$
MG = 911.6
m/z = 912.6 (+1)

OSO$_3$Na

$C_{59}H_{107}N_2NaSO_{19}$
MG = 1202.7
m/z = 1179.7 (−1)

OSO$_3$Na

$C_{67}H_{121}N_3O_{26}$
MG = 1383.8
m/z = 1382.8 (−1)

$C_{73}H_{131}N_3O_{31}$
MG = 1545.9
m/z = 1544.9 (−1)

OSO$_3$Na

$C_{73}H_{130}N_3NaSO_{34}$
MG = 1647.8
m/z = 1690.8 (−1)

$C_{84}H_{184}N_4O_{39}$
MG = 1836.97
m/z = 1857.9 (−1)

FIGURE 18.4 (Continued)

**FIGURE 18.4 (Continued)**    Emphasized region of the video image of a typical HPTLC plate showing characteristic ganglioside spots of a polar brain extract. The structures and *m/z* values of the most intense peaks detected in the MALDI/TOF mass spectra recorded directly from this HPTLC plate are also shown. Phospholipids (at the top of the HPTLC plate at the left) were not analyzed. The majority of compounds are more sensitively detectable as negative ions due to the presence of the *N*-acetylneuraminic acid residue or the sulfate residue. At the top of the figure, a typical ganglioside structure is shown, in which the different carbohydrate units are represented by geometric symbols as indicated at the top of the figure. According to the nomenclature of related cerebrosides (Cer), the number of carbons is used for structure assignments. Accordingly, the backbone of the shown compound would be termed Cer 18:0/18:1. (Reproduced from Fuchs, B. et al. 2008. *J. AOAC Int.*, 91: 1227–1236. With permission.)

of interest directly from the ice [43]. More information will be provided next in the context of GAG analysis.

IR MALDI is less common than UV MALDI because IR lasers are primarily available on homebuilt MALDI devices but commercially only on special request. Er:YAG (erbium-doped yttrium aluminum-Garret) IR lasers ($\lambda = 2.94$ nm) are normally used and have the considerable advantage that IR leads to a more significant ablation of the sample. Therefore, bringing the complete analyte from the inner of the plate to the TLC surface is less important in comparison to UV MALDI. Besides an IR laser, Dreisewerd and coworkers [44] used an orthogonal but not an axial system for glycolipid analysis. The orthogonal configuration has the significant advantage that irregularities of the surface of the TLC sample plate do not reduce the achievable mass accuracy significantly and there are only minor differences in comparison to a standard steel MALDI target when the spectra are desorbed from the TLC surface. It was shown that even minor gangliosides from a complex lipid mixture extracted from cultured Chinese hamster ovary cells can be unequivocally identified at these conditions.

The same authors [44] also provided evidence that the fluorescent dye "primuline" that is widely used in lipid research as it binds noncovalently to the fatty acyl residues of lipids [45] may be used as a nondestructive, TLC/MALDI-compatible staining agent. Similar data were independently obtained by another group that additionally introduced "vibrational" cooling [46]. The term "vibrational cooling" describes the desorption process in the pressure range, where "cooling" of the excess energy of the generated ions is achieved. At these conditions, fragmentation of labile analytes can be minimized. This is normally performed by introducing an inert gas (e.g., $N_2$) under a moderate pressure into the MS device.

In a recent study [47], 2,5-dihydroxybenzoic acid (DHB) in acetonitrile/water (1:1, v/v) was found very useful as matrix for the analysis of GSL because DHB is well soluble in this solvent mixture and the related solvents possess a relatively high surface tension leading to reduced analyte spreading. Sensitivities between 25 and 50 pmol could be obtained at these conditions. It should be noted that the application of highly concentrated matrix solutions is very important because a larger excess of matrix over the analyte in comparison to standard MALDI (i.e., the use of a stainless-steel target) is required for direct TLC/MALDI coupling in order to minimize fragmentation of the analyte. Although this has been established by using selected phospholipids, this seems to be valid for all compounds [48].

A combination between MALDI, TLC, and antibody detection was also recently suggested and is now a very hot topic in glycolipid research: the authors [49] used the following workflow: (1) TLC separation of cancer-associated GSL from human hepatocellular and pancreatic tumors; (2) their detection with oligosaccharide specific proteins; and (3) the direct *in situ* MS analysis of the GSLs previously detected by the antibody. Detection limits of less than 1 ng of immunostained GSLs could be obtained. It is a particular advantage of this approach that crude lipid extracts of biological origin can be directly used for TLC–IR–MALDI–MS and no laborious, previous GSL purification is needed. Such approaches can now be even automated, for instance, by using the recently established "PrimaDrop" method [50].

## 18.5 GLYCOSAMINOGLYCANS

Glycosaminoglycans (GAGs) are omnipresent in all vertebrates and of increasing interest because they possess important *in vivo* functions and are widely used in (bio)medicine. For instance, the only nonsulfated GAG, hyaluronan (which consists of alternating glucuronic acid and *N*-acetylglucosamine polymer-repeating units), has many important applications such as the enhancement of the viscosity of the synovial fluid from patients with inflammatory joint diseases [51]. HA is widely used in medicine and cosmetics because it is capable of binding huge amounts of water and possesses excellent gel-forming properties [52]. Chondroitin sulfate (CS) is an important food additive that is assumed to improve the quality of cartilage from people suffering from joint diseases. Finally, heparin (HE) has many biological applications and is particularly helpful in the clinics to suppress the clotting of blood, that is, it works as an anticoagulant. Careful heparin analysis is particularly important because of the heparin contamination crisis: some patients died because they were treated with oversulfated CS instead of heparin [53].

We will focus here on the analysis of HA and CS from the following reasons:

1. Both GAGs are most widely used and, thus, have the most significant biological significance.
2. Both GAGs are easily available and rather inexpensive.
3. HA is nonsulfated and CS is only moderately sulfated. This minimizes the separation problems occurring with higher sulfated GAGs considerably and overcomes problems with potential isomers.

The most serious problem of GAG (TLC) analysis is always the need of converting the polysaccharides into defined oligosaccharides because the native polysaccharides (with molecular weights in the 50 kDa–1 MDa range) can be neither separated by TLC nor successfully analyzed by MS methods [54]. It is highly recommended to apply GAG-specific enzymes such as chondroitinase (CSase) or hyaluronidase (HAase) instead of chemicals: although it is not a major problem to cleave the glycosidic linkages by chemical means, for instance, by treatment with strong bases or acids [55], this chemical fragmentation is always accompanied by unwanted site reactions, which particularly affect the N-acetyl side chain and the sulfate esters because these are the most labile chemical linkages within the polysaccharide. Therefore, specific enzymes are the better choice because they do not lead to unwanted fragmentation. Both CSase and HAase lead to the generation of defined oligosaccharides, whereby the tetra- and the hexasaccharides are generated in the highest yields when HAase is used. In contrast, CSase leads nearly exclusively to the generation of the disaccharide. The most pronounced difference between both enzymes is the introduction of a double bond in the uronic acid of the released oligosaccharides. This is of interest from the chemical point but does not affect the separation to a major extent. According to the best of our knowledge, normal phase silica gel thus far has been exclusively used. This is the reason why we will focus here on this type of stationary phase.

The negative ion MALDI–TOF mass spectra of selected GAGs (subsequent to enzymatic digestion and directly recorded from a TLC plate) are shown in Figure 18.5.

It is obvious from this figure [22] that separation of GAG oligosaccharides can be performed by TLC and high-quality mass spectra as well can be recorded directly from the TLC plate. Nevertheless, there is still one problem, which is coming from the use of high amounts of formic acid that are required for the separation of the GAGs on a normal phase TLC plate [56]: at these conditions, esterification occurs (detectable by the mass shift of 28) and, thus, a minor moiety of the GAG is only detectable as the corresponding formyl ester. This formylation occurs already at the TLC plate during the chromatographic run and can hardly be avoided at these experimental conditions. Of course, this problem could be overcome by using reversed phase TLC (instead of normal phase TLC) because under these conditions there would be no need to use highly polar solvents such as formic acid. However, to these authors' best knowledge, such investigations of GAG oligosaccharides have not yet been reported. However, Rothenhöfer et al. [57] performed comparable experiments on oligosaccharides of HA: these authors, however, did not use MALDI/MS but applied ESI/MS to monitor the oligosaccharides of interest, whereby the technique introduced by Luftmann [58] was used, that is, the sample was reeluted from the TLC plate prior to MS characterization.

## 18.6 CONCLUSIONS

We hope that we were able to provide sufficient evidence that TLC/MS is suitable for the characterization of a large variety of carbohydrates. Nevertheless, carbohydrate analysis is still a quite challenging task because (1) TLC analysis of carbohydrates is to a much lesser extent established in comparison to, for instance, lipids and (2) the achievable ion yields of sugars are also rather poor. This is a pity because the interest in carbohydrate analysis (not only of glycolipids) will massively increase in the future due to their (nowadays increasingly discovered) physiological relevance. It is expected that MALDI will play the leading role for the analysis of larger oligosaccharides with MW higher than about 500 Da. In contrast, ESI and DESI/MS will play a much more prominent role when smaller compounds are of interest. The future will show whether TLC/MALDI will become a real alternative method to LC/MS.

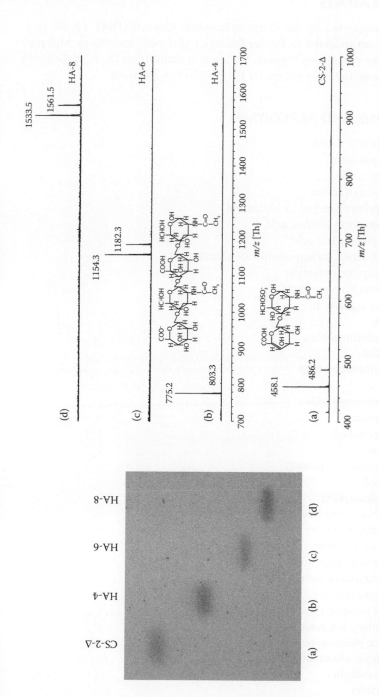

**FIGURE 18.5** Thin-layer chromatogram of selected commercially available GAG oligosaccharides on the left and the corresponding negative ion MALDI mass spectra (right) obtained directly from the TLC plate. The used oligosaccharides are (a) unsaturated chondroitin sulfate disaccharide (CS-2-Δ), (b) hyaluronan tetra- (HA-4), (c) hexa- (HA-6), and (d) octasaccharide (HA-8). The chemical formulae of two selected compounds are provided. Please note that high quality spectra can be obtained although there are normally also significant amounts of the formyl ester (mass shift of 28 amu). (Reproduced from Nimptsch, K. et al. 2010. *J. Chromatogr. A*, 1217: 3711–3715. With permission.)

## ACKNOWLEDGMENTS

This work was supported by the German Research Council (DFG TR 67, projects A2/A8). We are indebted to Bruker Daltonics (Bremen) and Merck Millipore (Darmstadt) for the continuous support. We are also thankful to Dr. Schnabelrauch and Prof. Rademann and their groups for the excellent cooperation.

## ABBREVIATIONS AND ACRONYMS

| | |
|---|---|
| CS | chondroitin sulfate |
| CSase | chondroitinase |
| Da | Dalton |
| DE | delayed extraction |
| DESI | desorption electrospray ionization |
| DHB | 2,5-dihydroxybenzoic acid |
| DNA | deoxyribonucleic acid |
| Er:YAG | erbium-doped yttrium–aluminum–Garret |
| ESI | electrospray ionization |
| FAB | fast atom bombardment |
| FT | Fourier transform |
| Fuc | fucose |
| GAG | glycosaminoglycan |
| Gal | galactose |
| GC | gas chromatography |
| Glu | glucose |
| GSL | glycosphingolipids |
| HA | hyaluronan |
| HAase | hyaluronidase |
| HE | heparin |
| LC | liquid chromatography |
| IR | infrared |
| LD | laser desorption |
| MALDI | matrix-assisted laser desorption and ionization |
| MS | mass spectrometry |
| $m/z$ | mass over charge |
| PI | phosphatidylinositol |
| PVDF | polyvinylidene difluoride |
| Rf | retardation factor |
| S/N | signal to noise |
| SIMS | secondary ion mass spectrometry |
| SPR | surface plasmon resonance |
| TLC | thin-layer chromatography |
| TOF | time-of-flight |
| UV | ultraviolet |

# REFERENCES

1. Gama, C.I. and Hsieh-Wilson, L.C. 2005. Chemical approaches to deciphering the glycosaminoglycan code, *Curr. Opin. Chem. Biol.*, 9: 609–619.
2. Lehmann, J. (Ed.). 1996. *Kohlenhydrate*, Georg Thieme Verlag, Stuttgart, Germany.
3. Maloney, M.D. 2005. Carbohydrates, In: *Handbook of Thin-Layer Chromatography*, 3rd ed., Sherma, J. and Fried, B. (Eds.), Marcel Dekker, Basel, Chapter 16, pp. 579–610.
4. Scherz, H. and Bonn, G. (Eds.). 1998. *Analytical Chemistry of Carbohydrates*, Georg Thieme Verlag, Stuttgart, Germany.
5. Ruiz-Matute, A.I., Hernández-Hernández, O., Rodríguez-Sánchez, S., Sanz, M.L., and Martínez-Castro, I. 2011. Derivatization of carbohydrates for GC and GC–MS analyses. *J. Chromatogr. B*, 879: 1226–1240.
6. Schiller, J. and Huster, D. 2012. New methods to study the composition and structure of the extracellular matrix in natural and bioengineered tissues, *Biomatter*, 2: 115–131.
7. Ruhaak, L.R., Zauner, G., Huhn, C., Bruggink, C., Deelder, A.M., and Wuhrer, M. 2010. Glycan labeling strategies and their use in identification and quantification. *Anal. Bioanal. Chem.*, 397: 3457–3481.
8. Siegenthaler, U. and Ritter, W. 1977. Eine rasche DC-Methode zum Nachweis von mono- and disacchariden in milchmischgetränken und joghurt. *Mitt. Gebiete Lebensm. Hyg.*, 68: 448–450.
9. Bergman, N., Shevchenko, D., and Bergquist, J. 2014. Approaches for the analysis of low molecular weight compounds with laser desorption/ionization techniques and mass spectrometry. *Anal. Bioanal. Chem.*, 406: 49–61.
10. Bosch-Reig, F., Marcote, M.J., Minana, M.D., and Cabello, M.L. 1992. Separation and identification of sugars and maltodextrines by thin layer chromatography: Application to biological fluids and human milk, *Talanta*, 39: 1493–1498.
11. Lewis, B.A. and Smith, F. 1969. Sugars and derivatives, In: *Thin-Layer Chromatography—A Laboratory Handbook*, 2nd ed., Stahl, F. (Ed.), Springer Verlag, New York, pp. 807–837.
12. Schneider, P., Ralton, J.E., McConville, M.J., and Ferguson, M.A. 1993. Analysis of the neutral glycan fractions of glycosyl-phosphatidylinositols by thin-layer chromatography, *Anal. Biochem.*, 210: 106–112.
13. Doner, L.W. and Biller, L.M. 1984. High-performance thin-layer chromatographic separation of sugars: Preparation and application of aminopropyl bonded-phase silica plates impregnated with monosodium phosphate, *J. Chromatogr.* 287: 391–398.
14. Klaus, R., Fischer, W., and Hauck, H.E. 1991. Qualitative and quantitative analysis of uric acid, creatine, and creatinine together with carbohydrates in biological material by HPTLC, *Chromatographia*, 32: 307–316.
15. Patzsch, K., Netz, S., and Funk, W. 1988. Quantitative HPTLC of sugars—Part 2: Determination in different matrices, *J. Planar Chromatogr.*, 1: 177–179.
16. de Jong, J.G., Aerts, J.M., van Weely, S., Hollak, C.E., van Pelt, J., van Woerkom, L.M., Liebrand-van Sambeek, M.L., and Wevers, R.A. 1998. Oligosaccharide excretion in adult Gaucher disease, *J. Inherit. Metab. Dis.*, 21: 49–59.
17. Zanetta, J.P., Timmerman, P., and Leroy, Y. 1999. Determination of constituents of sulphated proteoglycans using a methanolysis procedure and gas chromatography/mass spectrometry of heptafluorobutyrate derivatives, *Glycoconj. J.*, 16: 617–627.
18. Zhang, Z., Xiao, Z., and Linhardt, R.J. 2009. Thin layer chromatography for the separation and analysis of acidic carbohydrates, *J. Liq. Chromatogr. Relat. Technol.*, 32: 1711–1732.

19. Schiller, J., Süss, R., Fuchs, B., Müller, M., Petković, M., Zschörnig, O., and Waschipky, H. 2007. The suitability of different DHB isomers as matrices for the MALDI-TOF MS analysis of phospholipids: Which isomer for what purpose? *Eur. Biophys. J.*, 36: 517–27.

20. Caldwell, G.W., Masucci, J.A., and Jones, W.J. 1990. Indirect thin-layer chromatography-fast atom bombardment and chemical ionization mass spectrometry determination of carbohydrates utilizing simple and rapid microtransfer techniques, *J. Chromatogr.*, 514: 377–382.

21. Dreisewerd, K., Kölbl, S., Peter-Katalinić, J., Berkenkamp, S., and Pohlentz, G. 2006. Analysis of native milk oligosaccharides directly from thin-layer chromatography plates by matrix-assisted laser desorption/ionization orthogonal-time-of-flight mass spectrometry with a glycerol matrix, *J. Am. Soc. Mass Spectrom.*, 17: 139–150.

22. Nimptsch, K., Süss, R., Riemer, T., Nimptsch, A., Schnabelrauch, M., and Schiller, J. 2010. Differently complex oligosaccharides can be easily identified by matrix-assisted laser desorption and ionization time-of-flight mass spectrometry directly from a standard thin-layer chromatography plate, *J. Chromatogr. A*, 1217: 3711–3715.

23. Qureshi, M.N., Stecher, G., Sultana, T., Abel, G., Popp, M., and Bonn, G.K. 2011. Determination of carbohydrates in medicinal plants—Comparison between TLC, mf-MELDI–MS and GC–MS, *Phytochem. Anal.*, 22: 296–302.

24. Hay, I.D., Ur Rehman, Z., Moradali, M.F., Wang, Y., and Rehm, B.H. 2013. Microbial alginate production, modification and its applications, *Microb. Biotechnol.*, 6: 637–650.

25. Shimokawa, T., Yoshida, S., Kusakabe, I., Takeuchi, T., Murata, K., and Kobayashi, H. 1997. Some properties and action mode of (1→4)-alpha-L-guluronan lyase from Enterobacter cloacae M-1, *Carbohydr. Res.*, 304: 125–132.

26. Zhang, Z., Yu, G., Zhao, X., Liu, H., Guan, H., Lawson, A.M., and Chai, W. 2006. Sequence analysis of alginate-derived oligosaccharides by negative-ion electrospray tandem mass spectrometry, *J. Am. Soc. Mass Spectrom.*, 17: 621–630.

27. Suzuki, H., Suzuki, K., Inoue, A., and Ojima, T. 2006. A novel oligoalginate lyase from abalone, *Haliotis discus hannai*, that releases disaccharide from alginate polymer in an exolytic manner, *Carbohydr. Res.*, 341: 1809–1819.

28. van Houdenhoven, F.E., de Wit, P.J., and Visser, J. 1974. Large-scale preparation of galacturonic acid oligomers by matrix-bound polygalacturonase, *Carbohydr. Res.*, 34: 233–239.

29. Taki, T. 2012. An approach to glycobiology from glycolipidomics: Ganglioside molecular scanning in the brains of patients with Alzheimer's disease by TLC-blot/matrix assisted laser desorption/ionization-time of flight MS, *Biol. Pharm. Bull.*, 35: 1642–1647.

30. Taki, T. 2013. Bio-recognition and functional lipidomics by glycosphingolipid transfer technology, *Proc. Jpn. Acad. Ser. B: Phys. Biol. Sci.*, 89: 302–320.

31. Fuchs, B., Süss, R., Teuber, K., Eibisch, M., and Schiller, J. 2011. Lipid analysis by thin-layer chromatography—A review of the current state, *J. Chromatogr. A*, 1218: 2754–74.

32. Ellis, S.R., Brown, S.H., In Het Panhuis, M., Blanksby, S.J., and Mitchell, T.W. 2013. Surface analysis of lipids by mass spectrometry: More than just imaging, *Prog. Lipid Res.*, 52: 329–353.

33. Seng, J.A., Ellis, S.R., Hughes, J.R., Maccarone, A.T., Truscott, R.J., Blanksby, S.J., and Mitchell, T.W. 2014. Characterisation of sphingolipids in the human lens by thin layer chromatography–desorption electrospray ionisation mass spectrometry, *Biochim. Biophys. Acta*, 1841: 1285–1291.

34. Meisen, I., Mormann, M., and Müthing, J. 2011. Thin-layer chromatography, overlay technique and mass spectrometry: A versatile triad advancing glycosphingolipidomics, *Biochim. Biophys. Acta*, 1811: 875–896.
35. Guittard, J., Hronowski, X.P.L., and Costello, C.E. 1999. Direct matrix-assisted laser desorption/ionization mass spectrometric analysis of glycosphingolipids on thin-layer chromatographic plates and transfer membranes, *Rapid Commun. Mass Spectrom.*, 13: 1838–1849.
36. Griesinger, H., Fuchs, B., Süß, R., Matheis, K., Schulz, M., and Schiller, J. 2014. Stationary phase thickness determines the quality of thin-layer chromatography/matrix-assisted laser desorption and ionization mass spectra of lipids, *Anal. Biochem.*, 451: 45–47.
37. Domon, B. and Costello, C.E. 1988. Structure elucidation of glycosphingolipids and gangliosides using high-performance tandem mass spectrometry, *Biochemistry*, 27: 1534–1543.
38. O'Connor, P.B., Budnik, B.A., Ivleva, V.B., Kaur, P., Moyer, S.C., Pittman, J.L., and Costello, CE. 2004. A high-pressure matrix-assisted laser desorption ion source for Fourier transform mass spectrometry designed to accommodate large targets with diverse surfaces, *J. Am. Soc. Mass Spectrom.*, 15: 128–32.
39. Distler, U., Souady, J., Hülsewig, M., Drmić-Hofman, I., Haier, J., Denz, A., Grützmann, R. et al. 2008. Tumor-associated CD75s- and iso-CD75s-gangliosides are potential targets for adjuvant therapy in pancreatic cancer, *Mol. Cancer Ther.*, 7: 2464–2475.
40. Fuchs, B. and Schiller, J. 2009. Recent developments of useful MALDI matrices for the mass spectrometric characterization of apolar compounds, *Curr. Org. Chem.*, 13: 1664–1681.
41. Fuchs, B., Nimptsch, A., Süß, R., and Schiller, J. 2008. Analysis of brain lipids by directly coupled matrix-assisted laser desorption ionization time-of-flight mass spectrometry and high-performance thin-layer chromatography, *J. AOAC Int.*, 91: 1227–1236.
42. Rohlfing, A., Müthing, J., Pohlentz, G., Distler, U., Peter-Katalinić, J., Berkenkamp, S., and Dreisewerd, K. 2007. IR–MALDI–MS analysis of HPTLC-separated phospholipid mixtures directly from the TLC plate, *Anal. Chem.*, 79: 5793–5808.
43. Pirkl, A., Soltwisch, J., Draude, F., and Dreisewerd, K. 2012. Infrared matrix-assisted laser desorption/ionization orthogonal-time-of-flight mass spectrometry employing a cooling stage and water ice as a matrix, *Anal. Chem.*, 84: 5669–5676.
44. Dreisewerd, K., Müthing, J., Rohlfing, A., Meisen, I., Vukelić, Z., Peter-Katalinić, J., Hillenkamp, F., and Berkenkamp, S. 2005. Analysis of gangliosides directly from thin-layer chromatography plates by infrared matrix-assisted laser desorption/ionization orthogonal time-of-flight mass spectrometry with a glycerol matrix, *Anal. Chem.*, 77: 4098–4107.
45. White, T., Bursten, S., Federighi, D., Lewis, R.A., and Nudelman, E. 1998. High-resolution separation and quantification of neutral lipid and phospholipid species in mammalian cells and sera by multi-one-dimensional thin-layer chromatography, *Anal. Biochem.*, 258: 109–117.
46. Ivleva, V.B., Sapp, L.M., O'Connor, P.B., and Costello, C.E. 2005. Ganglioside analysis by thin-layer chromatography matrix-assisted laser desorption/ionization orthogonal time-of-flight mass spectrometry, *J. Am. Soc. Mass Spectrom.*, 16: 1552–1560.
47. Nakamura, K., Suzuki, Y., Goto-Inoue, N., Yoshida-Noro, C., and Suzuki, A. 2006. Structural characterization of neutral glycosphingolipids by thin-layer chromatography coupled to matrix-assisted laser desorption/ionization quadrupole ion trap time-of-flight MS/MS, *Anal. Chem.*, 78: 5736–5743.

48. Fuchs, B., Schiller, J., Süss, R., Schürenberg, M., and Suckau, D. 2007. A direct and simple method of coupling matrix-assisted laser desorption and ionization time-of-flight mass spectrometry (MALDI/TOF MS) to thin-layer chromatography (TLC) for the analysis of phospholipids from egg yolk, *Anal. Bioanal. Chem.*, 389: 827–834.

49. Souady, J., Soltwisch, J., Dreisewerd, K., Haier, J., Peter-Katalinić, J., and Müthing, J. 2009. Structural profiling of individual glycosphingolipids in a single thin-layer chromatogram by multiple sequential immunodetection matched with direct IR-MALDI-o-TOF mass spectrometry, *Anal. Chem.*, 81: 9481–9492.

50. Ruh, H., Sandhoff, R., Meyer, B., Gretz, N., and Hopf, C. 2013. Quantitative characterization of tissue globotetraosylceramides in a rat model of polycystic kidney disease by PrimaDrop sample preparation and indirect high-performance thin layer chromatography-matrix-assisted laser desorption/ionization-time-of-flight-mass spectrometry with automated data acquisition, *Anal. Chem.*, 85: 6233–6240.

51. Volpi, N., Schiller, J., Stern, R., and Soltés, L. 2009. Role, metabolism, chemical modifications and applications of hyaluronan, *Curr. Med. Chem.*, 16: 1718–1745.

52. Kogan, G., Soltés, L., Stern, R., and Gemeiner, P. 2007. Hyaluronic acid: A natural biopolymer with a broad range of biomedical and industrial applications, *Biotechnol. Lett.*, 29: 17–25.

53. Liu, H., Zhang, Z., and Linhardt, R.J. 2009. Lessons learned from the contamination of heparin, *Nat. Prod. Rep.*, 26: 313–321.

54. Schnabelrauch, M., Scharnweber, D., and Schiller, J. 2013. Sulfated glycosaminoglycans as promising artificial extracellular matrix components to improve the regeneration of tissues, *Curr. Med. Chem.*, 20: 2501–2523.

55. Riemer, T., Nimptsch, A., Nimptsch, K., and Schiller, J. 2012. Determination of the glycosaminoglycan and collagen contents in tissue samples by high-resolution $^1$H NMR spectroscopy after DCl-induced hydrolysis, *Biomacromolecules*, 13: 2110–2117.

56. Zhang, Z., Xie, J., Zhang, F., and Linhardt, R.J. 2007. Thin-layer chromatography for the analysis of glycosaminoglycan oligosaccharides, *Anal. Biochem.*, 371: 118–120.

57. Rothenhöfer, M., Scherübl, R., Bernhardt, G., Heilmann, J., and Buschauer, A. 2012. Qualitative and quantitative analysis of hyaluronan oligosaccharides with high performance thin layer chromatography using reagent-free derivatization on amino-modified silica and electrospray ionization-quadrupole time-of-flight mass spectrometry coupling on normal phase, *J. Chromatogr. A*, 1248: 169–177.

58. Luftmann, H. 2004. A simple device for the extraction of TLC spots: Direct coupling with an electrospray mass spectrometer, *Anal. Bioanal. Chem.*, 378: 964–968.

# 19 Spontaneous Chiral Conversion and Peptidization of Amino Acids Traced by Means of TLC–MS

*Agnieszka Godziek, Anna Maciejowska,*
*Mieczysław Sajewicz, and Teresa Kowalska*

## CONTENTS

## 19.1 SPONTANEOUS OSCILLATORY CHIRAL CONVERSION AND SPONTANEOUS OSCILLATORY PEPTIDIZATION OF AMINO ACIDS

In Reference 1, spontaneous oscillatory chiral conversion for the first time was reported for several propionic acid derivatives, stored for longer periods of time in 70% aqueous ethanol, based on the results originating from thin-layer chromatography (TLC) (and other instrumental techniques). Later, an analogous evidence of spontaneous chiral conversion obtained with use of high-performance liquid chromatography with diode-array detection (HPLC–DAD) was presented [2]. It was demonstrated that the oscillatory chiral conversion is a general property that characterizes the low-molecular weight carboxylic acids from the groups of profen drugs [1], amino acids [3], and hydroxyl acids [4], when dissolved in aqueous or nonaqueous solvents and stored for certain periods of time in solution. Chiral conversion of such compounds can occur according to two different pathways. In aqueous solutions, the general scheme is represented as [5] follows:

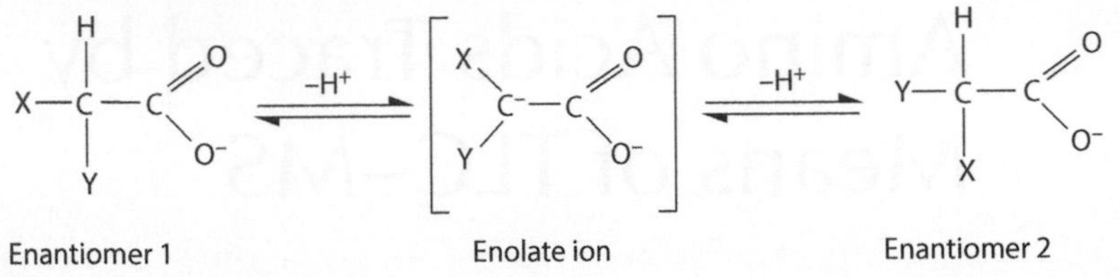

| Enantiomer 1 | Enolate ion | Enantiomer 2 |

where X: –R (aliphatic) and Y: –NH$_2$, –OH, or –Ar (aromatic).

In anhydrous media and in the presence of trace amounts of water, the probable mechanism of chiral conversion is [6] as follows:

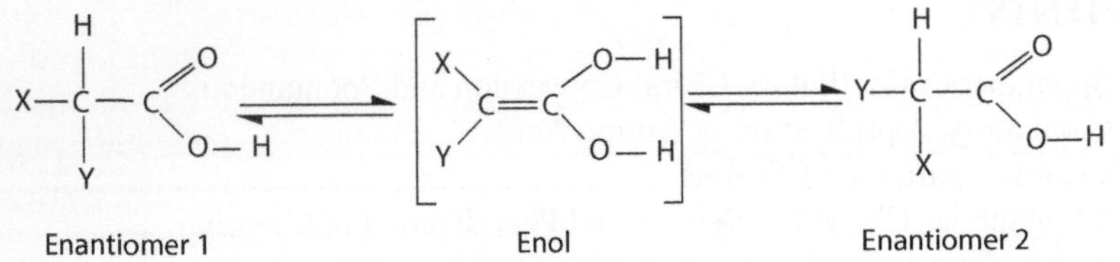

| Enantiomer 1 | Enol | Enantiomer 2 |

From our earlier investigations, it came out that the oscillatory chiral conversion of the low-molecular weight carboxylic acids occurs in parallel with the oscillatory condensation, which most probably has thermodynamic justification [2]. In Reference 7, the results were presented of spontaneous oscillatory peptidization for three amino acids (L-Met, L-His, and L-Ser) dissolved in water, and in References 8 and 9, the analogous results were given for three binary amino acid systems (L-Pro-L-Hyp, L-Pro-L-Phe, and L-Hyp-L-Phe) dissolved in aqueous organic solvents. The parallel processes of chiral conversion and peptidization of amino acids running in abiotic systems can be illustrated by the following scheme [10]:

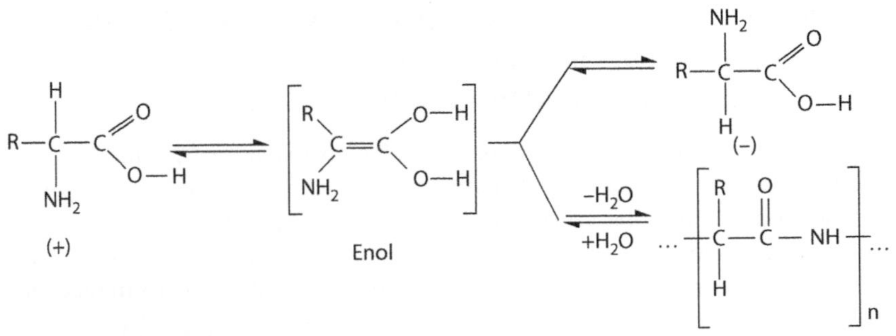

In Reference 8, a theoretical model of spontaneous nonlinear peptidization in the abiotic binary amino acid systems was developed, particularly focused on heteropeptide formation. This model assumes the following four different cases: (1) when two amino acids do not form heteropeptides and even in a binary solution they spontaneously produce homopeptides only; (2) when two amino acids of different nonlinear peptidization dynamics can form heteropeptides, and dynamics of faster peptidizing amino acid governs overall dynamics; (3) when two amino acids of different nonlinear peptidization dynamics can form heteropeptides, and dynamics of slower peptidizing amino acid governs overall dynamics; and (4) when two amino acids of different nonlinear peptidization dynamics can form heteropeptides according to cooperative mechanisms, where none of the two species governs the process dynamics.

Experimental evidence of the oscillatory chiral conversion and oscillatory condensation of amino acids (and of the other low-molecular weight carboxylic acids) is a challenging experimental task. For tracing dynamics of the oscillatory chiral conversion, both TLC and HPLC can be used (e.g., [1,2]), although each technique has its own advantages and shortcomings. For tracing dynamics of the oscillatory condensation, HPLC can be regarded as a technique of choice, due to high rates of the concentration changes, which could hardly be captured by means of TLC. If we, however, have no need to demonstrate the oscillatory nature of chiral conversion and peptidization, then TLC–densitometry proves handy for demonstration of chiral conversion, and TLC–MS proves equally handy for demonstrating peptidization. Unlike HPLC, where all separated species end up in an effluent tank, TLC is a good option that allows unconventional modifications of stationary and mobile phase, and an *in situ* preservation of the separated species for further examinations.

Spontaneous chiral conversion and peptidization of amino acids in abiotic systems means that in a certain way, these two parallel processes run out of control, although their dynamics certainly can be modified by external conditions (such as the solvent type, concentration, temperature, etc.). Thus far, the knowledge of the spontaneous nature of these two processes in abiotic systems has not yet become widespread among biochemists and life scientists in general, in spite of the growing importance of peptide nano- and microstructures for biotechnology. This modern technology branch is increasingly more interested in stable, or at least predictably behaving peptides, which can be employed in regenerative medicine, for delivery of bioactive therapeutics, as scaffolds in tissue engineering, etc. [11,12].

In this chapter, a brief overview is provided of our recent efforts in developing a novel thin-layer chromatographic method of the amino acid enantioseparation with use of chiral stationary phase (native cellulose) and with fortification of the amino acid sample just prior to the chromatographic analysis with the transition metal cation upon the example of Pro [13]. Then, an ability of two proteinogenic amino acids (i.e., Cys and Met) to undergo chiral conversion and peptidization is demonstrated with use of TLC–densitometry and TLC–MS [14,15]. It is shown how TLC–densitometry can provide evidence on spontaneous chiral conversion of amino acids taking place in the course of their storage in aqueous organic solutions. It is also shown how TLC–MS can be used to prove spontaneous peptidization of amino acids in the course of their aging, in spite of considerable and annoying background signals, which are hard to avoid, when the TLC–MS interface and the TLC–ESI–MS operation mode are used [16].

## 19.2 ENANTIOSEPARATION OF PROLINE

The choice of L-Pro (Scheme 19.1) for our studies was due to an important role of this proteinogenic amino acid as a building block of collagen, which is omnipresent in the connective tissues of mammals, and largely responsible for tissue architecture and strength. It was our aim to develop a novel approach to the enantioseparation of Pro (which might later be extended to the enantioseparation of other amino acids as well) because up to our best knowledge, direct enantioseparation of Pro by means of TLC has been done only once prior to our own research [17] (which reflects a difficulty of this supposedly easy analytical task). In fact, we revisited an old concept of the thin-layer chromatographic enantioseparations of amino acids on native cellulose adsorbents proposed decades ago (e.g., [18,19]), although introducing considerable modification to it.

Experimental evidence of successful enantioseparation of DL-Pro is given in Reference 13. As native chiral adsorbent, microcrystalline cellulose was used (the 20 cm × 20 cm commercial precoated glass plates; layer thickness, 0.10 mm; Merck; cat. # 1.05716). As the test samples, DL-Pro (for the purpose of the enantioseparation) and L-Pro (as an external standard) were used. Concentrations of both samples in 70% aqueous methanol were 1.0 mg mL$^{-1}$. In order to enhance the enantioseparation, equimolar amounts of Mn(II) acetate were added to each solution, in order to obtain complexes between the Mn(II) cation and Pro as a chelating agent. Enhancement of the enantioseparation process by fortifying the analyzed racemic mixture with different transition metal cations (e.g., Cu(II), Co(II), Ni(II), and Mn(II)) just prior to analysis proper was tested in our earlier studies focusing on DL-lactic acid [20,21] and positive results were obtained. Apart from enhancing the enantioseparation, complexation of transition metal cations with chiral low-molecular weight carboxylic acids plays one more important role. Namely, bonding of these acids as chelating ligands to the metal cation stops their oscillatory configuration changes and so to say "freezes" (i.e., stabilizes) their respective configurations [21]. Therefore, the concept was adopted in the discussed research also and the complexation mechanism is schematically given here:

$$\text{L-Pro} + \text{Mn(II)} \quad \Leftrightarrow \quad \text{L-Pro} \ldots \text{Mn(II)}; \quad K_1$$

$$\text{D-Pro} + \text{Mn(II)} \quad \Leftrightarrow \quad \text{D-Pro} \ldots \text{Mn(II)}; \quad K_2$$

the enantioseparation condition: $K_1 \neq K_2$

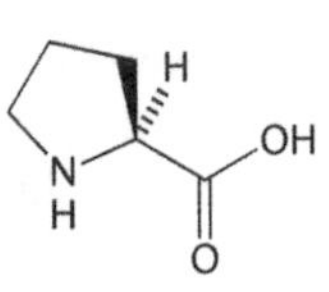

**SCHEME 19.1**   Chemical structure of Pro.

As mobile phase, 2-butanol–pyridine–glacial acetic acid–water (30:20:6:24, $v/v$) was used. The chromatogram was visualized by dipping the plate for 2 s in the 0.5% ninhydrin solution in 2-propanol, followed by heating for 5 min at 110°C.

As a result, the baseline enantioseparation was obtained, as shown in Figure 19.1a. Monomeric Pro is one of these rare amino acids, which develop yellow (and not bluish) color when visualized with ninhydrin. L-Pro used as an external standard (Figure 19.1b) confirmed the identity of the lower yellow spot number 2 as enantiomer L and the upper yellow spot number 3 as enantiomer D, as shown in Figure 19.1a. The respective $R_F$ values were $0.57 \pm 0.02$ and $0.74 \pm 0.02$. Brownish-purple spot number 1 ($R_F = 0.32 \pm 0.02$; Figure 19.1) apparently originates from the Pro-derived peptides and it is also fully separated from the monomeric L-Pro spot number 2. The presence of peptides in the two freshly prepared Pro samples witnesses to rapid peptidization of this amino acid (although contamination of the commercial monomeric DL-Pro and L-Pro samples with peptides cannot be excluded).

A method utilizing native cellulose adsorbent and the concept of the amino acid complex formation with the transition metal cation elaborated in Reference 13 was then applied to tracing spontaneous chiral conversion and spontaneous peptidization of the other amino acids, as presented in the forthcoming sections.

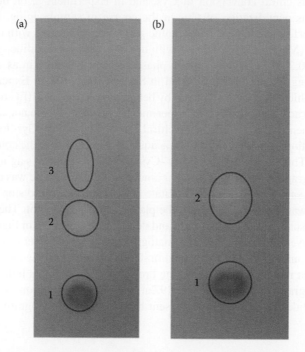

**FIGURE 19.1** Pictures of the chromatograms on the cellulose plates stained with ninhydrin and valid for (a) DL-proline and (b) L-proline; (1) proline-derived oligopeptide fraction; (2) L-proline; and (3) D-proline. Samples were applied to the plate in the aliquots of 5 μL, at the concentration of 1.0 mg mL$^{-1}$ amino acid (plus equimolar amount of Mn(II) acetate) and developed with 2-butanol + pyridine + glacial acetic acid + water (30:20:6:24, $v/v$). (From Sajewicz, M. et al. 2013. *J. Liq. Chromatogr. Relat. Technol.*, 36: 2497. With permission.)

## 19.3   SPONTANEOUS CHIRAL CONVERSION
## AND PEPTIDIZATION OF CYSTEINE

We focused our attention on L-Cys (Scheme 19.2) because of its importance as a sulfur-containing semiessential amino acid, which can be biosynthesized in humans and yet, due to its relatively low content in food, it is also used as a food additive (denoted as E920). L-Cys is an important building block of proteins that are used throughout the body, and it can physiologically be transformed to glutathione (a powerful antioxidant [22]), or taurine (essential for cardiovascular function, development and function of skeletal muscles, the retina, and the central nervous system [23]). Thus, the main aim of this study [14] was to employ TLC–densitometry and TLC–ESI–MS in order to demonstrate an ability of L-Cys to spontaneously undergo chiral conversion and condensation, when dissolved in 70% aqueous acetonitrile.

### 19.3.1   THIN-LAYER CHROMATOGRAPHY–DENSITOMETRY

Two thin-layer chromatographic experiments with densitometric detection were performed with Cys [14]. In Experiment 1, the main focus was on demonstration of spontaneous chiral conversion of Cys, and in Experiment 2, on demonstration of spontaneous peptidization of Cys in the course of sample aging. Both experiments were performed on chromatographic glassplates precoated with microcrystalline cellulose (Merck; cat. # 1.05716) with use of 2-butanol–pyridine–glacial acetic acid–water (30:20:6:24, v/v) as mobile phase and using ninhydrin as a visualizing agent (following the protocol described in Section 19.2 [13]). In Experiment 1, the chromatographic plates were activated by heating for 30 min at 110°C prior to applying the amino acid samples, and in Experiment 2, the plates were not activated.

In Experiment 1, L-Cys (for tracing chiral conversion) and DL-Cys (for proving the enantioseparation) were dissolved in 70% aqueous acetonitrile at the concentration of 0.7 mg mL$^{-1}$. The third sample was the L-Cys solution after 60 days aging. Just before the chromatographic analysis, equimolar amount of Mn(II) acetate was added to each of these three samples (in order to facilitate enantioseparation and stop oscillations). Each sample was spotwise applied to the plate in the 5-μL aliquot. The result in the form of the visualized chromatograms and densitograms is given in Figure 19.2.

In qualitative terms, all three chromatograms look similar, yet from a comparison of the chromatograms of L-Cys and DL-Cys, one can easily deduce that the blue spots represent monomeric Cys, and the brown and yellow spots hold for peptides. In all densitograms shown in Figure 19.2a(i–iii), the predominant peak originates from the peptide fraction and it is present both in the chromatograms of the fresh

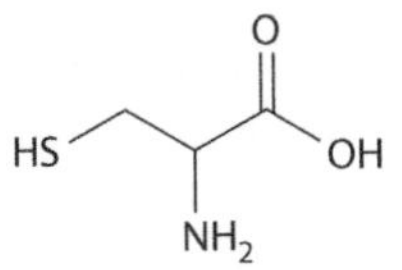

**SCHEME 19.2**   Chemical structure of Cys.

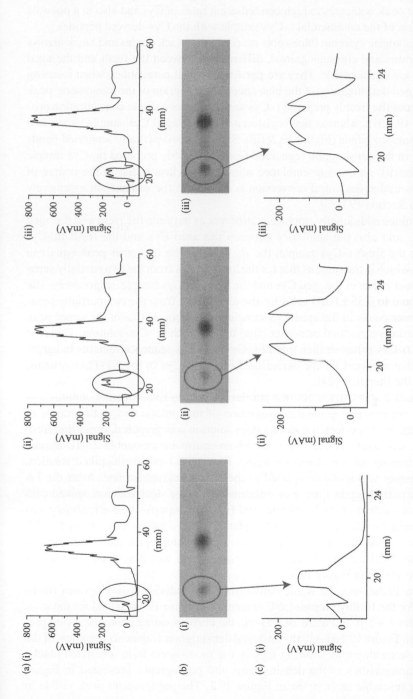

**FIGURE 19.2** Densitograms and chromatograms of Cys solution with equimolar addition of Mn(II) acetate. (i) Fresh prepared L-Cys solution; (ii) Cys solution after 60 days' aging; (iii) fresh prepared DL-Cys solution. (a) Densitometric scans of the whole chromatograms (i)–(iii). (b) Photographs of the whole chromatograms (i)–(iii). (c) Enlarged densitometric scans of the Cys bands (i)–(iii). Black circles and arrows indicate the Cys bands. (From Godziek, A. et al. 2015. *J. Planar Chromatogr.—Modern TLC*, 28: 144–151. With permission.)

samples (Figure 19.2a(i) and (ii)) and in that of the aged one (Figure 19.2a(iii)). This predominant peak witnesses to high condensation rates of Cys and also to a possible contamination of the commercial L-Cys sample with the Cys-derived peptides.

With monomeric cysteine (blue spots marked with black circles and black arrows on densitograms and chromatograms), differences between the fresh and the aged Cys sample are considerable. They are particularly well perceptible, when focusing on the enlarged densitograms of the blue spots. Densitogram of the monomeric peak registered from the freshly prepared L-Cys sample shows a single concentration profile (Figure 19.2c(i)), whereas that registered from the aged Cys sample shows two partially separated bands (Figure 19.2c(ii)). Similarly two partially separated bands can be seen in the densitogram registered from the freshly prepared DL-Cys sample (Figure 19.2c(iii)) and this resemblance allows a conclusion that in the course of aging, L-Cys undergoes chiral conversion according to the mechanism extensively discussed in Section 19.1.

The $R_F$ values additionally emphasize differences between the fresh and the aged Cys sample, and also the similarity between the aged Cys and the fresh DL-Cys sample. For the fresh L-Cys sample, the $R_F$ value of the monomer peak equals to $0.31 \pm 0.01$, which is the same as that for the lower peaks from the two partially separated monomer bands in the aged Cys and the fresh DL-Cys sample, respectively. The $R_F$ value (equal to $0.35 \pm 0.01$) valid for the upper peak from the two partially separated monomer peaks in the aged Cys sample is the same as that of the upper peak from the partially separated monomer band for the fresh DL-Cys solution. Thus, the $R_F$ value of D-Cys is higher than that of L-Cys, and this sequence remains in agreement with that reported for the derivatized L- and D-Cys in the NP-TLC systems, reported in the literature [24].

Experiment 2 was carried out in a similar manner to Experiment 1, although its aim was to demonstrate gradual consumption of monomeric Cys in the course of peptidization. To this effect, the stock L-Cys solution was prepared. From this fresh stock, 1 mL was withdrawn and spiked with an equimolar amount of Zn(II) nitrate, and the remaining lot was stored for aging. From this 1-mL fresh spiked solution, the 5-μL aliquot was spotwise applied to the chromatographic plate. After the 1-h long storage period, again 1 mL was withdrawn from the stock solution, spiked with an equimolar amount of Zn(II) nitrate, and from this sample the 5-μL aliquot was spotwise applied to the chromatographic plate. This procedure was repeated in 1-h intervals for 5 h. At the end, one and the same chromatographic plate with the Cys samples after 0-, 1-, 2-, 3-, 4-, and 5-h storage period was developed. The results obtained are shown in Figure 19.3.

In Figure 19.3a(i–vi), the whole densitograms of individual development tracks are shown for the freshly prepared L-Cys solution (Figure 19.3a(i)), and for the samples stored for 1 + 5 h. In Figure 19.3b(i–vi), the corresponding photographs are presented and in Figure 19.3c(i–vi), the enlarged densitogram fragments are given of the respective chromatograms showing Cys in the monomeric form (encircled black). General characteristics of the densitograms and photographs presented in Figure 19.3 largely resemble those given in Figure 19.2. The predominant peak visible in each densitogram (and the corresponding brown spot on the respective picture) holds for the main fraction of the condensation products, yet it is out of the scope of our

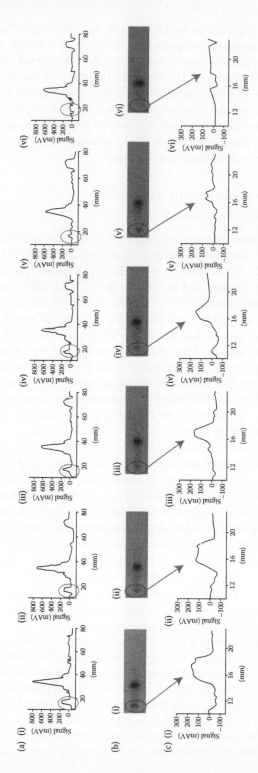

**FIGURE 19.3** Densitograms and chromatograms of L-Cys solution with equimolar addition of Zn(II) nitrate. (i) Fresh prepared L-Cys solution; (ii) Cys solution after 1 h aging; (iii) Cys solution after 2 h aging; (iv) Cys solution after 3 h aging; (v) Cys solution after 4 h aging; (vi) L-Cys solution after 5 h aging. (a) Densitometric scans of the whole chromatograms (i)–(vi). (b) Photographs of the whole chromatograms (i)–(vi). (c) Enlarged densitometric scans of the Cys bands (i)–(vi). Black circles and arrows indicate the Cys bands. (From Godziek, A. et al. 2015. *J. Planar Chromatogr.—Modern TLC*, 28: 144–151. With permission.)

discussion. We focus our attention on the blue spot of the monomeric Cys in Figure 19.3b(i–vi), and on the enlarged densitograms of this fragment in Figure 19.3c(i–vi). Initially, color intensity of the blue spot is high, yet in the 1-h interval, considerable lowering of its intensity is observed. The enlarged fragments of the densitograms additionally emphasize the bleaching effect with the blue spot. Namely, the intensity of the Cys monomer peak with the fresh prepared solution equals to 170 mAV and in the course of the 5-h lasting aging, it drops to the bare 36 mAV. In that way, relatively rapid disappearance of the monomeric Cys band is confirmed, which can only be due to the rapidly progressing spontaneous peptidization.

## 19.3.2 THIN-LAYER CHROMATOGRAPHY–ELECTROSPRAY IONIZATION–MASS SPECTROMETRY

The TLC–ESI–MS experiment was performed for the chromatograms obtained from Experiment 1, yet without using ninhydrin as a visualizing agent [14]. In this experiment, we employed a TLC–MS interface (CAMAG), which enabled direct elution of individual chromatographic bands from the plate to the LC–ESI–MS system. Elution of the target spots was carried out with 50% aqueous methanol. The employed LC–ESI–MS System Varian was equipped with the Varian ProStar model pump, the Varian 100-MS mass spectrometer, and the Varian MS Workstation v. 6.9.1 software for data acquisition and processing. This system operated under the following working conditions: The mobile phase was methanol–water (50:50, $v/v$) at the flow rate of 0.20 mL min$^{-1}$. Mass spectrometric detection was carried out in the ESI mode (extended ESI/MS scan from $m/z$ 100–3500, positive ionization, spray chamber temperature 50°C, drying gas temperature 350°C, drying gas pressure 25 psi, capillary voltage 50 V, needle voltage 5 kV).

In fact, we focused our attention on one spot with the highest retardation factor ($R_F = 0.60 \pm 0.02$), which appeared yellow on visualization and was attributed to the least retarded peptide fraction. For the sake of comparison, we registered mass spectra of the yellow spot originating from the freshly prepared DL-Cys solution (Figure 19.4a) and for that valid for the aged Cys solution (Figure 19.4b), as those which illustrate the sample aging issue in the most spectacular and also direct manner. The results presented in these two figures considerably differ. The primary difference consists in the intensity of the eluted liquid chromatographic signals. In the case of the aged Cys solution, this intensity is considerably higher and measured in MCounts (Figure 19.4b), whereas with the fresh DL-Cys solution, it is much lower and measured in kCounts only (Figure 19.4a). This is convincing evidence of the peptidization yields considerably growing in the course of aging.

Further evidence originates from a comparison of the respective mass spectra registered for the discussed target spots. The most intense peak (229 Counts) present in the mass spectrum of the fresh sample (Figure 19.4a) appears at $m/z$ 148 and it can be attributed to monomeric Cys (in the form of the [Cys + Na + He]$^+$ cation). The intensities of peptide signals originating from the fresh sample are much lower than that observed for the signal of the monomer. For the sake of example, let us consider certain peptide signals and the intensities thereof originating from the fresh sample, that is, those at 371 (133 Counts), 959 (55 Counts), and 1373 (37 Counts). The following

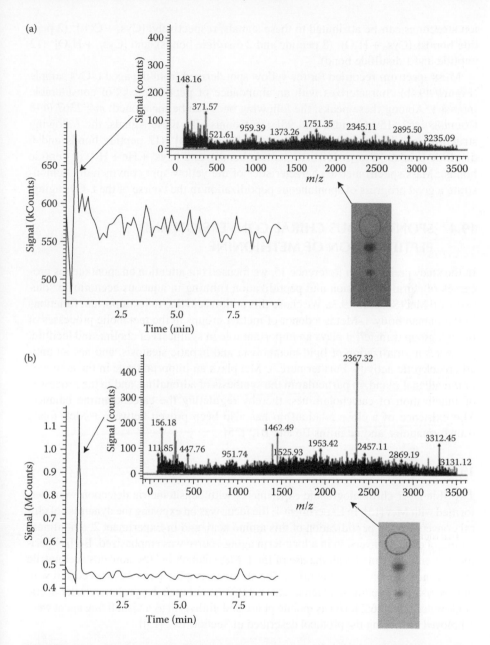

**FIGURE 19.4** Thin-layer chromatograms, signals of the chromatographic spots representing an oligopeptide fraction (black framed on the respective chromatograms), directly eluted from the chromatographic plates, and the respective mass spectra recorded for the (a) fresh DL-Cys sample and (b) aged L-Cys sample. (From Maciejowska, A. et al. 2015. *J. Liq. Chromatogr. Relat. Technol.*, 38: 1164–1171. With permission.)

ion structures can be attributed to these signals, respectively: $[Cys_3 + CO_2]^+$ (2 peptide bonds), $[Cys_9 + H_2O]^+$ (8 peptide and 2 disulfide bonds), and $[Cys_{13} + H_2O]^+$ (12 peptide and 1 disulfide bond).

Mass spectrum recorded for the yellow spot derived from the aged L-Cys sample (Figure 19.4b) characterizes with an abundance of peptide peaks of considerable intensity. Among these peaks, the following ones can be mentioned: $m/z$ 2367 (448 Counts), 1462 (159 Counts), and 951 (56 Counts). To these signals, the following structures can be attributed, respectively: $[Cys_{22} + Na]^+$ (17 peptide bonds and 6 disulfide bonds), $[Cys_{14} + H_2]^+$ (13 peptide bonds), and $[Cys_9 + He + H_2]^+$ (8 peptide bonds). Mass spectrometric characteristics of the yellow spot convincingly demonstrate a good progress of spontaneous peptidization in the course of the L-Cys aging.

## 19.4  SPONTANEOUS CHIRAL CONVERSION AND PEPTIDIZATION OF METHIONINE

In the study presented in Reference 15, we focused our attention on spontaneous processes of chiral conversion and peptidization running in aqueous acetonitrile solution of L-Met (Scheme 19.3). We chose this amino acid due to its important functions in the human body. L-Met is a donor of methyl groups in the metabolic processes of methyl group transfer; it plays an important role in synthesis of choline and lecithin, promotes normalization of lipid metabolism and hepatic steatosis, and has an anti-atherosclerotic activity. Furthermore, L-Met plays an important role in the activities of the adrenal gland, in particular in the synthesis of adrenaline, and in the processes of inactivation of catecholamines, thereby regulating the catecholamine balance. The existence of a close relationship has also been proven between L-Met, folate transformations, and vitamins B6 and B12 [25].

### 19.4.1  THIN-LAYER CHROMATOGRAPHY–DENSITOMETRY

Two thin-layer chromatographic experiments with densitometric detection were performed with Met [15]. In Experiment 1, the focus was on exposing the dynamics of chiral conversion and peptidization of this amino acid, and in Experiment 2, a nonlinear nature of chiral conversion in a long-term aging course was emphasized. Both experiments were performed with the use of the L-Met solution in 70% aqueous acetonitrile at the concentration of $1.0$ mg mL$^{-1}$. The chromatographic glassplates precoated with microcrystalline cellulose (Merck; cat. # 1.05716), 2-butanol–pyridine–glacial acetic acid–water (30:20:6:24, $v/v$) as mobile phase and ninhydrin as a visualizing agent were employed (following the protocol described in Section 19.2 [13]).

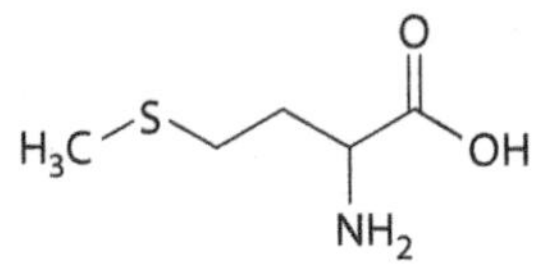

**SCHEME 19.3**  Chemical structure of Met.

In Experiment 1, the stock L-Met solution was first prepared. From this fresh stock, 1 mL was withdrawn and spiked with an addition of Zn(II) nitrate (the molar ratio of amino acid to Zn(II) nitrate was equal to 2:1, as suggested for an efficient chelating effect with the transition metal cations (e.g., in Reference 21), and the remaining lot was stored for aging. From this 1-mL fresh solution spiked with Zn(II) nitrate, the 5-μL aliquot was spotwise applied to the chromatographic plate. After the 1-h long storage period of stock solution again, 1 mL was withdrawn, spiked with an addition of Zn(II) nitrate, and from this sample, the 5-μL aliquot was spotwise applied to the chromatographic plate. This procedure was carried out in 1-h intervals for 5 h. At the end, the chromatographic plate with the Met samples deposited in it after 0-, 1-, 2-, 3-, 4-, and 5-h storage period was developed. The chromatogram was visualized with ninhydrin and densitometrically scanned (Figure 19.5).

In Figure 19.5a–f, six chromatographic lanes and the corresponding densitograms are shown. Figure 19.5a represents the chromatographic lane and the densitogram for the freshly prepared L-Met sample, whereas Figure 19.5b–f represents respective lanes and densitograms for the Met samples after from 1–5 h aging period. On the chromatograms shown in Figure 19.5a–f, an intense purple-bluish spot (number 2) corresponds

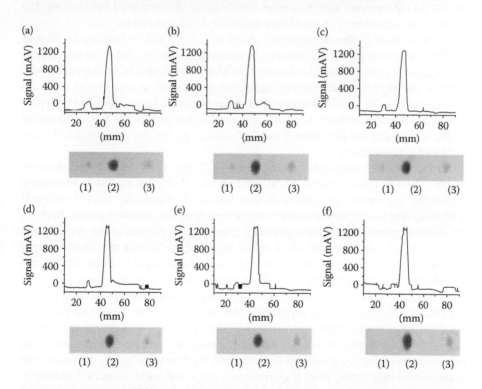

**FIGURE 19.5** Chromatographic lanes and densitograms of the L-Met solution with an addition of Zn (II) nitrate (molar ratio of L-Met to zinc (II) nitrate, 2:1). (a) Freshly prepared L-Met solution, and Met solution after (b) 1 h aging, (c) 2 h aging, (d) 3 h aging, (e) 4 h aging, and (f) 5 h aging. (From Maciejowska, A. et al. 2015. *J. Liq. Chromatogr. Relat. Technol.*, 38: 1164–1171. With permission.)

with monomeric L-Met, a less intense purple-bluish spot (number 1) corresponds with monomeric D-Met, and the yellow spot (number 3) represents peptide fraction. One advantage of using ninhydrin as a visualizing reagent is that it allows differentiating between blue or purple-bluish spots of monomeric amino acids and yellow or brown spots of peptide fraction. The intense purple-bluish spot number 2 ($R_F = 0.54 \pm 0.02$) originating from monomeric L-Met, characterizes with practically equal signal intensity in each densitogram. The presence of yellow spot number 3 on all chromatograms ($R_F = 0.92 \pm 0.02$) witnesses to considerable L-Met peptidization rate, although this spot becomes more distinct after 5-h sample aging only. The presence of the less intense purple-bluish spot number 1 originating from D-Met ($R_F = 0.30 \pm 0.02$) in the freshly prepared L-Met sample witnesses to the high rate of chiral conversion, yet its intensity drop in the course of the sample storage period is the most characteristic feature of Experiment 1. This intensity drops from 70.56 mAV for peak 1 in the freshly prepared sample to 55.89 mAV after a 2-h storage period, to 44.48 mAV after a 4-h storage period, and to 8.62 mAV after a 5-h storage period. A relatively short (5 h) storage period of the Met sample and a relatively long (1 h) sampling interval did not allow perceiving an oscillatory pattern of the amino acid chiral conversion. However, reappearance of the D-Met signal after 5 months' sample aging (demonstrated in Experiment 2) serves as an indication of an oscillatory nature of chiral conversion.

In Experiment 2, chromatographic plates were activated by heating for 30 min at 110°C prior to applying the amino acid samples. Just before the chromatographic analysis, Zn(II) nitrate was added to the two Met samples, that is, to the fresh L-Met solution and after 5 months' aging (again, the molar ratio of amino acid to Zn(II) nitrate was 2:1). On the development, the chromatograms were visualized with ninhydrin and densitometrically scanned. The results obtained for the freshly prepared L-Met sample and for that after 5 months' storage period are presented in Figure 19.6a and b, respectively.

Again, the chromatographic spots numbers 1–3 were detected in both chromatograms, with the intense purple-bluish spot number 2 originating from monomeric L-Met, the less intense purple-bluish spot number 1 originating from monomeric D-Met, and the yellow spot number 3 originating from the peptide fraction. Spots in the chromatogram and the corresponding concentration profiles in the densitogram were indicated pair-wise with black ovals. Signal of the intense purple-bluish spot number 2 originating from monomeric L-Met is the highest and its intensity does not considerably change in the course of the 5 months' storage period. Signal of the less intense purple-bluish peak number 1 (originating from monomeric D-Met) is very low (10.42 mAV) with freshly prepared L-Met sample, yet after the storage period of 5 months, it grows to 85.67 mAV. In Experiment 1, we saw a decrease of intensity of peak 1 in the course of the initial 5 h monitoring the process of aging, and now, we observe an intensity growth in the course of the 5 months' aging. A comparison of the results originating from Experiments 1 and 2 and valid for peak 1 indirectly points to a nonlinear pattern of chiral conversion of Met. Yellow spot number 3 in Figure 19.6b valid for the peptide fraction after 5 months' sample aging is more intense than spot number 3 in Figure 19.6a, valid for the freshly prepared L-Met solution. This is a direct proof that the process of sample aging results in gradual accumulation of peptides.

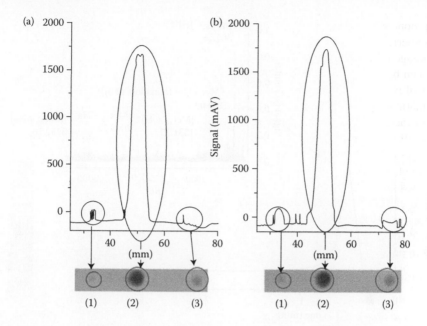

**FIGURE 19.6** Chromatographic lanes and densitograms for the L-Met solution with an addition of Zn (II) nitrate (molar ratio of L-Met to zinc (II) nitrate, 2:1). (a) Freshly prepared L-Met solution; (b) Met solution after 5 months' aging; (1) D-Met; (2) L-Met; (3) peptide fraction. (From Maciejowska, A. et al. 2015. *J. Liq. Chromatogr. Relat. Technol.*, 38: 1164–1171. With permission.)

### 19.4.2 THIN-LAYER CHROMATOGRAPHY–ELECTROSPRAY IONIZATION–MASS SPECTROMETRY

Important evidence on the reactions spontaneously occurring in the course of the L-Met aging was obtained with use of TLC–ESI–MS. The analyses were carried out for the chromatograms obtained according to the procedure assumed for L-Met in Experiment 2 and the results are presented in Figure 19.7. Figure 19.7a, c, and e shows the mass spectra recorded for spots numbers 1–3 from the chromatogram of the freshly prepared L-Met sample, and Figure 19.7b, d, and f shows the analogous mass spectra recorded from the chromatogram of the L-Met sample after 5 months' aging. Mass spectra valid for the freshly prepared and the aged Met sample evidently differ, in spite of an earlier recognized fact that with use of the TLC–MS interface considerable amounts of the background (noise) signals appear, which make interpretation of the spectra a challenging task [16]. Now, let us focus on the message extracted from Figure 19.7.

In Figure 19.7a, the chromatogram and mass spectrum recorded from the freshly prepared sample and valid for an intense purple-bluish spot of monomeric L-Met are given, and the predominant signal in this spectrum appears at $m/z$ 301, which can possibly be attributed to $[Met_9 + 4H]^{4+}$. However, peak of monomeric Met at $m/z$ 144 can also be seen, with a loss of 6 Da in fragmentation. Last but not least, more peaks originating from peptides are present in this spectrum, although their intensities are

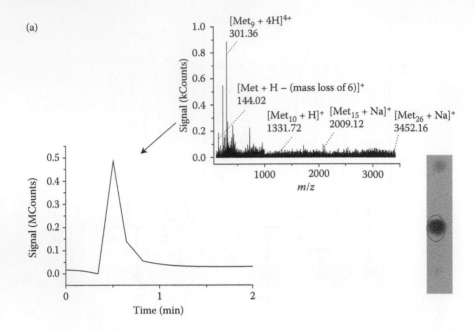

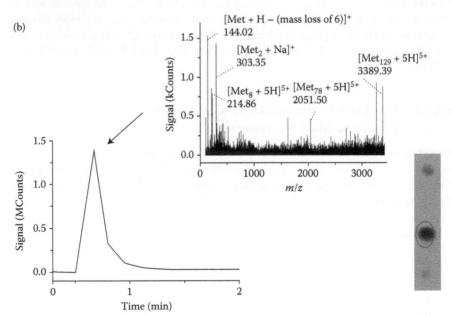

**FIGURE 19.7** Thin-layer chromatograms, signals of chromatographic spots marked with black ovals and directly eluted from the chromatographic plate, and the respective mass spectra recorded for L-Met fraction in (a) freshly prepared and (b) aged solution, peptide fraction in (c) freshly prepared and (d) aged solution, and D-Met fraction in (e) freshly prepared and (f) aged solution. (From Maciejowska, A. et al. 2015. *J. Liq. Chromatogr. Relat. Technol.*, 38: 1164–1171. With permission.)                                    *(Continued)*

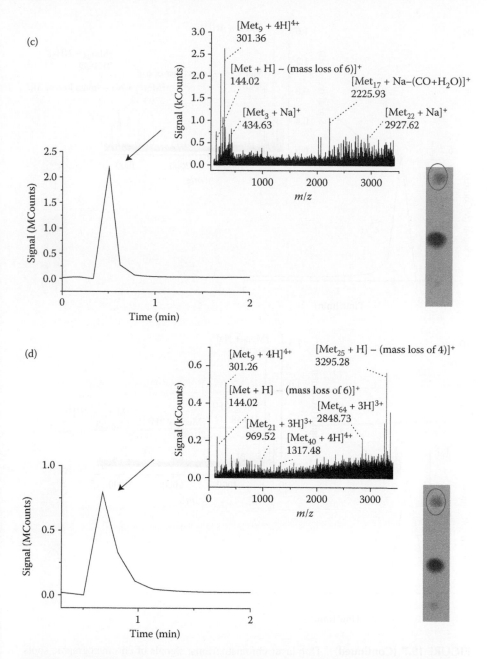

**FIGURE 19.7 (Continued)** Thin-layer chromatograms, signals of chromatographic spots marked with black ovals and directly eluted from the chromatographic plate, and the respective mass spectra recorded for L-Met fraction in (a) freshly prepared and (b) aged solution, peptide fraction in (c) freshly prepared and (d) aged solution, and D-Met fraction in (e) freshly prepared and (f) aged solution. (From Maciejowska, A. et al. 2015. *J. Liq. Chromatogr. Relat. Technol.*, 38: 1164–1171. With permission.) *(Continued)*

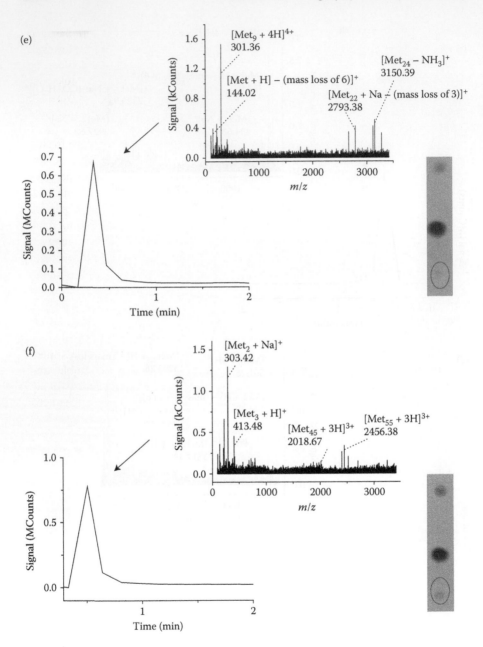

**FIGURE 19.7 (Continued)** Thin-layer chromatograms, signals of chromatographic spots marked with black ovals and directly eluted from the chromatographic plate, and the respective mass spectra recorded for L-Met fraction in (a) freshly prepared and (b) aged solution, peptide fraction in (c) freshly prepared and (d) aged solution, and D-Met fraction in (e) freshly prepared and (f) aged solution. (From Maciejowska, A. et al. 2015. *J. Liq. Chromatogr. Relat. Technol.*, 38: 1164–1171. With permission.)

quite low. In Figure 19.7b, valid for an intense purple-bluish spot of Met in the aged sample, the predominant signal at $m/z$ 144 represents monomeric Met. However, higher signals at, for example, $m/z$ 2051 and 3389 are also present, which can be attributed to $[Met_{78} + 5H]^{5+}$ and $[Met_{129} + 5H]^{5+}$, respectively. In fact, molecular weights of these two peptides are equal to 10,252 and 16,944 Da, respectively, which explains their low mobility in the employed thin-layer chromatographic system, and sticking to the monomeric fraction.

In Figure 19.7c, the chromatogram and mass spectrum recorded from the freshly prepared sample and valid for the yellow spot of peptide fraction are given. Again, signal at $m/z$ 301 is predominant, yet other signals originating from the peptides are also intense (e.g., those at $m/z$ 2225 and 2927, which might correspond with $[Met_{17} + Na - (CO + H_2O)]^+$ and $[Met_{22} + Na]^+$, respectively). The intense peptide signals recorded from the freshly prepared sample witness to an efficient and rapid peptidization process. In Figure 19.7d, chromatogram and mass spectrum are given valid for the yellow spot of peptide fraction in the aged sample. This mass spectrum confirms considerable progress of peptidization in the course of the 5 months' aging (as compared with that for the corresponding yellow spot from the freshly prepared sample; Figure 19.7c).

Data shown in Figure 19.7e refer to a less intense purple-bluish spot valid for monomeric D-Met, obtained through chiral conversion of L-Met in the freshly prepared solution. Due to rather low conversion yields, signal intensities in this spectrum are relatively low, yet the mass spectral pattern valid for this spot resembles that recorded for the monomeric L-Met in the freshly prepared solution (Figure 19.7a). In Figure 19.7f, valid for the less intense purple-bluish spot of D-Met in the aged sample, considerable intensity growth of the predominant peak representing D-Met is observed. This result confirms an efficient chiral conversion of L-Met in the course of the 5 months' aging and corresponds well with the thin-layer chromatographic results summarized in Figure 19.6.

Surprisingly, many peptides remained unresolved from the monomeric L-Met fraction (Figure 19.7a and b), and from the monomeric D-Met fraction as well. A persuasive evidence of this fact was confirmed by the photograph of the monomeric L-Met fraction taken from the back side of chromatographic plate (Figure 19.8). From this transparent glass backside, a "yellow eye" can be seen in the center of each purple-bluish spot, representing peptides (which remain invisible from the front side of the visualized adsorbent layer). In that way, clear explanation is given why

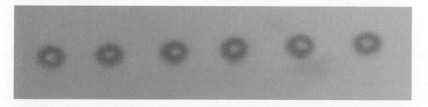

**FIGURE 19.8** Photograph of the back side of a chromatographic plate showing the purple-bluish spot of monomeric L-Met with the "yellow eye" of peptide fraction inside of it. (From Maciejowska, A. et al. 2015. *J. Liq. Chromatogr. Relat. Technol.*, 38: 1164–1171. With permission.)

mass signals originating from peptides were recorded from the purple-bluish spots of monomeric L-Met and D-Met. A more general comment can also be made that an imperfect separation performance of TLC is in certain cases rather incompatible with high sensitivity of mass spectrometry (thus considerably adding to an inconvenience of background signals of different origin, encountered in the TLC–ESI–MS technique and discussed in Reference 16).

## 19.5 CONCLUSIONS

1. TLC–ESI–MS has to be accompanied by TLC–densitometry and/or videoscanning (photography) of the developed chromatograms, in order to help localize separated chromatographic bands on the adsorbent layers, prior to their elution with use of the TLC–MS interface.

2. In the case of complex samples and the thin-layer fractionation thereof, mass spectra obtained by means of TLC–ESI–MS basically serve as fingerprints, providing information of qualitative or semiquantitative importance. This is due to an imperfect chromatographic separation and an additional eclipsing effect of background signals (extensively discussed in Reference 16), combined with high sensitivity of the mass spectrometric technique.

3. As a confirmation of the above statement, similar complex mass spectra of the fingerprint importance can be quoted, which have been recorded for medicinal plant extracts from the chromatographic thin layers and shown in papers [26–29].

4. In the research discussed in this chapter and dealing with spontaneous chiral conversion and peptidization of amino acids, fingerprint results obtained with use of the TLC–ESI–MS technique serve as convincing evidence of the chiral conversion and peptidization progress and furnish certain information on identity of the formed species.

## REFERENCES

1. Sajewicz, M., Piętka, R., Pieniak, A., and Kowalska, T. 2005. Application of thin-layer chromatography (TLC) to investigating oscillatory instability of the selected profen enantiomers, *Acta Chromatogr.*, 15: 131–149.
2. Sajewicz, M., Gontarska, M., and Kowalska, T. 2014. HPLC/DAD evidence of the oscillatory chiral conversion of phenylglycine, *J. Chromatogr. Sci.*, 52: 329–333.
3. Sajewicz, M., Kronenbach, D., Gontarska, M., Wróbel, M., Piętka, R., and Kowalska, T. 2009. TLC in search for structural limitations of spontaneous oscillatory in-vitro chiral conversion. α-hydroxybutyric and mandelic acids, *J. Planar Chromatogr.—Modern TLC*, 22: 241–248.
4. Sajewicz, M., Kronenbach, D., Gontarska, M., and Kowalska, T. 2010. TLC and polarimetric investigation of the oscillatory *in vitro* chiral conversion of r-β-hydroxybutyric acid, *J. Liq. Chromatogr. Relat. Technol.*, 33: 1047–1057.
5. Belanger, P., Atkinson, J.G., and Stuart, R.S. 1969. Exchange reactions of carboxylic acid salts; Kinetics and mechanism, *J. Chem. Soc. D: Chem. Commun.*, 1067–1068.
6. Xie, Y., Liu, H., and Chen, J. 2000. Kinetics of base-catalyzed racemization of ibuprofen enantiomers, *Int. J. Pharm.*, 196: 21–26.

7. Godziek, A., Maciejowska, A., Sajewicz, M., and Kowalska, T. 2015. HPLC monitoring of spontaneous non-linear peptidization dynamics of selected amino acids in solution, *J. Chromatogr. Sci.*, 53: 401–410. DOI: 10.1093/chromsci/bmu122.

8. Sajewicz, M., Dolnik, M., Kowalska, T., and Epstein, I.R. 2014. Condensation dynamics of L-proline and L-hydroxyproline in solution, *RSC Adv.*, 4: 7330–7339.

9. Sajewicz, M., Godziek, A., Maciejowska, A., and Kowalska, T. 2015. Condensation dynamics of the L-Pro-L-Phe and L-Hyp-L-Phe binary mixtures in solution, *J. Chromatogr. Sci.*, 53: 31–37. DOI: 10.1093/chromsci/bmu006.

10. Sajewicz, M., Matlengiewicz, M., Leda, M., Gontarska, M., Kronenbach, D., Kowalska, T., and Epstein, I.R. 2010. Spontaneous oscillatory *in vitro* chiral conversion of simple carboxylic acids and its possible mechanism, *J. Phys. Org. Chem.*, 23: 1066–1073.

11. Shoseyov, O. and Levy, I. (Eds.) 2008. *NanoBioTechnology: BioInspired Devices and Materials of the Future*, Humana Press, Totowa, NJ.

12. Castillo, J., Sasso, L., and Svendsen, W.E. (Eds.) 2013. *Self-Assembled Peptide Nanostructures: Advances and Applications in Nanobiotechnology*, Pan Stanford Publishing, Singapore.

13. Sajewicz, M., Matlengiewicz, M., Juziuk, M., Penkala, M., Weloe, M., Schulz, M., and Kowalska, T. 2013. Thin-layer chromatographic evidence of proline peptidization in solution and its thin-layer chromatographic enantioseparation, *J. Liq. Chromatogr. Relat. Technol.*, 36: 2497–2511.

14. Godziek, A., Maciejowska, A., Talik, E., Sajewicz, M., and Kowalska, T. 2015. Thin-layer chromatographic investigation of L-cysteine in solution, *J. Planar Chromatogr.— Modern TLC*, 28: 144–151.

15. Maciejowska, A., Godziek, A., Talik, E., Sajewicz, M., and Kowalska, T. 2015. Investigation of spontaneous chiral conversion and oscillatory peptidization of L-methionine by means of TLC and HPLC, *J. Liq. Chromatogr. Relat. Technol.*, 38: 1164–1171.

16. Morlock, G.E. 2014. Background mass signals in TLC/HPTLC–ESI–MS and practical advices for use of the TLC–MS interface, *J. Liq. Chromatogr. Relat. Technol.*, 37: 2892–2914.

17. Mack, M., Hauck, H., and Herbert, H. 1988. Enantiomeric separation in TLC with the new HPTLC pre-coated plate CHIR with concentration zone, *J. Planar Chromatogr.— Modern TLC*, 1: 304–308.

18. Fukuhara, T., Isoyama, M., Shimada, A., Itoh, M., and Yuasa, S. 1987. Resolution of six polar DL-amino acids by chromatography on native cellulose. *J. Chromatogr.*, 387: 562–565.

19. Fukuhara, T., Isoyama, M., Shimada, A., Itoh, M., and Yuasa, S. 1987. Resolution of all proteinic DL-amino acids on native cellulose chromatography, *Sci. Rep. Osaka Univ.*, 35: 11–21.

20. Sajewicz, M., John, E., Kronenbach, D., Gontarska, M., and Kowalska, T. 2008. TLC study of the separation of the enantiomers of lactic acid, *Acta Chromatogr.*, 20: 367–382.

21. Sajewicz, M., John, E., Kronenbach, D., Gontarska, M., Wróbel, M., and Kowalska, T. 2009. How to suppress the spontaneous oscillatory in-vitro chiral conversion of α-substituted propionic acids? A thin-layer chromatographic, polarimetric, and circular dichroism study of complexation of the Cu(II) cation with L-lactic acid, *Acta Chromatogr.*, 21: 39–55.

22. Valko, M., Leibfritz, D., Moncol, J., Cronin, M.T.D., Mazur, M., and Telser, J. 2007. Free radicals and antioxidants in normal physiological functions and human disease, *Int. J. Biochem. Cell Biol.*, 39: 44–84.

23. Huxtable, R.J. 1992. Physiological actions of taurine, *Physiol. Rev.*, 72: 101–163.

24. Bhushan, R. and Martens, J. 2010. *Amino Acids*, HNB Publishing, New York, pp. 76, 85.

25. Murray, R.K., Bender, D.A., Botham, K.M., Kennelly, P.J., Rodwell, V.W., and Weil, P.A. 2012. *Harper's Illustrated Biochemistry*, 29th ed., McGraw-Hill, New York.
26. Sajewicz, M., Wojtal, Ł., Hajnos, M., Waksmundzka-Hajnos, M., and Kowalska, T. 2010. Low-temperature TLC–MS of essential oils from five different sage (Salvia) species, *J. Planar Chromatogr.—Modern TLC*, 23: 270–276.
27. Sajewicz, M., Wojtal, Ł., Natić, M., Staszek, D., Waksmundzka-Hajnos, M., and Kowalska, T. 2011. TLC–MS versus TLC–LC–MS fingerprints of herbal extracts. Part I. Essential oils, *J. Liq. Chromatogr. Relat. Technol.*, 34: 848–863.
28. Sajewicz, M., Staszek, D., Natić, M., Wojtal, Ł., Waksmundzka-Hajnos, M., and Kowalska, T. 2011. TLC–MS versus TLC–LC–MS fingerprints of herbal extracts. Part II. Phenolic acids and flavonoids, *J. Liq. Chromatogr. Relat. Technol.*, 34: 864–887.
29. Sajewicz, M., Staszek, D., Natić, M., Waksmundzka-Hajnos, M., and Kowalska, T. 2011. TLC–MS versus TLC–LC–MS fingerprints of herbal extracts. Part III. Application of the reversed phase liquid chromatography systems with C18 stationary phase, *J. Chromatogr. Sci.*, 49: 560–567.

# Index

Printed and bound by CPI Group (UK) Ltd, Croydon, CR0 4YY

24/10/2024

01778302-0012